A Historical Review and Analysis of Army Physical Readiness Training and Assessment

by
Whitfield B. East

Combat Studies Institute Press
US Army Combined Arms Center
Fort Leavenworth, Kansas

Foreword

"The Drillmaster of Valley Forge—Baron Von Steuben—correctly noted in his "Blue Book" how physical conditioning and health (which he found woefully missing when he joined Washington's camp) would always be directly linked to individual and unit discipline, courage in the fight, and victory on the battlefield. That remains true today. Even an amateur historian, choosing any study on the performance of units in combat, quickly discovers how the levels of conditioning and physical performance of Soldiers is directly proportional to success or failure in the field.

In this monograph, Dr. Whitfield "Chip" East provides a pragmatic history of physical readiness training in our Army. He tells us we initially mirrored the professional Armies of Europe as they prepared their forces for war on the continent. Then he introduces us to some master trainers, and shows us how they initiated an American brand of physical conditioning when our forces were found lacking in the early wars of the last century. Finally, he shows us how we have and must incorporate science (even when there exists considerable debate!) to contribute to what we do—and how we do it—in shaping today's Army. Dr. East provides the history, the analysis, and the pragmatism, and all of it is geared to understanding how our Army has and must train Soldiers for the physical demands of combat.

Our culture is becoming increasingly "unfit," due to poor nutrition, a lack of adequate and formal exercise, and too much technology. Still, the Soldiers who come to our Army from our society will be asked to fight in increasingly complex and demanding conflicts, and they must be prepared through new, unique, and scientifically based techniques. So while Dr. East's monograph is a fascinating history, it is also a required call for all leaders to better understand the science and the art of physical preparation for the battlefield. It was and is important for us to get this area of training right, because getting it right means a better chance for success in combat.

Mark P. Hertling
LTG (Ret), US Army

Preface

The Combat Studies Institute is excited to publish this work on the history of physical readiness training in our Army by Dr. Whitfield B. East, a Professor in the Department of Physical Education at the United States Military Academy at West Point. This manuscript is part of CSI's series of works that bring the scholarship of our academics from the Army's schools into the larger discourse on military matters.

Dr. East's work provides the reader an interesting and detailed historical recounting of physical readiness training in our Army. In doing so, he makes the case for the further development of physical training programs with a greater emphasis on programs built from scientific research.

CSI – The Past is Prologue!

                                          Roderick M. Cox
                                          Colonel, US Army
                                          Director, Combat Studies Institute
                                          Fort Leavenworth, Kansas

Author's Introduction

> *"The strength of a nation, therefore, depends upon its material wealth, supported by the character and abilities of the people who compose it--their intelligence, sense of justice and responsibility, physical fitness, and moral stamina. When the people possess these qualities in high degree, they will make the nation, which they compose, a strong one."*

—*Studies in Citizenship for the Recruit*, US Army Training Manual No. 1

Through the process of critical review, the purpose of this monograph is to analyze the history of physical readiness training and assessment in the United States Army. Although the evolution of Army physical readiness training (PRT) doctrine begins during the pre-Colonial period in America, in order to fully understand this evolutionary process we must first understand the development of military physical training in Europe and its role in shaping the philosophy and doctrine of US Army PRT. After a short review of the role of physical training in antiquity, we will review in depth the growth of military "gymnastics" in Europe, especially Prussia, during the 19th century and the pathways of this doctrine and training to the United States and the US Army. A full understanding of the foundations of European military gymnastics is crucial to understanding the evolution of PRT in the US Army since European military gymnastics served as the touchstone for Army PRT. We will then explore the extrinsic and intrinsic forces that have shaped Army PRT doctrine since 1700 with particular attention to the influences of a changing economic, social, and political milieu and evolution of warfighter tactics and technology.

Acknowledgements

There were many faculty and staff at the United States Military Academy that make this project possible. Without the help of the library staff at the United States Military Academy Cadet Library at West Point this project would have been impossible. I would formally like to recognize Mr. Celeste Evans, Liaison for the Department of Physical Education. She consistently provided information and assistance and was vital to the completion of this project. I would also like to recognize Mr. Dan Pritchard, Associate Director – Information Gateway, Mr. Paul Nergelovic, Documents Librarian, and Ms. Suzanne Christoff, Special Collections. Finally this project could not have been completed without the assistance of Ms. Sharon Gillespie and Mr. Bob Sorce, USMA Interlibrary Loan Technicians, who were instrumental in procuring a significant number of obscure documents. I would also like to thank Colonel Lance Betros, Head, Department of History for his time, guidance, encouragement and assistance and Colonel Matthew Moten, Deputy Head, Department of History for his guidance and willingness to share his original materials pertaining to the time period from 1840 – 1885, especially as it pertained to the USMA curriculum review prior to the Civil War. Lastly, thanks to Colonel's Greg Daniels, Director, and Jesse Germain, Deputy Director of the Department of Physical Education. Without their patience, support, and forbearance I could not have completed this project.

I believe the graphic images significantly enhance the meaningfulness of this document. There were many individuals who gave their personal and/or corporate assistance and permission for use of these images. I would like to sincerely thank:

Mr. Marshall Gagne, who enlisted in the Army in 1967 and completed his basic training at Fort Knox in 1967. He served with the 82nd Airborne, was a on the Green Beret Sky Diving Team and was a proud member of the United States Army Parachute Team, the Golden Knights. Thank you for permission to use your personal Army Combat Basic Training photos from 1967.

Ms. Lena Dirbashi, International Media Relations Specialist for Encompass Digital Media, a component of the Defense Video & Imagery Distribution System (DVIDS). Their motto of "Connecting the Military to the World" is right on the mark. Thanks for your assistance in obtaining the photos from the US Third Army.

Mr. William Jones (through the assistance of Mr. John Turner-www.arthurjonesexercise.com) for granting permission to use the photo of his father, Mr. Arthur Jones. The photo was taken by Mr. Arthur Jones' wife Inge Cook Jones during 1975 at the Fort Collins, Colorado training site.

Mr. Warren Evans (a true American Army hero) for his permission to use the ranger photo taken of his squad as they trained in 1942 with British Commandos

Tricia Davies, Director/Curator, of the Clinton County Historical Association for their permission to use the c. 1917 photo of former President Theodore Roosevelt talking to General Leonard Wood (www.clintoncountyhistorical.org).

Mr. Andy Erickson from www.criticalpast.com for donating three still images taken from the Physical Combat Proficiency Test (1969).

Mr. Adam Watson, State Archivist of Florida for permission to use photo entitled "Soldiers Performing Training Exercises on the Beach during WWII-Miami Beach, Florida." This photo is part of a collection managed by the Florida Memory project.

Mr. Bill Miller, Friends of Rowing History for providing information concerning the photo of John B. Kelly. The photograph was originally published in the book, The Schuylkill Navy of Philadelphia, 1858-1937, which was compiled by Dr. Louis Heiland, and published by Drake Press (1938).

Ms. Jane Johnson, Librarian at the Charlotte Mecklenburg Library who granted permission to use the boxing photo (The Manly Art) taken at Camp Green prior to World War I (http://www.cmstory.org/ imagegallery/showimage.asp?pictureid=595). The photo is part of the "post card collection" of the Robinson-Spangler Carolina Room, Public Library of Charlotte and Mecklenburg County, 310 North Tryon Street, Charlotte, North Carolina 28202.

Steve Van Camp and Frank Palkoska – United States Army Physical Fitness School for sharing old PRT manuals and unpublished USAPFS archives.

Capt. Gregory A. Wolf, USMC, Media Officer, Division of Public Affairs for securing permission to use the photo of Cpl. Alvin "Tony" Ghazlo, the senior bayonet and unarmed combat instructor at Montford Point, NC in Figure 29.

Lou Tomasi and Ed Thomas, who were there at the start of the Soldier Fitness School, FT Ben Harrison, for sharing their oral history and a plethora of original Army PRT documents and research.

Michael Kates, Executive Director and Tina Achebe Visitor Services Manager at the FT Des Moines Museum for permission to use the WAC calisthenics photos in Figure 25. FT Des Moines was one of the largest basic training installations for WACs during WWII.

Jennifer Payne, Archives Assistant, Norwich University Archives & Special Collections for her assistance in obtaining obscure documents about the history of Norwich University and Alden Partridge, in particular the document "A Journal of an Excursion Made by the Corps of Cadets of the American Literary, Scientific, and Military Academy under Capt. Alden Partridge. June 1822; Concord, NH: Hill and Moore, 1822."

Christine Witzsche, Communications Manager, Cooper Aerobics, Health and Wellness for securing Dr. Cooper's permission to use the personal photo in Figure 39. The photo was taken of Kenneth H. Cooper, MD, MPH, Founder and Chairman of Cooper Aerobics at Cooper Clinic in Dallas in the 1970s.

Lastly I would like to thank Dr. Donald Wright, Research and Publications Chief, Combat Studies Institute for his guidance and encouragement through this process.

WBE

Contents

page

Foreword iii

Author's Introduction v

Acknowledgements vi

Chapter 1
Historical Infuences on Army Physical Readiness Training .. 1

Chapter 2
The Naissance of Army Physical Readiness Training in
America 21

Chapter 3
The Koehler Era 35

Chapter 4
World War I—The Princeton Years 49

Chapter 5
World War II—A Return to Combat Readiness 79

Chapter 6
The Cold War Era—Fomenting a National Fitness Policy .119

Chapter 7
Return to Combat—Focused Physical Readiness Training. ....
.... 179

Chapter 8
Summary, Analysis, and Discussion 197

Appendix A
Chronological Summary of Significant Activities for the US
Army Soldier Physical Fitness Center 227

Appendix B
Chronological Summary of Publications for US Army
Physical Fitness Training and Assessment 231

Bibliography 241

Figures Bibliography 267

Figures   *page*

Figure 1. Jahn's Turnplatz. 8

Figure 2. MacLaren's 12 Apostles (April, 1861)............................... 12

Figure 3. US Turnvereine Team—Frankfurt 1880. 35

Figure 4. USMA Physical Education under Herman Kohler. 39

Figure 5. Kohler's First Manual for the Army (1892). 40

Figure 6. Milwaukee Bundesturnfest—1893. 41

Figure 7. Roosevelt and Wood at Plattsburg Training Camp (1916)... 50

Figure 8. WWI Recruiting Posters for Plattsburg and the Army (1917).. 53

Figure 9. Secretary of War Newton Baker drawing the first Draft Number (1917)... 55

Figure 10. WWI Army Physical Training Formation........................ 56

Figure 11. Boxing Instruction and Contests—WWI Training Camps. 58

Figure 12. WWI Combat Readiness Training. 59

Figure 13. Post WWI PRT Manuals (Raycroft-Koehler). 61

Figure 14. Obstacle Course Run. 65

Figure 15. Studies in Citizenship for Recruits................................... 67

Figure 16. Renault Light Tank (1917). 68

Figure 17. John B. Kelly, Chair—National Physical Fitness Council.. 81

Figure 18. Physical Efficiency Matrix. 84

Figure 19. WWII Physical Readiness Training. 85

Figure 20. Obstacle Course Test (1941)... 86

Figure 21. Rescuing Soldiers during the Normandy Invasion (1944).. 87

Figure 22. Colonel Theodore Paul "Ted" Bank................................. 88

page

Figure 23. Victory through Fitness—The Victory Corps. 93

Figure 24. Women's Army Corps Fitness (1943). 94

Figure 25. Women's Army Corps (WAC) Physical Training. 95

Figure 26. WAC Combat Readiness Training. 96

Figure 27. Army Air Corps Physical Training (Miami Beach, c.1943). 100

Figure 28. WWII Combat Readiness Training............................... 105

Figure 29. Bayonet and Unarmed Combat Instruction.................. 106

Figure 30. Exercises from the Kraus-Weber Test........................... 121

Figure 31. US Physical Fitness Training Program manual (1963). 128

Figure 32. Army Special Forces Rappel Training (1963). 131

Figure 33. Physical Readiness Training (1967)............................... 132

Figure 34. Strength Circuit in Basic Combat Training (1967)........ 134

Figure 35. Combat Readiness Physical Training (1967)................. 135

Figure 36. Combat Obstacle Course Training (1967)..................... 136

Figure 37. Physical Combat Proficiency Test (1969)...................... 138

Figure 38. Combatives Training during Basic Training (Fort Knox, 1967). 142

Figure 39. Kenneth Cooper and Arthur Jones (c. 1975)................. 143

Figure 40. Women's Army Corp PRT (FM 35-20, 1975)................. 145

Figure 41. WAC Combat Readiness Training (FM 35-20, 1975). ... 148

Figure 42. Message from Ronald Reagan—PAM 350-18 (1983). ... 151

Figure 43. Introduction to DA PAM 350-18 (1983)......................... 157

Figure 44. Ranger-Athlete-Warrior-Task Matrix. 187

Figure 45. OEF/OIF Physical Readiness Training.......................... 190

Figure 46. OER/OIF Combat Readiness Training.......................... 192

page

Figure 47. Physical Work Capacity Continuum. 208
Figure 48. Unit Formation Run. 211

Chapter 1
Historical Infuences on Army Physical Readiness Training

> ...when physical training ceased to be a national characteristic, and the men of brawn were succeeded by creatures of luxury, the decadence of national prosperity followed.[1]
>
> —James E. Pilcher

Antiquity to the Middle Ages

The Spartans were perhaps the most tenacious warriors in the history of mankind. Their entire civilization revolved around the safety and security of the State. In many if not most of their military conflicts the Spartans were significantly outnumber by their opponents. This was certainly true in their engagements with the Romans and the Persians. The foundation of their military strategy was to leverage physical conditioning and toughness as a force multiplier for combat effectiveness. "Sparta needs no other bulwarks than the bodies of her sons."[2]

Although battle-focused physical training can be traced to well before the Greek civilization of the 1st Century B.C., the Greeks are most noted for refining and utilizing systematic physical training to prepare Soldiers for war. The Spartans, perhaps more than all others, took the physical training of its citizen soldiers to the most extreme. Around age seven, Spartan males were sent to a military and athletic school where they learned toughness, discipline, endurance of pain, and survival skills. At the age of 20, after 13 years of physical and military training, a Spartan joined the standing Army as an adult citizen warrior.[3] The Spartans also trained an elite special force called the Krypteia, which was composed of 18 year old males who exhibited exceptional military and physical skills.[4] By training the elite fighting soldier of their time, Sparta prided itself on fielding a small, mobile, lethal force capable of engaging much larger forces as occurred at the Battle of Thermopylae. In 480 B.C. a force of approximately 7,000 Spartan soldiers engaged the Persian Army estimated to be in the hundreds of thousands. The small Spartan force held out for seven days.

Rather than conducting simulated assessments of physical readiness, the Greeks chose a more authentic form of assessment – the sport festival. Most events in the ancient Greek Olympic festival such as running, javelin, wrestling, boxing, and riding focused on warrior tasks and battle drills. Two contests were more directly linked to basic combat skills:

the pankration—a freestyle combination of boxing and wrestling where victory was secured by knockout, submission, or death, and the 400 to 800m sprint in armor (generally consisting of helmet, shield, and greaves weighing about 50 lbs.). There was little separation in Greek civilization between the physical training required for war and sport. Strength, mobility, speed and stamina were all keys to success on the battlefield and in the stadion. The Greeks also valued the health-related aspects of gymnast exercises as Galen declared "him to the best physician who was the best teacher of gymnastics.[5]

The more you sweat in peace, the less you bleed in war.

—Sun Tzu

During the 1st and 2nd Centuries A.D. Roman legions carried on the warrior traditions refined by the Greeks. Legionnaires may well be characterized as the first professional soldiers, who were trained and certified to serve in the army. Some of the key physical skills were marching at speed, running, swimming; use of the sword, bow, javelin; lifting/carrying heavy burdens. The Roman historian Vegetius tells us that it was of the utmost importance for a legionnaire to be able to march at speed, especially when moving to contact. Much of the Roman tactical phalanx strategy depended on a swift and precise deployment of forces as an integrated unit. It was inherently problematic to the tactical strategy when soldiers "fell out" of a movement to contact. Therefore "during the summer months the soldiers were to be marched twenty Roman miles, which had to be completed in five hours.[6] Soldiers generally trained under full combat load, which weighted approximately 50-60 lbs. A further part of basic military training was organized physical exercises...running, long jump, high jump and carrying heavy packs."[7] Physical readiness was an integral part of the training and development of Roman soldiers;

> Every soldier is every day exercised...with great diligence, as if it were in time of war, which is the reason why they bear the fatigue of battles so easily...nor would he be mistaken that should call those their exercises unbloody battles, and their battles bloody exercises.[8]

During the Middle Ages, the "soldier" class was primarily filled by lower class nobility called knights. Knights served in a variety of capacities, as home guard, policemen, enforcers, and Soldiers. As part of the "melee," knights often fought from a mounted or standing position, using heavy armor to protect themselves from the sword, mace, and lance. Thought to weigh between 40-60 pounds, a knight's armor required him to possess great strength, power, and agility. The scholar, clergyman, and teacher Johannes Rothe sought to capture the essence of the late middle age knight's education in his work *Der Ritterspiegel* (The Knight's Mirror).[9] As opposed to the broad-based studies in the septem artes liberals (seven liberal arts), Rothe described the knight's educational curriculum as the septem artes probitates.[10] The seven knightly arts (skills) were: horseback riding—fast in and out of the saddle, swimming, shooting—cross-, arm-, and handbows, climbing—especially ladders, ropes, and poles, mounted fighting—jousting; ground fighting—wrestling and fencing; and socializing with dance and courtly manners. "From a practical point of view, the nobleman's life depended on his physical skills and endurance."[11] As Europe moved inexorably into the Modern Age, significant changes in technology such as the refinement of the arbalest and introduction of gunpowder made heavy body armor a liability and so ended the era of knighthood.[12]

The Renaissance and Physical Culture

Throughout the Middle Ages there were relatively negligible changes in the essence of warfare and the physical training of Soldiers. With changes in technology, which accompanied the dawning of the Renaissance, mobility and endurance gained increased significance in combat readiness. At the same time educators, philosophers and theologians sought to reestablish the contribution of physical development to the Greek tripartite of mind-body-spirit, primarily as a way of improving physical health and vigor. One of the more impactful Renaissance writers relative to the application to exercise to combat skills was the French monk and physician François Rabelais. Rabelais used two novels *Pantagruel* and *Gargantua*, published in 1533 and 1535 respectively, to espouse the physical nature of the human spirit and the physical needs of war. The protagonist, Gargantua, was provided with an apt tutor, "a young man from Touraine, named "Esquire Gymnast," who provided training in vaulting, hand to hand combat, running, swimming, gymnastics, and lifting "leaden" weights."[13] Gargantua's physical exercises epitomized Rabelais's ideal of physical culture through his extensive recitation of nearly all known gymnastic exercises.[14] All of Gargantua's physical training was in preparation for the "gentleman's occupation"—war.[15]

Approximately 20 years later the Italian writer Hieronymus Mercurialis, made significant contributions to the development and application of gymnastic exercises. Mercurialis was a physician and philosopher, who became the first to document the benefits and application of physical exercise when he published *De Arte Gymnastica* (1569). Mercurialis divided exercises into three categories: legitimate (used for general health), military and athletic (dangerous).[16] He was the first Renaissance writer to directly address the hygienic and medical benefits of exercise and the application of exercise in preparation for war. Indulging in a bit of hyperbole, Mercurialis selected the name "medicine ball" for the weighted balls used for gymnastic exercise.

In the early 18th Century, Dr. George Turnbull (1698–1748), the Scottish philosopher, was well known for incorporating exercise and sport into his holistic educational model. Significantly influenced by the work of John Locke, Turnbull advocated the "necessity of corporal exercise to invigorate the soul as well as the body… to produce courage, firmness, and manly vigour in the latter." He also linked the benefits of physical exercise to successful for military service:

> Hardy exercises were reckoned by the ancients…in the formation of a liberal character…no doubt, the better adapted the exercises of youth are to this end [preparation for war], the better will they serve the general purpose of exercises, with the additional advantage of fitting youth for the arts and toils of warfare…young men were…not only initiated in warlike discipline, and trained to arms, but likewise accustomed to watch and keep guard.[17]

In 1762, another of Locke's protégés, Jean Jacques Rousseau, published his seminal work *Emile*. Rousseau wrote "Give his body constant exercise…everyone who has considered the manner of life among the ancients, attributes the strength of body and mind by which they are distinguished from the men of our own day to their gymnastic exercises."[18] Rousseau was influential in developing the scheme of modern gymnastics. "The body must be vigorous to obey the soul…the weaker the body, the more it commands; the stronger the body, the more it obeys."[19]

The first practical application of Rousseau's theories on exercise came to fruition a decade later. In 1774 Johann Bernhard Basedow created an educational institution in town of Dessau called the Philanthropin.[20] Although its primary mission was to educate the children of well-to-do Prussian families, it was in the Philanthropin where Basedow formally realized Rousseau and Locke's dream of integrating the education of the mind and the body. In his 1774 prospectus outlining the educational opportunities at the Philanthropin, Basedow promised "that if the numbers are sufficient and the ages suitable there will be drill in military positions and movements, and frequent marches on foot."[21] It was in Dessau that physical education and the modern gymnastic (exercise) movement came to life. During the early years of the Philanthropin one of Basedow's instructors was Christian Gothilf Saltzman. In 1784 Salzmann left the Dessau Philanthropin to start a new school in Schnepfenthal. Although Salzmann did little to advance the causes of gymnastic education, in 1785 he hired a young instructor named Johann GutsMuths, "and to him confided the direction for gymnastics."[22] Perhaps the singular most defining change in physical training for soldiers began in late 1778 with the birth Johann Friedrich GutsMuths. His seminal work *Gymnastik für die Jugend* would lay the foundation for the refined gymnastics systems of Frederick Jahn and Pehr Ling. Following in Saltzman's footsteps, "as early as 1804 he [GutsMuths] urged the introduction of gymnastic training into the schools as a means of increasing the military efficiency of future recruits."[23]

Emergence of Military Gymnastics in Europe

By the dawn of the 19th century, the health-related and performance benefits of German gymnastics were spreading throughout Europe. "The great importance and even absolute necessity of a regular and systematic course of exercise for the preservation of health and confirming and rendering virtuous the constitution, I presume, must be evident to the most superficial observer."[24] In Denmark Franz Nachtegall, a strident disciple of GutsMuths was profoundly influenced by *Gymnastik für die Jugend*. In 1798 he started a gymnastics club in Copenhagen and a year later founded a private gymnasium. As his reputation grew, Nachtegall's efforts came to the attention of the Crown Prince. Believing that gymnastics would be useful for military training, the Crown Prince created the Institute of Military Gymnastics on 25 August 1804.[25] Nachtegall was named the director of the institute where officers and NCOs were trained in the art of military gymnastics. These officers/NCOs became gymnastics subject matter experts (SMEs) for their units. By 1828 Denmark passed a law requiring the introduction of physical training in all Danish elementary schools.[26]

Pehr Henrik Ling, the Father of Swedish Gymnastics, began his journey to prominence in the gymnastics world as a young man traveling through Europe. During his travels he worked with Franz Nachtegall at his gymnastics school in Copenhagen, where he was introduced to GutsMuth's system of gymnastics. Ling also learned to fence at the local university. He was impressed with the physical benefits of gymnastic training, but was particularly take with the health-related benefits. When Ling returned to Sweden around 1804, he had a "broken constitution and a suggestion of the usefulness of physical training."[27] Using his fledgling knowledge of gymnastics, Ling "secured his own recovery to health." Shortly thereafter he was appointed the fencing master at the University of Lund, where he continued to study physiologic health and pathology of disease.

Around 1813 Ling convinced the Swedish Board of Education on the idea of teaching gymnastics in schools. His program received such positive attention that in 1814 the King commissioned the Royal Central Institute of Gymnastics to serve both the public education and the military.[28] "Not only is great care taken with the physical education of the army at large, but non-commissioned officers displaying especial aptitude receive particular attention to qualify them for service as instructor, while cadets at the Royal Military School who displayed exceptional expertness are made assistant instructors at the school, in order to train them for special duty in connection with physical training upon receiving their commissions."[29] The Swedish military also utilized the unit subject matter expert model to provide trained gymnastic instructors for army units.

Don Francisco Amoros et Ondeano (Father of Physical Training in France) began his military career as a soldier in the Spanish army, where he acquired extensive combat experience. In 1806 he was named the director of the Pestalozzian Institute in Madrid. Through war, rebellion, and political intrigue Amoros was forced to immigrate to France, where he became a naturalized citizen in 1816. With little more than his military and gymnastics background to trade upon, he opened a gymnasium, which came to the attention of the French Minister of War in 1819. In 1820 the *Gymnase Normal Militaire* opened and Amoros was promptly named the director.[30] The chief objective of the military gymnastic school was to train teachers of gymnastics for the Army and secondarily to provider individual training to the infantry regiments of the Royal Guard. Amoros later published the *Manuel d'Education Physique, Gymnastique et Moral* in 1830. As a result of his profound effect on the physical training practices of French Army, Amoros was memorialized in the foundation of the Ecole de Joinville (school for military training with gymnastics) in 1852.[31]

While GutsMuths laid the foundation for the renaissance of gymnastic education throughout Europe, Frederick Ludwig Jahn took the science and art of gymnastics to the next level for the Prussian Army. Jahn studied theology and philosophy during the early 1800's at Halle University, where he was introduced to the works of Nachtegall and GutsMuths. Upon graduation from the University, Jahn's fledgleing career as a teacher was forestalled by Napoleon I's invasion of Prussia. Following the decisive defeat of the Prussian Army at the Battle of Jena 14 October, 1806, Jahn, the enthusiastic nationalist, enlisted in the Prussian Army where he fought for three years. In 1809 Jahn left the army and moved to Berlin where he began a career as a teacher. One of his additional duties was to "supervise" his male students two afternoons a week following academic classes. Finding it difficult to maintain the level of attention and discipline to which he was accustomed in the army, Jahn introduced a myriad of the exercises and games to the afternoon program. In an attempt to find a constructive use for their energy he took the boys to a nearby empty field where they practiced jumping, climbing, vaulting, and throwing and played chasing and "war" games.[32]

Following the crushing defeat by the French at Jena (1806) the task of rebuilding the Prussian army fell to General Gerhard von Scharnhorst. In some ways von Scharnhorst reflected the nationalistic views of Jahn as it pertained to the composition and development of the Army. He opened the officer's ranks to the common people and utilized performance based standards for promotion. Scharnhorst believed that the only way to revitalize the Prussian Army was to open higher military ranks to the middle class and establish universal conscription.[33] If every citizen was to be considered for service in the army, it was incumbent upon the nation to educate and train the populace. In order to develop the physical skills and level of fitness required for military service, Scharnhorst "strongly advised secondary schools to introduce physical education according to the teaching of Johann Christopher Friedrich GutsMuths."[34] In 1808 Chief of Staff von Scharnhorst urged that fencing, swimming, leaping, etc be taught in schools as a means of building a national army with the physical capacity to defend the nation.[35]

In an attempt to combat the demoralization influence of Napoleon's victory at Jena and in keeping with von Scharnhorst's physical training plan, Jahn developed a new physical training program called "turnen" (gymnastics), ostensibly to revitalize the German national "spirit."[36] Rather than focusing on elite performance, Turnen focused on the whole body, to improve the fitness level of young males in preparation for war.[37] Often known as the Turnvater–father of modern gymnastics, Jahn opened the first open-air Turnplatz in Berlin in 1811 and initiated a society of gymnastics called the Turnvereine. The Turnvereine movement was a "modern revival of the Greek ideal of building manhood in a harmonious development of body, mind and character."[38] When Napoleon once again invaded Prussia, Jahn joined in the famous Lutzow Jager Freikorps of the Prussian Army as a battalion commander and served from about 1813–1815. Many of his "students" from the Turnplatz followed him into the Lutzow Freikorps. After numerous engagements his unit received national and international recognition for their physical prowess and discipline in battle. Jahn attributed his unit's military success to the utilization of turnen as a physical training model.[39] Almost 15,000 Turners fought in combat during the Franco-Prussian War. Following his military successes, Jahn became consumed by the need "to develop the 'perfect German', physically prepared for life and war."[40] Following the final defeat of Napoleon at the Battle of Waterloo (June, 1815) that resulted in Germany's independence, Jahn turned his attention to the publication of his most important work *"Die Deutsche Turnkunst"* (German Gymnastics).[41]

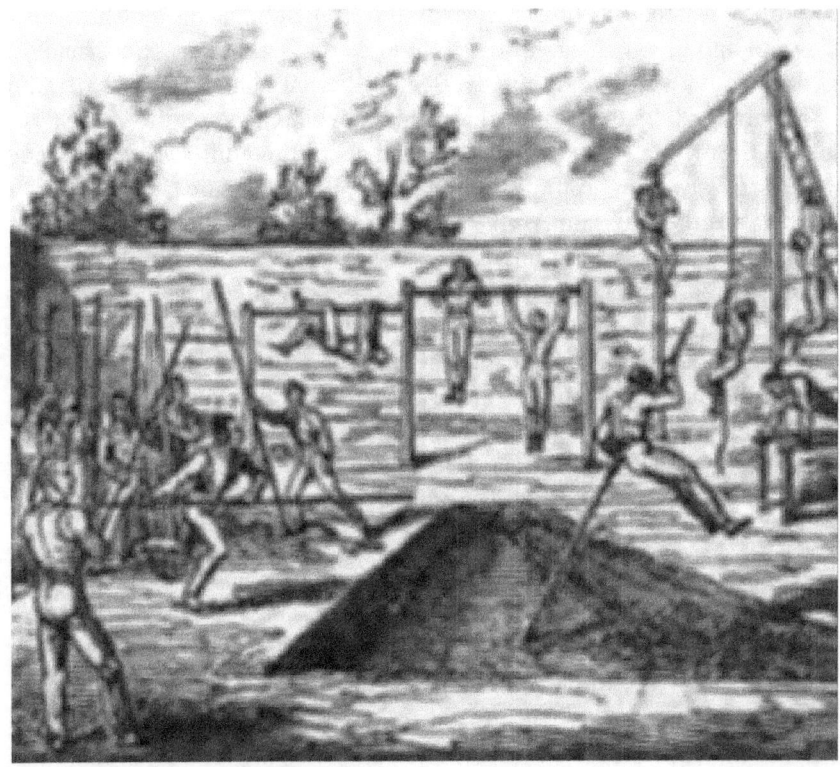

Figure 1. Jahn's Turnplatz.

While Prussia, Denmark, and Sweden were in the process of militarizing gymnastic training during the early 19th Century, around 1791 an American-born Swiss immigrant, Phokion H. Clias, left his native Boston with his father (a former officer in the Continental Army) to be educated in Holland. After tiring of school Clias spent nearly 10 years traveling throughout Europe where he was introduced to the benefits of gymnastic exercises. Following the death of his wife in 1809, Clias returned to Bern, Switzerland where he joined the Swiss Army. While serving as an Artillery Officer in 1814, Clias found it difficult to keep his troops occupied and "out of mischief." His solution was to introduce several physical exercises such as vaulting, swimming, and wrestling to his soldiers.[42] His exercises were so popular that Clias was appointed the "Government Professor of Gymnastics" at the Academy of Bern, where in 1816 he published a treatise entitled *Elements of Gymnastics*.[43] From 1817-1819 Clias traveled to Paris and enrolled in the "Gymnase Normal Militaire" where he studied gymnastics under Amoros.[44] In 1819 Clias returned to Bern and introduced a variety of "medical" gymnastic exercises to the public and to the military. It so happened that his gymnastic instruction came to the attention of a group of visiting British Army officers, who made his program of instruction know to the English minister of war.

In 1822 Clias was called to England where the King conferred upon him the rank of Captain in the Army and he was appointed Professor of Gymnastics, Superintendent of Physical Training, with responsibility for all physical training for the Army and Navy and the Royal Military College at Sandhurst, Royal Military Academy at Woolwich, the Royal Military Asylum at Chelsea, and the Royal Naval Asylum at Greenwich.[45] In 1825 Clias published a seminal work Elementary Course of Gymnastics Exercises, which from a classical Swedish or German gymnastics perspective was rather unsophisticated; however from a military physical training perspective it was quite remarkable. Clias wrote that "modern Gymnastic Exercises, as well as mutual instruction, is one of the improvements of the present age."[46] He placed into clear context the principle of exercise "progression" and its benefits to injury prevention:

> As the continuation and the rapidity of running depend absolutely on the power of the lungs, the suppleness of the hips, and the agility and strength of the thighs, legs, and feet…before undertaking things too difficult…when the powers are once well developed, young persons may make, without inconvenience, many violent exercises, which would be injurious to them, if they were allowed to practice them too soon.[47]

Of particular note in the gymnastic exercise treatise was his discourse on "running." Clias use "balancing" drills as a precursor to running drills to promote proper running form. He described five levels of running drills: (1) low intensity runs at a 9:00-10:00 minute pace for sedentary students; (2) running games and drills like circle, square, and sinuous running; (3) running moderately (pace runs), where students run a mile in 9:00 minutes and continue to double that distance while lowering the pace until young scholars "can run the distance of six miles in 50 minutes;" (4) prompt running, which cover distances up to 1000 yards in 2 minutes; and (5) precipitate running–high intensity interval runs (for adults a distance of 400 yards was recommended).[48] Clias also provided a rather detailed discussion of wrestling and swimming and their application to the military arts:

> Of all Gymnastic exercises…walking easily and erectly, running, and jumping deserve the preference; because they are the most natural movements of man, and those which he has most frequently occasion to use. If we consider the physical qualities of military life, where the success of the greatest enterprises depends oftener on the rapidity with which they are executed, than the quality of force employed, we shall be convinced that walking, running and jumping, carried to a certain degree of perfection, must overcome many obstacles in military expeditions.[49]

Efflorescence of Military Gymnastics in Europe

History shows that among communities where physical education has been either neglected or misused, a general enervation has prevailed, causing even the ruin of the nation itself.[50]

—Karl Heinrich Schaible, 1892

The nascent works by GutsMuths, Amoros, Jahn, and Clias, establishing the foundations of gymnastic education and their application to physical training in the military, set the stage for a dramatic surge in the militarization of gymnastic education throughout Europe during the mid-19th century. As a result of the ensuing civil unrest that followed the murder of the German official August von Kotzebue by Karl Sand (a known Turner and member of the Burschenschaft) on 23 March, 1819, in January 1820, the Prussian government banned Turning and closed many of the primary gymnastic schools, particularly in cities like Berlin. These actions triggered the first migration of Prussian Turners to the United States. By the mid 1830's the adverse effects on health and fitness to the loss of gymnastic education were felt throughout Germany. In 1836 a Germany physician, Dr. Karl Lorinser published a pamphlet entitled *For the Protection of Health in Schools.*[51] Lorinser attributed the significant decline in personal hygiene in German schools to the lack of physical activity. In 1842 the German Minister of Education, supported by the ministers from the Departments of War and Interior, recommended that physical training in the form of *"turnen"* be required for all high school boys. In June of 1842, King Friedrich Wilhelm IV decreed that "bodily exercises" should be recognized as an integral and indispensible part of a male's education. The King also formalized gymnastic training in Brigade and Division Schools in the Army. These two actions elevated military gymnastics to a place of prominence in Prussia and the Prussian military.[52]

With "turnen" was once again approved as a system of physical training, the Prussian Army immediately "pushed their system of military physical training to a high degree of efficiency."[53] In Berlin and Hannover hundreds of company-grade officer and NCOs were annually qualified as instructors in gymnastic exercises. In the infantry alone over 230,000 officers and soldiers were "under constant instruction" in physical training. Dissatisfied with interruptions in training due to weather the Germans initiated the construction of large buildings so training could continue throughout all seasons. In the program of instruction the infantry were trained on five basic exercises: "exercises without apparatus, gymnastics with weapons, gymnastics with apparatus, and applied gymnastics." New recruits, from the German peasantry, soon filed the barracks "with figures that would put to shame the most exaggerated cartoons of the comic papers. The awkward fellows, whose neglected carriage makes them look like a set of botched-up images, try hard, but in vain, to stand erect...So, before teaching them a single movement of the military drill...they are taught gymnastic exercises, advancing progressively and gently from the easier to the more advanced, until finally they have command over their muscles and joints."[54] Exercises for new recruits began at the lowest level of effort and skill and progressed as the recruit developed mastery over his "muscles and joints." The results of the military gymnastic training were so remarkable as to cause Prince Hohenlohe to remark "the recruit acquires a more symmetrical development, a natural and erect carriage, and a methodical gait; he has learned to subordinate his muscles to his will, and at the same time he has insensibly learned to submit his will to the word of command."[55]

Meanwhile, following the leadership of Francisco Amoros, the French incorporated gymnastic training into military training in 1847. In 1852 the Central School of Gymnastics at Vincennes was established to support the needs of the military. The initial focus of the French system was on basic callisthenic exercises designed to give the soldier control over his muscles. Once "control" was mastered at a satisfactory level, the soldier would move on to applied exercises like gymnastics, boxing, wrestling, and swimming. However, their system was "essentially Gallic in character, gratifying the national taste for graceful recreation."[56]

As was so often the case when a charismatic leader gave up the reins of physical training leadership, interest in gymnastics training at the Royal Military Academies dwindled following the Superintendency of Phokion Clias. It was not until the late 1850's that interest in military physical training was revitalized when after action reviews of the Crimean War revealed a serious lack of fitness among British soldiers.[57] In 1858 a Scottish gymnastics teacher named Archibald MacLaren opened a private gymnasium in Oxford, England and at the same time began teaching classes at Oxford University. "Some progressive mind in the War Office came to the conclusion that the physical welfare of the soldier—even some form of physical fitness training—should be introduced into the military curriculum."[58] Twelve hand-picked NCO's under the leadership of Major Frederick Hammersley were selected to attend a 6-month course in gymnastics at Oxford University taught by Archibald MacLaren.

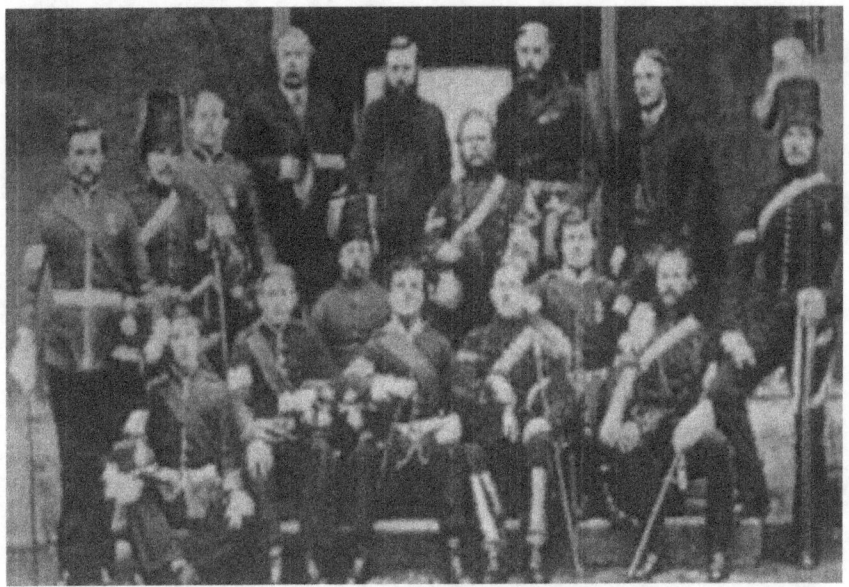

Figure 2. MacLaren's 12 Apostles (April, 1861).

Simultaneously several officers were sent abroad to study the gymnastic systems employed by other armies in Europe. In 1860 MacLaren was asked to develop a system of military gymnastics for the British Army, which resulted in the publication of *A Military System of Gymnastics Exercises for the Use of Instructors* (1868).[59] The success of the Hammersley cohort and positive reports on the contributions of military gymnastics in Europe stimulated the construction of the gymnastic training school at Aldershot in 1861.[60] MacLaren was named the director of the Army Gymnastics Staff (which later became the Army Physical Training Crops) and Hammersley was named the first "Superintendent of Gymnasia." A cadre of non-commissioned officers trained by MacLaren were selected as instructors of gymnastics at the military gym at Aldershot. MacLaren later published the *System of Physical Education* (1869), in which he stated that although "systemized exercise is valuable to all…the power of the man and the serviceability of the soldier are inseparable conditions."[61] When you physically train a soldier "you endow him with the power to overcome all difficulties against which such qualities can be brought to bear, against all difficulties requiring strength, activity, energy, dexterity, presence of mind, tenacity, and endurance."[62] "There is no change in any art or branch of science…common to ancient or modern times, so great as in these systems of bodily Exercise."[63] "It is found that no other form of drill [other than gymnastics] so rapidly converts the recruit into the trained soldier."[64] MacLaren goes on to laud the benefits of gymnastic training to the Prussian Army; "since the soldiers' period of service is so short (three years), that every agent to hasten his efficiency must be seized."[65]

MacLaren was one of the few 19th century practitioners who focused on progressive physical development.[66] Relative to training soldiers, he contrasted the exercise focus of the "ancients"—make the strong stronger (the cultivation of individual energy, strength and courage) to that of the 18th century gymnasts—"do them good" (effortless precision of a well-directed machine). MacLaren proposed that a military system of physical development should: (1) cultivate the body to the highest attainable capacity, and (2) apply this physical power to 'professional purposes' (i.e., functional fitness). "A military system of bodily training should be so comprehensive that it should be adapted to all stages of professional career of the soldier."[67] Physical training should be gradual, uniform, and progressive giving rise to "elasticity to his limbs, strength to his muscles, mobility to his joints…and stimulate to healthy activity those organs of the body…under all circumstances of trial, privation, or toil…to strengthen the man in order to perfect the soldier…military authorities have been the first to recognize the importance of systematized bodily training… and thus will every soldier in depot, camp, or garrison, be provided with the means of bodily exercise, in the most complete form."[68] "By getting soldiers out of the barracks, canteens and brothels and into the gymnasium and onto the games field, officers believed that they could improve the fighting capabilities of their men while also improving their minds, morale and moral fiber."[69]

Following the initial gymnastics training of MacLaren's "twelve apostles," the British Army used the training academies to develop cohorts of military gymnastics instructors for the Army. "After undergoing this selection process, would-be gymnastics instructors attended a six-month course of gymnastics and physical training, including long distance cross-country running, fencing, boxing, and various conditioning drills involving rope-climbing, trapeze work, and the negotiation of obstacles while carrying packs and rifles."[70] Gymnastic training for all new soldiers lasted for the first three months and generally took president over all other training. Instructors were trained and certified at Aldershot and were under the supervision of a senior officer who was also a trained instructor.

Leading up to the Franco-Prussian War in 1870, the conceptualization and doctrine of physical readiness training took quantum leaps forward in the Prussian Army. As found in the *Die Vorschriften uber das Turnen fur der Infanterie (Gymnastic Instructions for the Infantry)*, published in 1876, the Prussian Army fully inculcated military gymnastic exercises into their military training programs. "Gymnastic exercises constitute an essential factor in the military training of the individual man. They should not only increase the strength, agility, and endurance of the body, but should strengthen his will power, resolution, self-confidence and courage, and call forth a health spirit of emulation."[71] Exercises in the Prussian physical training program were divided into three categories: (1) free- and weapon exercises, (2) exercises with gymnastic machines, and (3) exercises in applied gymnastics. Balance was a key principle of Prussian physical training; "In the course of every hour devoted to gymnastics, all parts of the body are…to be brought equally into play."[72] They considered the free movements to be the foundation of bodily training for soldiers and should be arranged in groups, "so that head, arms, back, legs, and feet shall be exercised in equal measure."[73]

During his travels throughout Europe, Dr. Edward Hartwell established further evidence of the use of military gymnastics in the training and development of German soldiers and officers. "Gymnastic exercises constitute a considerable and important part of the preliminary training of officers in the cadet and war schools, and of the drill to which recruits and soldiers in the Army are subjected."[74] Most of the gymnastics training of Prussian recruits and soldiers was done by "under-officers" who were trained and supervised by officers. Much of the success of the gymnastic training was attributed to the extensive training of the officer corps. All infantry officers were required to be familiar with the principles of military gymnastics and a select cadre of approximately 200 infantry officer attended a 5-month course at the Militarturnanstalt in Berlin each year.

Medical officers provided lectures in anatomy and physiology. "Practical instruction is given in free gymnastics, heavy gymnastics, jumping, sword-play, bayonet exercise, and in…'applied military gymnastics' (*Hindernissturnen*)," which were squad-level exercises related to clearing ditches and scaling walls and spiked fences.[75]

When Napoleon III of France attacked Prussia in 1870, the Prussian Army was prepared for war. In a little less than two months the Prussian Army routed the French Army and captured Napoleon III. Many historians attribute the Prussian victory to superior rail transportation and the introduction of breech-loading artillery and rifles.[76] However, others give much of the credit for victory to the physical training and discipline of the Prussian soldiers, which was generally attributed to the rise of physical and gymnastics education (*Turnen*) in German schools. The application and benefits of physical readiness training to combat was made clearly evident during the Franco-Prussian War (1870 War). "When the superior physical training of one of the parties to so great a contest as the Franco-Prussian War is known to have been the force that turned the tide of victory in its favor, the United States cannot afford to reject it."[77]

Notes

1. James E. Pilcher, "The Building of the Soldier." *The United Service Magazine*: 4 (April, 1892): 322; Pilcher's comments were in reference to the fall of the Roman Empire.

2. Pilcher, "The Building of the Soldier," 322.

3. J.T. Hooker, *The Ancient Spartans*, (London: J.M. Dent, 1980), 137; Paul Cartledge, *Spartan Reflections*, (Los Angeles: University of California Press, 2001), 85-88.

4. Cartledge, *Spartan Reflections*, 88.

5. J.C. Boykin, "Physical Training," in *Report of the Commissioner of Education for The Year 1891-1892* (Washington: Government Printing Office, 1894), 459.

6. 20 Roman miles is equivalent to 18.4 miles; 18.4 miles in 300 minutes equals a 16:18/mile pace.

7. Online at www.roman-empire-net/army/training.html (accessed February 2, 2011).

8. Josephus Flavius, from *The War of the Jews* (78 AD), Book 3 (From Vespasian's *Coming to Subdue the Jews to the Taking of Gamala*), Chapter 5 (A Description of the Roman Armies and Roman Camps and of Other Particulars for Which the Romans Are Commended), 1, available at: http://www.sacred-texts.com/jud/josephus/index.htm (accessed 11 April 2012).

9. Jan Broekoff, "Chivalric Education in the Middle Ages." *Quest* 11 (1968): 27.

10. The seven liberal arts are: rhetoric, grammar, dialectics, arithmetic, geometry, astronomy, and music.

11. Broekoff, "Chivalric Education in the Middle Ages," 28.

12. In the Battle of Agincourt of 1415, marching through muddy terrain in heavy armor so severely fatigued the French army that they lost the battle to a much smaller and lighter armored English force.

13. Dore, Gustave, trans., *The Works of Rabelais* (with notes and illustrations)—Book 1: Gargantua and His Son Pantagruel, (Derby: The Moray Press, 1894), Book 1, Chapter 1.23, unnumbered; later translated into English by Sir Thomas Urquhart of Cromarty and Peter A. Motteux.

14. Boykin, "Physical Training," 473.

15. Fred E. Leonard, *History of Physical Education* (Philadelphia: Lea & Febiger, 1923), 52.

16. Edward Ford, "The "de Arte de Gymnastica" of Mercuriale: *Australian Journal of Physiotherapy* :1 (October 1954): 32; The complete analysis of "De Arte Gymnastica" by Hieronymus Mercuralis (1569).

17. George Turnbull, *Observations upon Liberal Education, In All Its Branches*. (London: A Milar, 1742), 295-6.

18. Rousseau, Jean-Jacques, *Emile (On Education)*, Foxley, Barbara, trans., (The Project Gutenberg EBook Series, 18 July 2002), 64.

19. Rousseau, Jean-Jacques, *Emile (On Education)*, Foxley, Barbara, trans., 16; Boykin, *Physical Training*, 482.

20. Fred E. Leonard, "The Beginning of Modern Physical Training in Europe," *American Physical Education Review*:2 (1904): 90.

21. Leonard, *History of Physical Education*, 68.

22. Boykin, "Physical Training," 483; Johann GutsMuths is widely acknowledged to be the father of modern physical education.

23. Pilcher, "The Building of the Soldier," 325.

24. Alden Partridge, "Lecture on Education," in *The Art of Epistolary Composition and Discourse on Education*, ed. Francois Peyre-Ferry's (Middletown, Conn.: E & H. Clark, 1826), 265.

25. Fred E. Leonard, *Pioneers of Modern Physical Training*. (New York: Association Press, 1915), 23-24.

26. Leonard, "The Beginning of Modern Physical Training in Europe" 98; Leonard, *Pioneers of Modern Physical Training*, 25-26.

27. Pilcher, "The Building of the Soldier," 324.

28. Leonard, "The Beginning of Modern Physical Training in Europe," 99; Fred E. Leonard, "Per Heinrich Ling, and His Successors at the Stockholm School of Gymnastics," *American Physical Education Review*:4 (1904): 226; Leonard, *Pioneers of Modern Physical Training*, 27.

29. Pilcher, "The Building of the Soldier," 324.

30. Leonard, "The Beginning of Modern Physical Training in Europe," 99-102.

31. Leonard, "The Beginning of Modern Physical Training in Europe," 100; Gertrud Pfister, "Cultural Confrontations: German *Turnen*, Swedish *Gymnastics* and English Sport—European Diversity in Physical Activity from a Historical Perspective," *Culture, Sport, Society*:1 (2003): 80.

32. Pfister, "Cultural Confrontations," 65.

33. Michael Schoy, "*General Gerhard Von Scharnhorst:* Mentor of Clausewitz and Father of the Prussian-German General Staff," (unpublished, March, 1809): 1.

34. Ulrich Hesse-Lichtenberger, *Tor! The Story of German Football*. (London: WSC Books Ltd, 2003), 16.

35. Edward Hartwell, "Physical Training in American Colleges and Universities," in *Report to the Commission of the US Stated Bureau of Education, No. 5-1885*, (Washington: Government Publishing Office, 1886), 158.

36. Gunars Cazers, and Glenn A. Miller, "The German Contribution to American Physical Education: A Historical Perspective," *The Journal of Physical Education, Recreation & Dance*:6 (2000): 344.

37. Pfister, "Cultural Confrontations," 65; Gertrud Pfister, "The Role of German Turners in American Physical Education," *International Journal of the History of Sport*:13 (2009): 1896.

38. Ralph D. Paine, "The Gospel of the Turn Verein," *Outing*:2 (May, 1905): 174.

39. Charles Henry Schaible, *An Essay on the Systematic Training of the Body* (London: Trubner and Co., Ludgate Hill, 1878), xvi.

40 Hesse-Lichtenberger, *Tor! The Story of German Football*, 17.

41. Fredrik Jahn and Ernst Eiselen, (Berlin: Preis and Thaler, 1816); Schaible, *An Essay on the Systematic Training of the Body*, xvi, 57; Pfister, "Cultural Confrontations," 66.

42. Schaible, *An Essay on the Systematic Training of the Body*, 58; Hartwell, "Physical Training in American Colleges and Universities," 94.

43. Schaible, *An Essay on the Systematic Training of the Body*, 59.

44. Leonard, "The Beginning of Modern Physical Training in Europe," 102.

45. Hartwell, "Physical Training in American Colleges and Universities," 94.

46. Phokion H. Clias, *An Elementary Course of Gymnastic Exercises*, 4th ed. (London: Sherwood, Gilbert, And Piper, 1825), vii; Leonard, "The Beginning of Modern Physical Training in Europe," 103; Leonard, *Pioneers of Modern Physical Training*, 50.

47. Clias, *An Elementary Course of Gymnastic Exercises*, 52-3.

48. Clias, *An Elementary Course of Gymnastic Exercises*, 54-56.

49. Clias, *An Elementary Course of Gymnastic Exercises*, 19.

50. Schaible, *An Essay on the Systematic Training of the Body*, 3.

51. Hartwell, Hartwell, "Physical Training in American Colleges and Universities," 161-2; Schaible, *An Essay on the Systematic Training of the Body*, 63.

52. Hartwell, "Physical Training in American Colleges and Universities," 161-3; Pilcher, "The Building of the Soldier," 325; Schaible, An Essay on the Systematic Training of the Body, 64.

53. Pilcher, "The Building of the Soldier," 325.

54. Pilcher, "The Building of the Soldier," 325-326.

55. Pilcher, "The Building of the Soldier," 326.

56. Pilcher, "The Building of the Soldier," 326.

57. Pilcher, "The Building of the Soldier," 327.

58. E.A.L. Oldfield, *History of the Army Physical Training Corps*, (Aldershot: Gale & Polden LTD, 1955): 1.

59. Fred E. Leonard, and George B. Affleck, *A Guide to the History of Physical Education*, (Philadelphia: Lea & Febiger, 1947), 206; Oldfield, *History of the Army Physical Training Corps*, 1-2; J.D. Campbell, "Training for Sport Is Training for War: Sport and the Transformation of the British Army, 1860-1914," *International Journal of the History of Sport*: 4 (2000): 27.

60. Hartwell, "Physical Training in American Colleges and Universities," 94.

61 Archibald MacLaren, *A System of Physical Education–Theoretical and Practical*, (Oxford: Clarendon Press Series, 1869), 75.

62. MacLaren, *A System of Physical Education,* 75-76.

63. MacLaren, *A System of Physical Education*, 79-80.

64. MacLaren, *A System of Physical Education*, 80.

65. MacLaren, *A System of Physical Education,* 79-80.

66. Archibald MacLaren, *A Military System of Gymnastic Exercises, and a System of Fencing, for the Use of Instructors*, (London: Her Majesty's Stationary Office, 1868), 33.

67. MacLaren, *A Military System of Gymnastic Exercises, and a System of Fencing, for the Use of Instructors,* 90.

68. MacLaren, *A System of Physical Education*, 90.

69. Campbell, "Training for Sport Is Training for War ," 27.

70. Oldfield, *History of the Army Physical Training Corps*, 2; Campbell, "Training for Sport Is Training for War," 29.

71. *"Die Vorschriften uber das Trunen der Infanterie, 1876"* (direct translation in Hartwell, 1886), 179.

72. *"Die Vorschriften uber das Trunen der Infanterie,"* 179.

73. *"Die Vorschriften uber das Trunen der Infanterie,"* 180.

74. Hartwell, "Physical Training in American Colleges and Universities," 178.

75. Hartwell, "Physical Training in American Colleges and Universities," 179.

76. Jonathan House, *Toward Combined Arms Warfare: A Survey of 20th-Century Tactics, Doctrine, and Organization*, (Fort Leavenworth, KS: US Army Command and General Staff College, 1984), 16.

77. Pilcher, "The Building of the Soldier," 336

Chapter 2
The Naissance of Army Physical Readiness Training in America

Colonial and Revolutionary War Periods in America

As the colonization of America progressed into the 18th Century, settlers were mostly preoccupied with providing the basic needs of food, shelter, and security. Physical exercise was limited to the strenuous manual labor required to provide these basic needs and to defend the often small, remote settlements. Most colonial settlements adopted the European "militia model" of self defense. As early as 1692 the Massachusetts Bay Colony sent a fully formed and equipped militia on the Salem expedition.[1] These constabularies were used to fend off attacks from Indians and marauders and to protect crops and hunting grounds. Those who joined the local militia were often the strongest, most fit citizens who were most capable of defending the settlement. Speed, strength, and stamina were among the most beneficial physical characteristics of colonial militiamen.

During the early 1700s a myriad of émigrés and American-born citizens initiated a national discussion concerning the structure and function of public education and how education informs the national ethos. Benjamin Franklin was a significant figure in the early development of public education and was the first American to propose that physical training be a part of the curriculum of an educational institution. In the early 1740's Franklin traveled frequently to England where he was introduced to the works of Renaissance writers such as Milton, Locke, and Turnbull. Franklin's perceptions of universal education were further influenced by his love for swimming and participation in a variety of other physical activities. Significantly influenced by Turnbull's *Observations on a Liberal Education* (1742), Franklin penned his own theories of education entitled *Proposals Relating To The Education Of Youth In Pensilvania* (1747). In this treatise Franklin outlined the need for an "academy" in which the youth of Pennsylvania might "receive the Accomplishments of a regular education." Along with the three "R's," Franklin recommended "That to keep them in Health, and to strengthen and render active their Bodies, they be frequently exercis'd in Running, Leaping, Wrestling, and Swimming, &c."[2] As a national political figure, Franklin's treatise would find broader application to the training of soldiers in the national interest.

Throughout the colonial period militia and armies of the United States primarily utilized the military and training strategies appropriated from Europe. "The Continental Army was the product of European military science, but like all [American] institutions..., its origins were modified by the particular conditions of American experience."[3] Although improvements in rates of fire and the mobility of artillery had begun to change the training and deployment of infantry, there was no real effort to physically train soldiers during the colonial period in the United States. With the outbreak of the American Revolutionary War, it was readily apparent to colonial military leaders that the militias could not match up with the British Army with respect to—arms, tactics, manning, or discipline. Initially the Colonial Army resorted to guerilla style tactics, which increased the need for speed, mobility, and stamina. On 26 October 1774 the Massachusetts Provincial Congress adopted a comprehensive military program based upon the militia format. With little knowledge of or predilection for physical readiness training, rather than developing a systematic physical training program designed to prepare Soldiers for combat, military leaders chose to assign Soldiers to special units based upon preexisting physical skills and abilities. Military leaders divided their militia into "regular" units (about 75% of the force) and "minute men" units (about 25% of the force). The "minute men" companies were rapid response units composed of about 50 men who could turn out fully armed "in a minute's notice:"[4]

> Minutemen were a small hand-picked elite force, which were required to be highly mobile and able to assemble quickly...typically 25 years of age or younger, they were chosen for their enthusiasm, reliability, and physical strength.[5]

An extension of the "minutemen" concept was the "hit and run" guerrilla tactics used by many smaller Continental forces. Through his strategic vision as a gifted administrator and logistician, Georgia Statesman and Revolutionary War General William Few (1748-1828) utilized these small force tactics in his defense of the South. "Experience and innate common sense enabled him to develop patience, preserve his forces for key attacks, and then pick his time and place to defeat small enemy parties without unduly risking the safety of his men. Most important, he displayed the raw physical stamina required to survive the serious hardships of guerrilla warfare."[6]

A singularly important event relative to future physical training in the USArmy was the arrival of Frederick von Steuben at Valley Forge in February 1778. Impressed with von Steuben's credentials, General George Washington directed him to prepare a system of "discipline, maneuvers, and evolutions, regulations for guards."[7] Von Steuben took a demoralized and defeated colonial army and turned it into an effective fighting force during the summer of 1778. He utilized a variety of lessons (to include the "train the trainer" model) he learned at Prussian Military College. He instilled a sense of order and discipline into a sick, cold, and hungry cabal. More important than the training protocols themselves, was the historical implications of adopting training strategies from more experienced European countries—especially Prussia.

Following in the footsteps of his longtime friend Benjamin Franklin, Thomas Jefferson became an influential force in the development of the mind-body-spirit continuum in the United States. Jefferson was an avid outdoorsman, traveled extensively, and promoted education of the mind and body through physical activity and exercise. While serving as the minister to France from 1784-1789, Jefferson had an extended opportunity to study European physical culture.[8] Two of Jefferson's more pertinent pronouncements that demonstrated his commitment to health and physical activity were: "If the body be feeble, the mind will not be strong. The sovereign invigorator of the body is exercise, and of all the exercises walking is best….Not less than two hours a day should be devoted to exercise, and the weather should be little regarded."[9] "Dispositions of the mind, like limbs of the body, acquire strength by exercise."[10]

In 1790 during the post-Revolutionary war review, Secretary of War Henry Knox developed a staffing proposal for a "national system of defense." His plan required all able-bodied men to serve in the defense of the nation. Knox proposed three service "corps," the advanced corps (soldiers in training; ages 18-20), the main corps (ages 21-46) and the reserve corps (ages 46-60). In outlining an initial training program Knox proposed that: "No amusements should be admitted in camp but those which correspond with war: the swimming of men and horses, running, wrestling, and such other exercises as should render the body flexible and vigorous."[11] Although Congress failed to adopt Knox's plan for a defense force, "the need of a well-trained militia had been sharply and abundantly emphasized by the events of the revolutionary war."[12]

Over the next 10 years military and political leaders debated the need for a trained and educated officer corps. Following an extensive report filed by Secretary of War James McHenry, on 16 March 1802 President Thomas Jefferson signed the Military Peace and Establishment Act directing the establishment of the USMilitary Academy at West Point. The primary mission of the Academy was to establish a professional officer training program that would develop Army officers in the academic, military and physical domains.[13] During his first year as USMA Superintendent, Jonathan Williams undertook the development of the first organized physical education/training program.[14] "Physical training held a notional position in the curriculum of the United States Military Academy at West Point soon after its 1802 inception, reflecting some awareness of emerging European practices."[15] Williams' appreciation of the importance of physical education and athletics to combat readiness was demonstrated in an 1802 letter to President Jefferson requesting that a sword master and head-riding instructor be added to the USMA academic faculty.[16] That request was not fulfilled until 1816 when Alden Partridge (USMA Superintendent 1815-1817) bestowed the title of "Master of the Sword" on West Point's first fencing instruction, Pierre Thomas.[17]

The United States Military Academy was generally under resourced and little more than a token organization until the War of 1812 galvanized Army and political leaders to make better use of the Academy. This evolutionary period coincided with the appointment of Captain Alden Partridge as Superintendent in 1815. He was the first Superintendent to advocate a comprehensive officer training program, which placed significantly greater emphases on physical development. In his paper "Lecture on Education" (1826), Partridge declared that "Another defect in the present system is the entire neglect, in all our principle seminaries, of physical education. The great importance or even absolute necessity of a regular and systematic course of exercise for the preservation of health and confirming and rendering vigorous the constitution, must be evident to the most superficial observer."[18] As a vigorous proponent of physical education, Partridge developed and implemented a systematic program of physical training for military officers. He promoted a myriad of physical activities to include fencing, swimming, skating, hiking and marches, boxing, rowing and football.[19] Although Partridge resigned his commission in 1818 and left the Academy under somewhat dubious circumstances, he moved back to his native Northfield, Vermont to found the American Literary, Scientific, and Military Academy (better known today as Norwich University). Following in the footsteps of Benjamin Franklin, Partridge was one of America's first exercise enthusiasts and strident proponent of physical education as an integral part of a multidisciplinary educational curriculum. "That a youth may, by means of a regular system of exercise, preserve all his bodily activity and vigor, and at the same time apply himself most assiduously to study, I have never had any doubts; but if I had, the facts developed since the establishment of this seminary, would have dispelled them."[20] As part of his "academy" curriculum, Partridge often led his cadets on hiking expeditions in the local mountains of New England. On one excursion during the summer of 1822, over eight days (no physical activity was allowed on the "Sabbath") Partridge and a group of cadets hiked 145 miles from 14-22 June, averaging over 18 miles per day:[21]

> Many of my pupils...walk with facility forty miles per day. In the summer of 1823, several of them left Norwich at day-break in the morning, walked to the summit of Ascutney mountain, and returned to Norwich about 9 o'clock in the evening of the same day—the whole distance forty-six miles: which considering the fatigue and difficulty of ascending and descending the mountain, (upwards of 3,000 feet high,) may reasonable be estimated as equivalent to sixty miles on the usual roads of the country.[22]

> But, my fellow citizens, be not deceived by the syren song of peace, peace, when in reality, there is no peace, except in a due and constant preparation for war...so long as mankind possess the dispositions which they now possess, and which they ever have possess, so long they will fight.[23]

The period from 1817 to 1833 at the United States Military Academy was marked by significant grow in the academic programs resulting from the leadership of Sylvanias Thayer. Academic departments were formed with the intent of "perfecting and broadening its scope," to the general exclusion of military drill and physical education.[24] The singular focus on academic work did not escape the attention of the 1826 USMA Board of Visitors (BOV): "the undersigned are persuaded, that a Riding-School and Gymnastic Exercises are much wanted here; and they recommend that a building be erected, fitted for these purposes...."[25] The BOV later stated that "Gymnastic Exercises, too, or a thorough physical education, seem to the undersigned to be of great importance in an Institution like this, destined to furnish officers and engineers to the civil as well as military service, to whom a hard constitution and the easy and dexterous use of all their physical powers is indispensable for professional success."[26] "A thorough and careful physical education is more important to a military officer than to any other person... and is indispensable for professional success."[27]

Civil War Period in America

Despite the efforts of military leaders such as Alden Partridge and Winfield Scott to establish a standardized physical training program for the Military Academy and for the Army, the physical training doctrine for recruits and soldiers remained disordered and decentralized throughout the early 1800's. Recruits were often transported to military posts directly from recruiting depots with no physical or military training and little knowledge of their future duties and responsibilities. From 1837-1841 Joel Roberts Poinsett, Secretary of War in the Van Buren administration, attempted to remedy this training problem. In the early 1800's Poinsett had traveled extensively in Europe where he was introduced to the organization and regime of the French army under Napoleon, to include the constitution and duties of the general staff and improvements in artillery.[28] Poinsett instituted a program of initial military training by turning recruit depots into initial training centers. The first organized recruit training began in 1837 when the "War Department ordered all infantry recruits to Fortress Monroe (the name was soon changed to Fort Columbus) on Governor's Island for training and, in 1838, dragoon recruits to Carlisle Barracks for daily instruction and drills."[29] Although these early "drills" generally consisted of practicing facing movements, order of arms, and marching, during some drill periods recruits participated in what was known as "fatigue drill" or "fatigue duty."[30] These duties included hard manual labor such as clearing fields, digging pits or trenches, building enforcements, and loading/unloading supplies. Although the duty day for Army soldiers was generally dawn to dark, there were some free periods where soldiers were permitted to read, play games, swim, wrestle and box.[31]

While the science and application of gymnastic exercises were steadily evolving throughout England and Europe, from the late 1820's through the late 1840's the advancement of gymnastics, physical education, and sport developed exponentially in the United States due primarily to the influx of immigrants from Germany, Sweden, and England. In 1848, following the failure of a relatively bloody revolution designed to formalize the democratic nation of Germany, many of the more liberal Turners found it expedient to leave Germany. Many immigrated to the United States where they quickly re-established the Turnen gymnastics model. Turnvereine were established throughout the central United States from Ohio to Wisconsin. "The Turn Verein movement...is a modern revival of the Greek ideal of building manhood in a harmonious development of body, mind and character." It tries to do what organized athletics have partly failed to do...because the eagerness to win...have put into the background the benefits to be derived from the exercise...."[32] One of the more successful Turnvereine was established by George Brosius in Milwaukee, Wisconsin, who directly and indirectly played a crucial role in the development of USArmy physical training doctrine shortly following the Civil War.

Meanwhile, following a significant period of neglect primarily as a result of the academic predilection of Superintendent Silvanus Thayer (1817-1833), physical education at West Point had degenerated into a program of simple military drill; even recreational sports were viewed as nuisance activities.[33] As early as 1842 acting Surgeon-General Henry Heiskell recommended to the Secretary of War that a regular course in "gymnasticks" be established at West Point.[34] The first significant change that affected the physical training program at West Point since the Partridge Superintendence occurred on November 2, 1847 when Superintendent Henry Brewerton (1845-1852) issued Special Orders, No. 120. He directed cadets to form cricket clubs "as highly conducive to physical development…as another means of recreation during the winter, it is intended to arrange the riding and fencing halls for gymnastics and other exercise…"[35] These small steps set the stage for a more significant progressive period in the West Point physical program, which was marked with the reappointment of Richard Delafield in 1856 as the 11th Superintendent of the United States Military Academy.

From April of 1855 until mid-1856, Major Delafield traveled extensively throughout Europe under orders from the Secretary of War (Jefferson Davis-1853-1857) to study changes in military operations during the Crimean War.[36] Per his orders Majors Delafield and Mordecai, and Captain George McClellan traveled to Russia by way of Prussia, Austria, France and England. The product of this year-long venture was two reports: (1) *The Art of War in Europe* in which Major Delafield mostly outlined changes in European military tactics, armament, and fortification; and (2) *The Seat of War in Europe* by Captain McClellan.[37] Although they spent most of their time reviewing fortifications and maneuvers, Delafield and McClellan had numerous opportunities to view training, especially in France. McClellan described the French manual of gymnastics (*The System of Gymnastics*-1847) and training sessions at the gymnastic school near Vincennes, "to which one sergeant or corporal is sent from every regiment and independent battalion" for six months of training. The six month course contained instruction in gymnastics, scaling walls, swimming, fencing, etc. "The agility and skill exhibited by the pupils was really wonderful. The efficiency of the French infantry is in no small degree attributable to the great attention paid to these points throughout the army."[38]

Over a 20-year period Congress and Army leaders attempted to gain "control" over the curriculum at West Point. Finally in October 1858 Secretary of War John Buchanan Floyd appointed a board of officers to review the entire West Point curriculum to include physical training.

Based upon his observations of the benefits of the military gymnastics programs in France and Germany, Superintendent Richard Delafield was receptive to the reformation of the physical training curriculum. He appointed Lieutenant John C. Kelton, who was currently an instructor of gymnastics in the Department of Tactics, to review the physical education program as part of the Secretary Floyd's mandated curriculum review. To expand the scope of the physical program review, Delafield sent Kelton to Europe from 15 June 1859 to 24 April 1861 to "acquire by observation a knowledge of the progress and condition of this [gymnastics] and other field of professional usefulness."[39]

John Kelton conducted a thorough professional review and recommended comprehensive changes in the physical education program. He proposed a curriculum that included instruction in gymnastics, calisthenics, swimming, and fencing. Kelton also recommend specific physical standards for cadets and officers including the ability to: scale a fifteen foot wall without instruments, vault a horse fifteen hands high, leap a ditch ten feet wide, run a mile in eight minutes or two miles in eighteen minutes, walk four and one half miles in one hour, and walk three miles in one hour carrying a knapsack weighing twenty pounds with arms and equipment.[40] Kelton also recommended that each cadet be able to swim a mile and repeat, dive and remain three-quarters of a minute under water swimming, dive head foremost from a height of eight feet, and to leap into the water from a height of twenty feet. He additional recommended requirements for use of the foil, sword, and bayonet. Kelton designed and implemented the first professional physical education curriculum at West Point.[41]

With the failed reelection bid by Franklin Pierce in 1857, Jefferson Davis, resigned as Secretary of War and returned to his native Mississippi to run for Congress. He was elected and began his term of service in 1858. In an attempt to follow-through on his initial efforts to revise military training for the US Army, Davis requested the creation of a Congressional "Commission on the US Military Academy." Davis served as the president of the commission, which conducted another extensive review of the entire USMA curriculum. During the review, which was published on December 13, 1860, John Kelton again had the opportunity to promote his "new" physical education program to the Commission. As presented in Appendix B1, Kelton recommended that a standardized course in "military gymnastic exercises" be offered as instruction to the 5th and 4th Class cadets. When properly executed, these exercises would develop the "physique," aid in the skillful use of military weapons, develop self reliance and confidence, learn to estimate the exertion men are capable of enduring, and to "fit" him for the hardships of military service.[42]

Unfortunately Kelton's extensive work to develop and implement an innovative physical education curriculum at West Point was abruptly interrupted by the start of the Civil War. As with all wars the Civil War brought new technology and military tactics to the battlefield with improvements in the accuracy and rate of fire for rifles and artillery. The increased lethality of breech-loading firearms, such as the Spencer and the Gatling gun, triggered the need for changes in infantry tactics and ultimately changes in physical readiness training. One of the most poignant examples of the benefits of physically fitness to maneuver and fire came through the command of Confederate General Stonewall Jackson. Jackson trained his men to be the fastest, toughest marchers in the Army, "and time after time surprised Union troops who did not believe he was anywhere within miles of them."[43] "Within four weeks this army has made long and rapid marches, fought six combats and two battles... the severe exertions to which the commanding general called the army... is now given, in the victory of yesterday."[44] The physical work required to move great distances at fast paces, to provide cover and concealment, to dig entrenchments and fortifications, etc. significantly increased the work capacity needs of infantrymen.

Civil War commanders witnessed the futility of frontal assaults against linear defensive positions, such as Pickett's Charge during the Battle of Gettysburg. With over 200,000 combat deaths and almost 300,000 non-combat deaths, the United States Army was forced to reflect on ways to improved soldier health, fitness, and survivability on the battlefield. In several after action reports, military leaders discussed the poor physical condition of their soldiers and what affects that had on combat and non-combat casualties.[45] Although West Point had served as the nexus for physical training and doctrine development for the Army, with the start of the Civil War, virtually all efforts to enhance physical readiness training doctrine were lost.

Ironically, in comparison to the US Army the post Civil War period was a time of dynamic growth in the science of physical exercise and physical training for schools, communities, and colleges throughout the United States. This movement was fueled in part by the failure of the popular revolt in Germany (1848) and the immigration of large number of German Turners to the United States. By the 1860's the Turnverein movement was firmly rooted into the physical culture of the United States as witnessed by the development of "Normal Schools" from Pennsylvania to Wisconsin. Although Turners were not particularly interested in

American values or political goals, they wisely understand the need to contribute to the development of their new nation. As such the Turners set about to systematically introduce their physical culture (Turnen) into the American educational and military training systems. It was estimated that approximately 6,000 Turners joined the Union Army at the start of the Civil War (almost 2/3 of the entire Turner population in the US). Publications such as S.W. Mason's *Gymnastic Exercises for Schools and Families* (1863), J. Madison Watson's *Manual of Calisthenics* (1864), William Wood's *Manual of Physical Exercises* (1867), and J. Laughlin Hughes *Manual of Drill and Calisthenics* (1879) demonstrated the Turner influence on exercise and sport in the United States and Canada.[46]

From 1861-1882 organized physical training in the form of gymnastic exercises were discontinued at West Point.[47] There were small resurgences of military doctrine through this period like the 3 February 1866 publication in the *Army and Navy Journal*, Manual of Military Gymnastics. This short article, offered "to officers who needed some discipline of this kind," proposed exercises to work muscles that were not exercised during drill and manual labor. The unknown author suggested that these exercises, which were "being used in a number of army units…will be found of essential assistance in forming an athletic, well balanced, physically developed soldier."[48] The exercises were comprised of calisthenic and gymnastic exercises such as toe raises, stretching lunges, arm/shoulder exercises, knee bends, and ballistic jumps.

During the superintendency of Major General John M. Schofield the West Point physical program was to embark upon a 50 year renaissance that would change the nature of physical readiness training at United States Military Academy and in the Army. In 1877 Schofield began a reformation of the USMA curriculum. Among the many changes was the revitalization of systematic instruction in gymnastic exercises and swimming. On 20 January 1881 Major General Oliver O. Howard was appointed the 20th Superintendent of the United States Military Academy. Over concerns with the performance of the current Master of the Sword (Antone Lorentz) during academic year 1881, Howard related in his annual report (1881) that since "these [gymnastic] exercises and those of the fencing and sword exercise…did not prove this year to be as creditable as other performances of the cadets, the commandant has now placed [them] under the more direct and immediate control of one of his skillful tactical officers."[49] The skillful tactical officer was a young infantryman named Edward Samuel Farrow—an 1876 Academy graduate. After several deployments to the "frontier" and multiple commendations for his leadership and bravery fighting Indians, Second Lieutenant Farrow returned to USMA in

February, 1881 where he was assigned as an instructor in the Department of Tactics. Farrow was a prolific writer and had already published a book on marksmanship in 1879. During his first year at USMA as an instructor in infantry tactics, Superintendent Howard directed Farrow to prepare a "system of gymnastic exercises" and formal instruction for the "swimming baths."[50] On 4 November 1881, Farrow published *A System of Military Gymnastic Exercises and a System of Swimming* (1881). Much of his work was creatively influenced by the works of Ravenstein and Hully (English citizens of German descent who published *A Handbook on Gymnastics and Athletics* (1867) and Donald Walker (who published *British Manly Exercises*, London, 1834). However, much of Farrow's "inspiration" came directly from Archibald MacLaren's 1869 publication *A System of Physical Education*. Farrow continued to serve in the Department of Tactics until the spring of 1882. Although Antonio Lorentz (1858-1884) retained the title of Master of the Sword, Farrow served as the titular Master of the Sword from 1882-1884 when he was reassigned. Based upon the strides made by Farrow and subsequent death of Lorentz Antone Lorentz 1884, USMA initiated a comprehensive search for a new Master of the Sword with a pedagogical and performance background in gymnastics.

Notes

1. Robert K. Wright, *The Continental Army* (Washington, DC: Center for Military History, 1983), 11.

2. Benjamin Franklin, "Proposals Relating to the Education of Youth in Pensilvania," (National Humanities Center Resource Toolbox, *Becoming American: The British Atlantic Colonies, 1690-1763, 1774*), 3; J.C. Boykin, "Physical Training," in *Report of the Commissioner of Education for The Year 1891-1892*, (Washington: Government Printing Office, 1894), 496.

3. Wright, *The Continental Army*, 3.

4. Gregory J.W. Urwin, *United States Infantry: An Illustrated History 1775-1918*, (New York: Sterling Publishing Company, 1988), 13.

5. Online at www.ushistory.org (accessed 22 June, 2010).

6. Online at www.constitutionday.com/constitution-founding-fathers.html (accessed 27 April, 2011).

7. Von Stueben was actually retired from the Prussian Army as a Captain, however Benjamin Franklin felt he would not be taken seriously as a company grade officer; Franklin "manufactured" credentials for Von Steuben that identified him as a lieutenant general. Wright, *The Continental Army*, 140; John Laurens wrote: "I have since had several long conversations with the Baron Steuben, who appears to me a man profound in the science of war, and well disposed to render his best services to the United States." John Laurens, *The Army Correspondence of Colonel John Laurens in the Years 1777-8* (New York: Bradford Club, 1867), 130. Laurens, *The Army Correspondence of Colonel John Laurens in the Years 1777-8*, 134-41; Wright, *The Continental Army*, 141; Von Steuben's document of discipline and order was commonly known as "The Blue Book."

8. Jefferson suceeded his friend and mentor Benjamin Franklin as the Minister to France in 1884.

9. Letter from Thomas Jefferson to Thomas Mann Randolph, 27 August 1786; www.monticello.org (accessed 12 October, 2011).

10. Letter from Thomas Jefferson to Robert Skipwith, Aug. 3, 1771; www.monticello.ogr (accessed 12 October, 2011).

11. Edward Hartwell, "Physical Training in American Colleges and Universities," in *Report to the Commission of the US Stated Bureau of Education, No. 5-1885*, (Washington: Government Publishing Office, 1886), 96.

12. Hartwell, "Physical Training in American Colleges and Universities", 96.

13. Hartwell, "Physical Training in American Colleges and Universities", 97.

14. Jonathan Williams was the grandnephew of Benjamin Franklin and served with Franklin in France from 1776-1785; due to his relationship with Franklin Williams no doubt came in contact with Thomas Jefferson, who replaced Franklin as the US Minister to France; back in the United States Williams again come to the attention of Jefferson while serving in the Philadelphia judicial system; Jefferson would ultimately appoint him as the first Superintendent of the US Military Academy.

15. Jeffery A. Charlston, "Disorganized and Quasi-Official but Eventually Successful: Sport in the US Military, 1814-1914," *International Journal of the History of Sport*:4 (2002): 71.

16. Robert Degen, "The Evolution of Physical Education at the United States Military Academy" (Master thesis, University of Wisconsin, 1967), 18.

17 Michael J. Reagor, "Herman J. Koehler: The Father of West Point Physical Education, 1985–1923." *Assembly*: 3 (January 1993): 3.

18. Alden Partridge, "Lecture on Education," in *The Art of Epistolary Composition and Discourse on Education*, ed. Francois Peyre-Ferry's (Middletown, Conn.: E & H. Clark, 1826), 265.

19. Charlston, "Disorganized and Quasi-Official but Eventually Successful", 71; Degen, "The Evolution of Physical Education at the United States Military Academy," 18-19; Webb, 1965, 199; McClary, 2001, 18.

20. "American Literary, Scientific, and Military Academy," *The American Journal of Education*: 82 (1872): 860; This document contained significant portions of Alden Partridge's direct personal reflections, which clearly pre-dated the publication.

21. "American Literary, Scientific, and Military Academy": 860; Most of Partridge's cadets were 12-18 years of age.

22. Alden, *A Journal of an Excursion Made by the Corps of Cadets of the American Literary, Scientific and Military Academy* (Concord: Hill and Moore, June, 1822), 34-35.

23. Partridge, "Lecture on Education", 271-2.

24. Herman J. Koehler, "The Physical Training of Cadets," in *The Centennial of the United States Military Academy at West Point, New York-1802-1902* (Washington: Government Printing House, Volume I, 1904), 896.

25. *Annual Report of the Board of Visitors to the United States Military Academy*, (Washington: Government Printing Office, 1826), 13; Koehler, "The Physical Training of Cadets", 896.

26. *Annual Report of the Board of Visitors* (1826), 13.

27. Koehler, "The Physical Training of Cadets", 896.

28. Charles J. Stille, "The Life and Services of Joel R. Poinsett, The Confidential Agent In South Carolina of President Jackson during the Nullification Troubles of 1832," reprinted from *The Pennsylvania Magazine of History and Biography* (1888): 1,4,8,17; Edward Coffman, *The Old Army: A Portrait of the American Army in Peacetime, 1784-1898*, (New York: Oxford University Press, 1986), 156.

29. Coffman, *The Old Army*, 156.

30. Coffman, *The Old Army*, 157.

31. Coffman, *The Old Army*, 157.

32. Ralph D. Paine, "The Gospel of the Turn Verein," *Outing* 46:2 (May, 1905): 174.

33. Reagor, "Herman J. Koehler", 5-6.

34. James E. Pilcher, "The Building of the Soldier." *The United Service [Magazine]*:4 (April, 1892): 327.

35. Charlston, "Disorganized and Quasi-Official but Eventually Successful", 72.

36. *Annual Report of the Association of Graduates* (1858), 184.

37. Richard Delafield, *Report on the Art of War in Europe in 1854, 1855, 1856*, (Washington: George W. Bowman, Printer, 1860), v.

38. George B. McClellan, "The Seat of War in Europe" Report to the Secretary of War, (Washington: A.O.P. Nicholson, Printer, 1857), 44.

39. *Annual Reunion of the Association of Graduates,* 1894, 12; Charlston, "Disorganized and Quasi-Official but Eventually Successful", 73; David J. Yebra," Colonel Herman J. Koehler: The Father of Physical Education at West Point," Paper written for LD 720: American Military History, United States Military Academy, 1998, 5-6.

40. Kelton, "USMA Curriculum Committee Report, 1858-59."

41. Yebra, Colonel Herman J. Koehler, 3-5; "Reports of a Curriculum Study - USMA, 1858-1895;" *Annual Reunion of the Association of Graduates, 1894*, 10.

42. "Report of the Commission, Appointed under the eighth section of the act of Congress of June 21, 1860, to Examine into the Organization, System of Discipline, and Course of Instruction, West Point,": United States Military Academy, 13 December 1860, 217-219.

43. Will Lang, "Lucian Truscott," *Life* (2 October 1944): 106.

44. "General Order, No. 53," *The American Annual Cyclopedia and Register of Important Events of the Year 1862,* Volume II (by order of Major General Jackson on 28 May, 1862), (New York: D. Appleton & Company), 107.

45. Reagor, "Herman J. Koehler", 7.

46. Gertrud Pfister, "The Role of German Turners in American Physical Education," *International Journal of the History of Sport*:13 (2009): 2-3.

47. Koehler, "The Physical Training of Cadets", 898.

48. *Manual of Military Gymnastics,* 1866, 376-7.

49. *Annual Report of the Superintendent of the United States Military Academy*, (Washington: Government Printing Office, 1881), 160.

50. *Annual Report of the Superintendent* (1881), 160.

Chapter 3
The Koehler Era

"The germ of such physical training as exists at present in many of our colleges came from abroad, and was planted by German exiles in New England soil."[1]

After the Civil War the Turner's influence grew steadily in the United States and culminated in 1880 with a first place finish at the 5th General German Turnfest (25-28 July, 1880) in Frankfurt, Germany. The US team featured a young second generation German-American named Herman John Koehler, who took second prize. Koehler studied under George Heintz (later hired to teach physical education and military gymnastics at the United States Naval Academy) at the Normal School of the Turnerbund of Milwaukee, where his uncle George Brosius was the headmaster. Shortly after their return from Frankfurt, the Milwaukee Turners were "big news" throughout the country, but especially in the northeast. This attention did not escape the notice of the Army leadership, who thanks to the work of Edward Hartwell were well aware of the growing popularity of "gymnastic" training in universities and colleges throughout the United States and Armies throughout Europe.

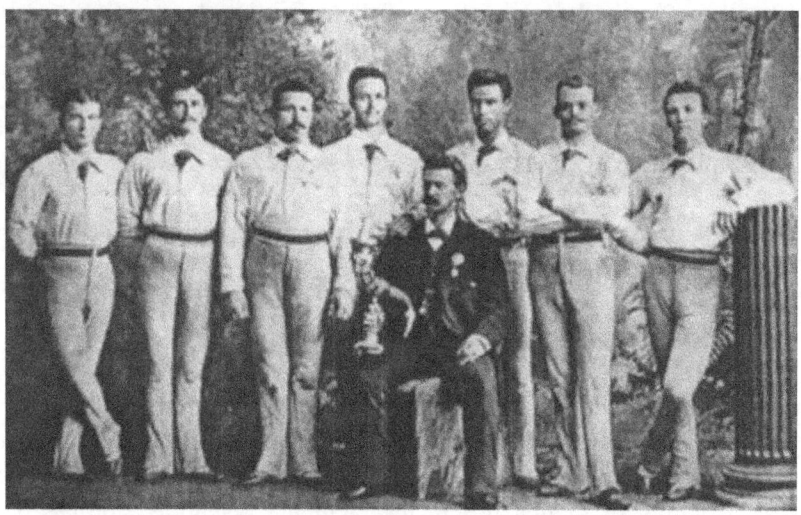

Figure 3. US Turnvereine Team—Frankfurt 1880.[2]

In 1881 the United States Military Academy began to revitalize the physical education program under the leadership of Lieutenant Edward

Farrow (1881–1884). Farrow developed and maintained a system of instruction in gymnastic exercises and swimming, which he published as a text entitled *A Military System Of Gymnastic Exercises And A System Of Swimming*. This systematic program of instruction revolutionized physical training at USMA. Although Farrow engaged his duties with significant ardor, he was a "rotating" military faculty only temporarily assigned to USMA. Recognizing the need for long-term continuity in the physical education program, in the 1884 Annual Report of the Superintendent Superintendent Wesley Merritt wrote: "A permanent assistant instructor from civil life, will be a lasting benefit to this important part of the training of cadets."[3]

The military and health-related benefits of physical training had garnered new attention in the US following the Franco-Prussian War. Many countries sent educators and scientists to Germany to study the use of gymnastics in military training. In 1884 the Commissioner of the United States Bureau of Education tasked Dr. Edward Hartwell, M.D. to develop a report on the status of physical training at American colleges and universities. Hartwell was one of the most powerful and influential scholars of the late 19th Century. He was broadly educated (M.D. from Cincinnati's Miami Medical College and Ph.D. in biology from Baltimore's Johns Hopkins University) and widely traveled. "His extensive formal education was enhanced by several visits to Europe to investigate medicine and, especially, physical training."[4] At every turn Hartwell touted the benefits of physical exercise and education. Gerber declared that he "should be considered one of the forefathers of physical education in the United States."[5]

In 1885 Hartwell travelled to Germany, Austria, and Sweden where he was introduced to the Swedish gymnastic system of Pehr Ling and the German gymnastic system of Friedrich Jahn. Hartwell was deeply impressed by the "German system" and believed that the European systems of physical training were far superior to physical education in the United States.[6] "Prussia's commanding position in science and politics is due to the perfection of her educational and military systems."[7] Hartwell was convinced that military superiority was predicated on the physical fitness of the individual soldier and that soldier fitness began at an early age through public school physical education and training. In his review of *Physical Training in Germany*, Hartwell quoted an extract from a circular on the teaching of gymnastics in the elementary schools, addressed to the superintendents and inspectors of schools in the District of Lieguitz, Province of Silesia (1871):

> It is acknowledged everywhere by soldiers and civilians that the astonishing accomplishments of our armies in the late war, especially their thorough discipline, exhibited in the most cheerful and self-sacrificing manner, their skill in overcoming natural and artificial obstacles in the enemy's country, their courage and calmness in battle, the resolution with which they bore pain and privation, must, in a large measure, be attributed to the gymnastic training of the rank and file.[8]

Hartwell concluded that in the interval between Jena and Sedan, Prussia "demonstrated most clearly and strikingly the power and worth of comprehensive and scientific [physical] training."[9]

The US Army was clearly aware that European countries had made significant progress in the physical readiness training of soldiers through the incorporation of gymnastic training.[10] When Antone Lorentz died in late 1884 (he had served as the Master of the Sword for 27 years) the Army leadership acknowledged the need for a trained "professor" of physical education at the United States Military Academy. Army leaders met with George Brosius (former Civil War Officer and "coach" of the 1880 American Turnfest team) and offered him the position of "Master of the Sword."[11] Although tempted, Brosius felt USMA needed a younger instructor with more experience in fencing (someone comparable to George Heintz, another Brosius protégé, who had recently been hired by the United States Naval Academy). He recommended his protégé and nephew, Herman John Koehler for the position of Master of the Sword to further the development of a professional gymnastics curriculum that was started by John Kelton and Edward Farrow.[12]

On February 1, 1885 the United States Military Academy hired Herman Koehler as the 10th "Master of the Sword." Koehler was USMA's first pedagogically trained physical educator.[13] He was a graduate of the Milwaukee Normal School of Physical Training (1880) and had previously served as the Director—School of Gymnastics in Oshkosh, Wisconsin. Koehler wasted little time implementing the gymnastics exercises from his Turner roots, which had an immediate and profound impact on the physical development of cadets and therefore the Army. Koehler was a gifted athlete and trained physical educator who understood how strength, speed, agility and endurance enhanced a soldier's effectiveness and survivability on the battlefield.[14] He also used his position at West Point to further the growing national efforts in physical education. As reported by William G. Anderson, M.D., the recording secretary of the newly formed American Association for the Advancement of Physical Education (AAAPE), the relatively young Herman Koehler attend the inaugural meeting of American Association for the Advancement of Physical Education (AAAPE) held on November 16, 1885 at Adelphi Academy in Brooklyn, N.Y. Although he had only completed his studies a few short years before, and was in the presents of such early physical education pioneers as D. A. Sargent, M.D., Rev. Edward Thwing Ph.D., Edward Hitchcock, M.D., and Dio Lewis, Koehler was named to the Council of Officers at this first meeting. Lieutenant Henry Kirby also attended from West Point representing the Department of Tactics:[15]

> Despite the fact that the military profession has not hesitated to impress almost every known science into its service, in an effort to successfully overcome man's endurance… the trained man has demonstrated his ability to hold his own against these almost unbelievable odds, and in the end it will be discovered that it is the carefully trained and conditioned man who alone can make victory possible.[16]

By 1887 Koehler had published the first of many military training manuals for USMA and the Army: *A System of Calisthenic Exercises: for use in School of the Soldier*. A few years later, Koehler morphed his "system of callisthenic exercises" into the US Army's first army-wide manual on physical training. In an attempt to codify combat physical training and provide guidance on developing physical fitness, the US Army published the *Manual of Calisthenic Exercises* (1892) written by Herman Koehler. This manual stressed the use of classical "Jahnian" gymnastics as the proper exercises to develop combat soldiers. Koehler stated that the West Point "system of training should be composed of exercises that will promote health, and at the same time develop strength, grace, agility, precision, self-reliance, courage and endurance."[17] Perhaps one of the more understated, yet critical, events in the rise of physical fitness training in the Army occurred in 1889. In recognition for the quality and scope of work Koehler had accomplished at West Point, he was commissioned as a First Lieutenant—Army Infantry as Master of the Sword, Instructor of Gymnastics and Swimming. Koehler's commissioning significantly increased his credibility with regular Army Officers and Soldiers. In 1892, after formalizing the USMA physical education curriculum and after years of persistent effort, Koehler convinced USMA leaders to appropriate funds for the construction of a new physical development center. The new facility contained a large gymnasium, running track, fencing rooms, dressing rooms, bowling alley, office, and a swimming tank. Koehler argued that the gymnastics equipment was "superior to any in the world."[18]

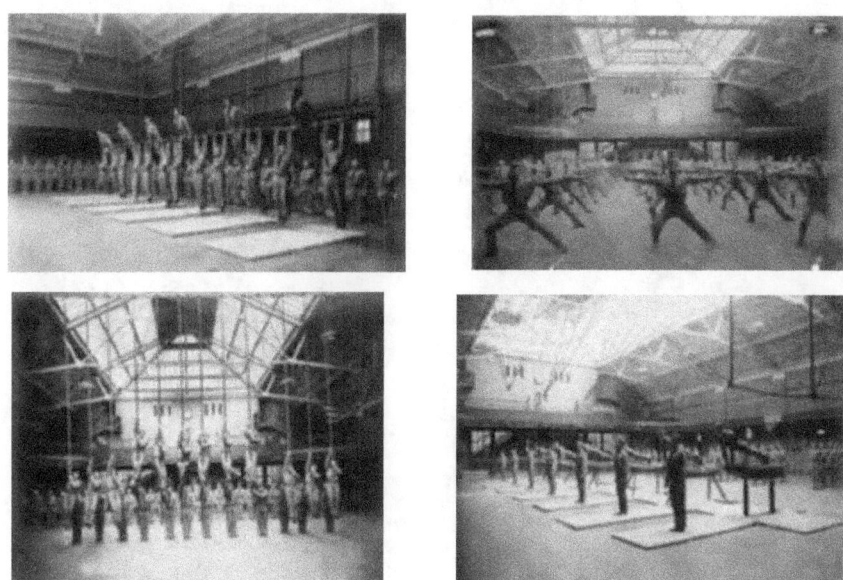

Figure 4. USMA Physical Education under Herman Kohler.

During the 1890's the full effect of Koehler's influence on physical training in the Army came to fruition. With Army physical training gaining momentum Lieutenant Colonel Alfred A. Woodhull, US Army Department of Medicine published *Notes on Military Hygiene for Officers of the Line* in 1890 (a revised edition was published in 1898). Woodhull concluded that "The whole military fabric rests upon the physical character of the individuals composing it. The recruits must be trustworthy in physique before the military character can be developed."[19] In 1892 Captain James E. Pilcher (US Army Medical Department) published a seminal history of physical readiness training entitled "The Building the Soldier" in Volume VII of the journal *The United Service—A Monthly Review of Military and Naval Affairs*. Through Koehler's influence Captain Constantine Chase, 4th Artillery, wrote a manual on Physical Drill for Foot Troops, which was published by the US Army in 1897. Chase proposed specific training in close order drills with weapons, bayonet, and Indian clubs. Finally in 1898 Major Edmund J. Butts published the *Manual of Physical Drill*, United States Army.[20] This extensive 175 page manual presented materials on rifle drills, dumb bell and barbell drills, calisthenics, gymnastics, and athletic games and contests.

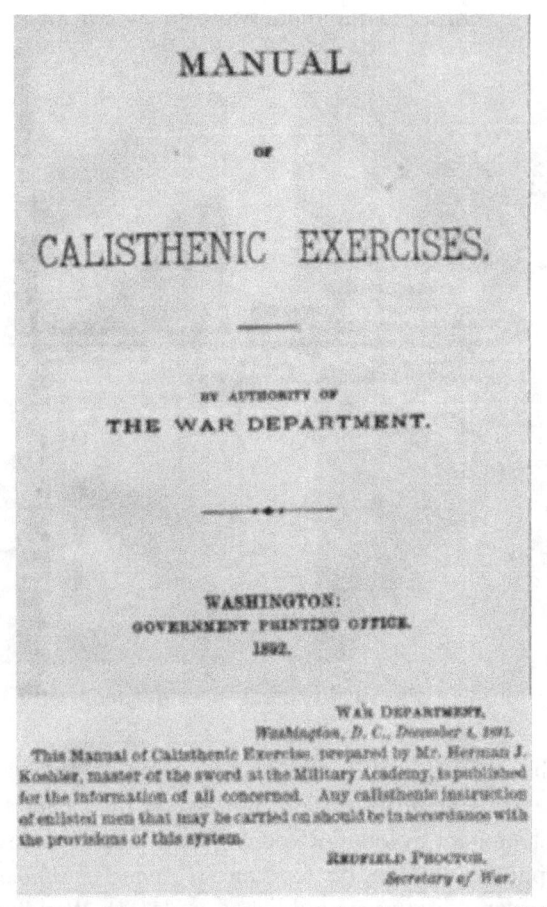

Figure 5. Kohler's First Manual for the Army (1892).

Shortly after the turn of the century Army physical readiness training experienced the perfect storm. First, Koehler's physical training program at West Point was rapidly gaining traction throughout the Army. His publications allowed large numbers of officers to learn how to develop and execute physical training/gymnastics programs. Koehler was appointed to the rank of Captain in 1906.[21] Second, the United States was in the process of implementing the lessons learned from the Spanish American War, which ended with the Treaty of Paris in 1898. Third, Theodore Roosevelt was elected President in 1901 and brought his commitment to physical fitness and exercise and combat leadership experiences to the White House. Fourth, J. Franklin Bell was appointed as the Army Chief of Staff in July 1906 and brought his pedagogical training in exercise and sport and combat leadership experiences to Army physical readiness training. These four events served to move physical readiness training into the mainstream of individual and unit training for the Army.

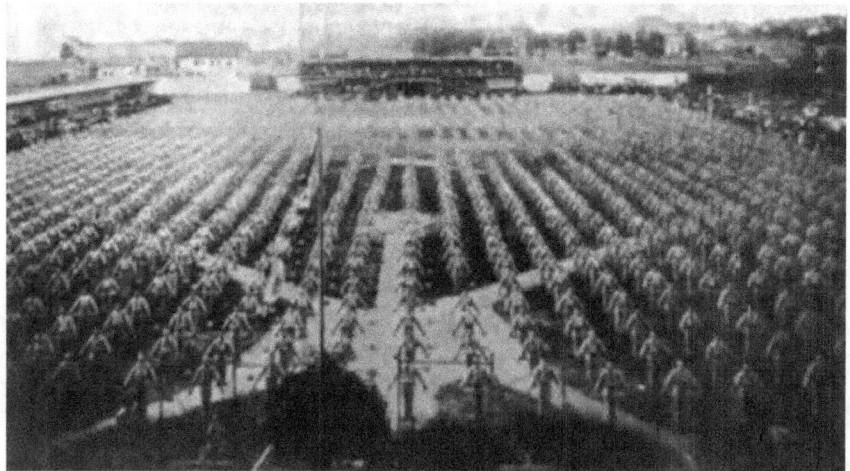

Figure 6. Milwaukee Bundesturnfest—1893.

As the Army entered the 20th Century, Koehler continued his efforts to develop an Army school designed to train officers in the proper techniques and procedures of physical training. The article "Physical Training in the Army" was published in the *Infantry Journal* and reprinted in the preface of Koehler's third *Manual of Exercises—Prepared for Use in Service Gymnasiums* (1904). Koehler reiterated his position on physical training:

> What the service requires is a system of training based upon proper educational principles, the chief object of which is to raise the physical standard of all…Physical training has been adopted by all the large armies of the world chiefly on account of economy…they have found that the efficiency of an army was directly dependent upon the physical fitness of all of its members…the physical training of the soldier is considered paramount to everything else in his development.[22]

He went on to identify two major issues with Army-wide physical training: proper facilities and proper instruction.

During the early 1900's the Army provided funds to construct gymnasia on most installations. With the "facility" problem solved, Koehler proposed a solution to the "instructional" problem: "it has been proposed to detail a number of specially fitted young officers to West Point from June 15 to September 1 to receive special instruction which will fit them to take charge of the service gymnasiums. This course of instruction to embrace the practice and theory of military and educational gymnastics, swimming, fencing, athletics, physiology, anatomy, and the physiology of exercise and anthropometry."[23] Koehler succinctly outlined what would become the resident "master fitness trainer" curriculum that would not come to fruition until 1983. There is no evidence that Koehler's "train the trainer" program, which had been so popular among armies throughout Europe during the 19th Century, gained support from the US Army.

With the recognition that war is a tough, physical business, where illness and deprivation were often more deadly than bullets, the United States Army renewed its attention to the importance of physical fitness.[24] Based upon his combat experiences during the Indian Wars and the Spanish-American War, J. Franklin Bell (West Point Class of 1878) emerged as a strong advocate for rigorous, realistic physical training.[25] Although born in Kentucky, Bell was exposed to "turner" gymnastics during his days at West Point and as the instructor of military science at Southern Illinois University from 1886-1889. During the summer of 1887, Bell seized the opportunity to studied physical culture and training at Harvard University under the direction of Professor Dudley Sargent (MD, Ph.D.), arguably the foremost authority in the field of physical culture in the United States at that time.[26] In 1905, while serving as Commandant of the General Staff College—Fort Leavenworth, Brigadier General Bell visited France to observe first-hand French maneuvers and training. "He was impressed with the physical fitness and rapid movement of the French infantrymen, reinforcing his determination to establish similar standards in the US Army."[27] His combined educational experiences at Harvard, combat experience during the Indian and Spanish-American Wars, and observations of the French Army maneuvers ingrained in Bell the inexorable relationship between physical fitness and combat readiness/ survivability. On March 6 1906 General Orders No. 44 was published. Although signed by J.C. Bates, Lieutenant General, Chief of Staff, most credit the text of General Order No. 44 to Bell and he was clearly the driving force behind its implementation. As the incoming Chief of Staff, Bell was widely noted for confronting organizational and fitness issues in the Army as was noted in the 24 May 1908 New York Times article where he was quoted as saying: "we have not an army fit to go to war with a first-class nation."[28]

General Order No. 44 established the first systematic program of unit physical training for the Army and specified requirements for garrison and non-garrison training programs. "Garrison training will include gymnastics and outdoor athletics, bayonet and kindred exercises....the hygiene care of the person...swimming, and generally all needful instruction."[29] In addition, troops were required to conduct weekly marches of 12 miles for the infantry and 18 miles for the horse-mounted artillery and cavalry. A three-day 90-mile riding test (on horseback) for artillery/cavalry and 45-mile marching test for infantry was initiated to assess the benefits of the new physical training program. There was much opposition to Bell's efforts to physically transform the Army due to the poor physical condition of many senior Army leaders.[30]

Based upon his personal predilection for physical fitness and combat experiences as an officer during the Spanish-American War, President Theodore Roosevelt understood the importance of physical fitness as a force multiplier in combat. After several illnesses as a youth, Roosevelt became obsessed with physical fitness and "became a leading proponent of a philosophy that became known as the 'cult of strenuosity.'"[31] "Throughout his life he was surrounded by the paraphernalia of bodybuilding: boxing gloves, weights, dumbbells, and horizontal bars."[32] Working with then Secretary of War Elihu Root, Roosevelt directed the armed services to develop and challenge the physical stamina of its soldiers. On 9 December 1908, President Theodore Roosevelt issued Executive Order 989, "Prescribing Regulations for Physical Examinations for Marine Corps Officers." Executive Order 989 required all Marine officers to march 50 miles in three days (in not greater than 20 hours marching time). Company-grade officers were required, during one of the marching periods, to double-time 200 yards, rest 30 seconds, double time 300 yards, rest 30 seconds and sprint the last 200 yards as proof of their physical fitness. As directed earlier that year all field officers were required to ride 90 miles over a 3-day period as a measure of physical stamina and cavalry skills.

Ever one to lead from the front, Roosevelt, with Bell by his side, set the fitness standard for Army Officers. He firmly believed that Soldiers must be fit and prepared to engage the enemy in combat at all times. In February 1908 Bell challenged the President to the Muldoon 15-mile test (8 mile walk and a 7 mile jog).[33] Although Bell won this contest, Roosevelt vowed to prevail in their next physical encounter. In November 1908 Roosevelt and Bell addressed the General Staff and Officers at the Army War College. President Roosevelt presented his views on the "desirability of officers keeping in fit condition at all times." Following General Bell's address the President "invited" General Staff and War College students to "join him in a stroll." Everyone who knew the President knew that a "stroll" meant vigorous exercise at a pace more rapid than Army "double-time." Departing from Boulder Bridge at 1500 that afternoon Roosevelt,

Bell, Secretary Garfield, and 58 Officers trekked through dense forest, forded deep streams, and free-climbed a 200 foot pitch. While Roosevelt thought it was a "bully walk," many officers were left "nursing their tired muscles…and wondering if they will escape pneumonia."[34] "The President's activity in regards to physical exercise for the army officers is in line with a movement…to establish a physical culture institution like Muldoon's at the army school at Fort Leavenworth."[35]

Notes

1. Edward Hartwell, "Physical Training in American Colleges and Universities," in *Report to the Commission of the US Stated Bureau of Education, No. 5-1885*, (Washington: Government Publishing Office, 1886), 17.

2. This is a photograph of the USTurnverein team that competed in the "Fifth General Frankfurt Turn Festival (Germany) in 1880; Professor George Brosius (head coach) is seated in the center and Mr. Herman Koehler is standing 3d from the right; Herman Koehler placed 2d overall in the Turnfest. George Brosius, *Fifty Years Devoted to the Cause of Physical Culture, 1864-1914* (Milwaukee: Germania Publishing, 1914), 28.

3. *Annual Report of the Superintendent of the United States Military Academy*, (Washington: Government Printing Office, 1884), 140.

4. Roberta J. Park, "Research Note: Edward M. Hartwell and Physical Training at the Johns Hopkins University, 1879-1890." *Journal of Sport History*:1 (1987): 108.

5. Ellen Gerber, *Innovators and Institutions in Physical Education*, (Philadelphia: Lea & Febiger, 1971), 318; Park, "Research Note: Edward M. Hartwell and Physical Training," 108.

6. Gertrud Pfister, "The Role of German *Turners* in American Physical Education," *International Journal of the History of Sport*:13 (2009): 1906.

7. Hartwell, "Physical Training in American Colleges and Universities,," 158.

8. Hartwell, "Physical Training in American Colleges and Universities," 180.

9. Hartwell, "Physical Training in American Colleges and Universities," 180.

10. Richard Delafield, *Report on the Art of War in Europe in 1854, 1855, 1856*, (Washington: George W. Bowman, Printer, 1860), v; Hartwell, "Physical Training in American Colleges and Universities," 17; George B. McClellan, "The Seat of War in Europe," Report to the Secretary of War, Washington: A.O.P Nicholson, Printer, 1857, 44.

11. Brosius, *Fifty Years Devoted to the Cause of Physical Culture*, 27.

12. Brosius, *Fifty Years Devoted to the Cause of Physical Culture*, 27.

13. *Annual Report of the Superintendent of the United States Military Academy*, (Washington: Government Printing Office, 1885), 191; Jeffery A. Charlston, "Disorganized and Quasi-Official but Eventually Successful: Sport in the US Military, 1814-1914," *International Journal of the History of Sport*:4 (2002): 77.

14. Department of the Army, FM 21-20 *Physical Readiness Training* (Washington, DC: US Government Printing Office, 1957), 8; Charlston, "Disorganized and Quasi-Official but Eventually Successful," 77; Robert Degen, "The Evolution of Physical Education at the United States Military Academy," Master thesis, University of Wisconsin, 1967, 32; Herman J. Koehler, "The Physical Training of Cadets," in *The Centennial of the United States Military Academy at West Point, New York – 1802-1902* (Washington: Government Printing House, Volume I, 1904): 898; David J. Yebra, "Colonel Herman J. Koehler: The Father of Physical Education at West Point," (Paper written for LD 720: American Military History, United States Military Academy, 1998), 7-8.

15. William G. Anderson, "The Early History of the American Association for HPER then Called the AAPE. *Journal of Health and Physical Education* 12(1) (1941): 61.

16. Herman J. Koehler, *Koehler's West Point Manual of Disciplinary Training,* (New York: E. P. Dutton & Company, 1919), 2.

17. Koehler, "The Physical Training of Cadets," 899.

18. Koehler, "The Physical Training of Cadets," 901.

19. Major Edmund Butts graduated in the West Point Class of 1890, which would have made him a Plebe (freshman) during Herman Koehler's second year as the Master of the Sword. Koehler's influence is self evident throughout Butts' drill manual.

20. Alfred A. Woodhull, *Notes on Military Hygiene for Officers of the Line* (New York: John Wiley & Sons, 1898), 1.

21. *Official Register of the Officers and Cadets of the United States Military Academy, 1905,* 5; *Official Register of the Officers and Cadets of the United States Military Academy,* 1906, 9.

22. Herman J. Koehler, *Manual of Gymnastic Exercises: Prepared for Use in Service Gymnasiums* (Washington DC: Government Printing Office, 1904), 10-12.

23. Koehler, *Manual of Gymnastic Exercises,* 14.

24. Leland & Oboroceanu reported for the Army there were 2,446 casualties during the Spanish-American War: 385 combat casualties and 2,061 casualties from accidents and disease. See Anne Leland, and Mari-Jana Oboroceanu, "American War and Military Operations Casualties: Lists and Statistics," *Congressional Research Service 7-5700, RL32492* (26 February 2010): 2.

25. Michael D. Krause, "History of US Army Soldier Physical Fitness," in *National Conference on Military Physical Fitness-Proceedings Report,* ed. Lois A. Hale (Washington, DC: National Defense University, 1990), 21; Major General Franklin Bell had extensive combat experience to include the Indian Campaigns of the early 1880's, and the 1890 Battle of Wounded Knee; he fought in the Spanish-American War, to include the attack on Manila in 1898 where he received the Medal of Honor; "Medal of Honor for Colonel Bell," *New York Times,* 29 November 1899; "General Bell's Career," *New York Times,* 26 March, 1917.

26. Krause, "History of US Army Soldier Physical Fitness," 21.

27. Krause, "History of US Army Soldier Physical Fitness," 21.

28. (28). Krause, "History of US Army Soldier Physical Fitness," 21.

29. *War Department. General Orders and Circulars-1906* (Washington: Government Printing Office, 1907), 251 (page 1 of General Order No. 44).

30. Krause, "History of US Army Soldier Physical Fitness," 21.

31. Monys Hagen, "Sport, Domestic Strength, and National Security," in *Work, Recreation, and Culture,* ed. Martin H. Blatt and Martha K. Norkunas (New York: Garland Publishing Inc., 1996), 73.

32. Nathan Miller, *Theodore Roosevelt: A Life* (New York: Quill-William Morrow, 1992), 50.

33. "Bell Beats Roosevelt," *New York Times*, 5 February 1908.

34. "Roosevelt Led 60 on a Bully Tramp," *New York Times*, 8 November 1908.

35. "Roosevelt Led 60 on a Bully Tramp," 5 February 1908; William Muldoon was a professional wrestler who competed in the late 19th Century. He retired to White Plains, NY and opened a training camp and "sanitarium" to develop physical fitness and treat health issues. Secretary of State Elihu Root and General Franklin Bell spent several weeks at "Muldoon's" to "cure" physical exhaustion from overwork. Muldoon's treatment "prescribed…a big glass of warm water on rising, practice with the medicine ball, then breakfast, which was followed by a long horseback ride… The afternoon was spent reading the sports pages…taking gymnastics and other exercises"; in an interview describing Root's treatment at Muldoon's, Mr. Muldoon stated that we "rode 18 miles on horseback, walked three more miles, and then boxed for 15 minutes," "Muldoon Curing General Bell," *New York Times*, 14 October 1907.

Chapter 4
World War I—The Princeton Years

In 1912 Woodrow Wilson was elected the 28th President of the United States. During his formative and college years Wilson was reasonably athletic and committed to a physically active lifestyle.[1] After college Wilson worked in a myriad of public administration jobs. From 1902-1910 he served as the 13th President of Princeton University and from 1910 to 1912 he served one term as the Governor of New Jersey. His athletic lifestyle and experiences at Princeton clearly informed his philosophy as president that good athletes make good soldiers. When Wilson assumed the Executive Office of the President on 4 March 1913, hostilities between Germany and other European countries were fomenting throughout Europe. As a liberal Democrat, Wilson took an unambiguously neutral stance relative to the United States' involvement in a European conflict.

As part of a two-phase process to improve the "preparedness" of the US Army, on 20 February 1914 the Army published a new doctrinal manual entitled *U.S. Army Manual of Physical Training*. The manual replaced Koehler's prior two PRT manuals published in 1892 and 1904. When addressing the importance of physical training, Major General Wood wrote in the preface: "there is nothing in the education of the soldier of more vital importance than this [physical fitness]."[2] The new manual clearly espoused the Turners' model of physical training. It was produced by a working group of three officers that included Lieutenant Colonel Fred W. Sladen, Captain Herman Koehler, and First Lieutenant Philip Mathews. As outlined in the preface, physical training should development the physical attributes of every soldier to the fullest extent possible. The objectives, in order of importance, should be: (a) general health and bodily vigor, (b) muscular strength and endurance, (c) self reliance, and (d) smartness, activity, and precision. Through the 1914 manual, Koehler's exercise and gymnastics programs quickly permeated the Army and served as the basis for physical readiness training for World War I.[3] As the Master of the Sword of the United States Military Academy from 1885 to 1923, Koehler established and/or significantly influenced all physical training in the Army through WWI.[4]

Woodrow Wilson's isolationist position was decidedly not the position of members of the "preparedness movement," which consisted of a vocal group of current and former US leaders including former President Theodore Roosevelt, former Secretaries of War Elihu Root and Henry Stimson, and the Chief of Staff—Army, Major General Leonard Wood.[5] As part of phase two of Wood's plan, the "preparedness movement" pressed forward with the development of military training camps throughout the Unites States. As early as 1913 these training camps provided physical, military, and disciplinary training for potential Soldiers and Officers. From 1913 to 1915, with little support from the Army, the charismatic Wood personally supervised the staffing and training in numerous "summer training camps," primarily designed to give college students and business men "a taste of army life," in the pursuit of officership."[6] He was unabashedly supported by President Roosevelt, who, as early as 1915, used his bully pulpit as the 26th President to call for aggressive and comprehensive preparation for war. Considering his penchant for personal fitness, Roosevelt believed that "Every officer and man should be kept to the highest standard of physical and moral fitness. The unfit should be ruthlessly weeded out."[7] Although President Wilson was still reticent about involving the United States in a foreign conflict, he did maintain that the camps would be "enormously beneficial to the United States because of the physical upbuilding and habits of discipline that would accrue to the attendants."[8] With the sinking of the Lusitania in May 1915 and continuing U-boat activity throughout the Atlantic Ocean, US neutrality was a continuing problem for Wilson. In the summer of 1915, with Wilson's failure to act in any preemptive manner vice military readiness, the "preparedness movement" seized the initiative by expanding the military-style training camp at Plattsburgh, NY where soldiering became a strenuous form of recreation.

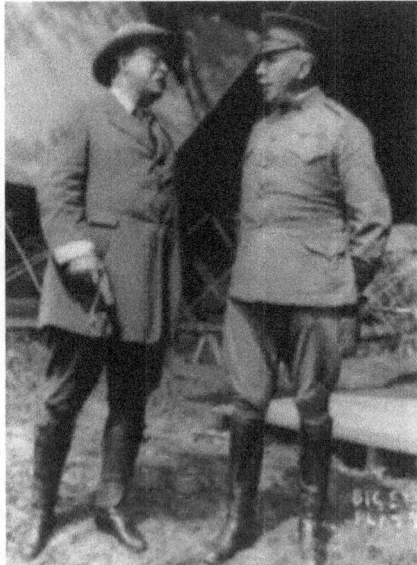

Figure 7. Roosevelt and Wood at Plattsburg Training Camp (1916).

In addition to the issues with his "isolationist" platform and the conflict in Europe, Wilson had growing border problems with Mexico. With the financial support of German agents, who gave millions of dollars to the Mexican "rebels," on 9 March 1916 hostilities escalated when Francisco "Pancho" Villa crossed the Rio Grande and attacked the US Army garrison at Columbus, New Mexico.[9] Although the garrison was quicly secured, during the summer of 1916 Soldiers from the National Guard were deployed to assist regular Army troops in patrolling the border with Mexico between Texas and Arizona.[10] Following this mobilization, "complaints began to pour into Washington about the evil and demoralizing conditions surrounding the camps. The newspapers carried lurid stories of lack of discipline, drunkenness and the rise of venereal disease. Newton Baker, who had only recently been appointed Secretary of War, was much disturbed...."[11] There were "allegations that the guardsmen were not sufficiently of properly fed, that their camps were not sanitary, and that they were poorly transported."[12] In July, 1916 Baker asked a former colleague and lifetime public servant Raymond B. Fosdick "to go to the Mexican border as his personal representation and found out just what the situation was."[13] Fosdick spent five weeks traveling the Mexican border, reviewing training camp conditions and formulating a solution to the ever-present problems of crime, dereliction, and deprivation. "There was nowhere for the men to go and forget the weariness, the homesickness, the loneliness, that prevailed…in the summer of 1916. There was nowhere to go and get away even for a short time from the monotony of drill and the almost unbearable heat."[14] Fosdick recounted that saloons and whorehouses abounded, yet there was no answer for "what we are going to substitute for the things we want to drive out…there was no athletic equipment of any kind—no baseballs, bats or mitts, no footballs, no basketballs, no playing fields or courts of any kind."[15] The ruminations on this problem sowed the seeds for what would become the largest "athletics" program the nation had ever witnessed when Fosdick was asked to solve this problem again a year later in WWI training camps.

Although "Pancho" Villa's incursion was quickly rebuffed, poor troop morale and a burgeoning alliance between Germany and Mexico created more problems for Wilson. "If the European war were to end and we were to continue to dilly-dally with Mexico, we would have to fight a veteran European army on Mexican Soil within a few months…"[16] It was increasingly evident that the United States was being inexorably drawn into the war in Europe and that the Army was unprepared for a full-scale military conflict.[17] In part to prepare the US for war and also to diffuse the growing political furor incited by Roosevelt, Wood, and the "preparedness movement," in May 1916 Wilson engineered the passage of the National Defense Act of 1916 (the Hay Act), which was signed into law on 3 June 1916. The provisions of the National Defense Act increased the peace-time Army to 175,000, increased the National Guard to over 400,000, created an Officer and Non-Commissioned Officer Reserve Corps, and created the Reserve Officer Training Corps (ROTC).

By early 1917 the Plattsburg Military Training Camp had become the nexus of the "preparedness movement." "Probably for the first time in history, an attempt was to be made to crowd into three months the training essential to a full-fledged and competent officer of the line."[18] To facilitate this process several "military training" manuals were developed to guide the physical training of citizens attending the Plattsburg Camp. *The Plattsburg Manual–A Handbook for Military Training* was published in Mach 1917 by Captains Ellis and Garey based upon their experiences during the summer of 1916 as instructors at the Camp. The "foreward" was written by Major General Wood. Chapter II addressed the physical requirements of soldering and citizens were encouraged to "read this chapter as soon as you decide to attend a Camp."[19] Recruits were encouraged to "let down on your smoking" and to purchase and break in a high quality pair of hiking boots so they would arrive at camp with "hardened legs and broken in shoes." Ellis and Garey identified five "setting up" exercises to help recruits prepare for the physical rigors of the Plattsburg Camp.

On 23 December 1917 Captain James Cole and Major Oliver Schoonmaker, of the 17th Provisional Training Regiment, Plattsburg, NY, published the second "Plattsburg" training manual entitled *Military Instructors Manual*. Chapter 3 was entitled "Physical Training" and began with the assertions that "Only the carefully trained and conditioned man can make victory possible. For this reason the first and most important concern of a nation at war is the physical training of its soldiers."[20] The exercise period should begin with setting-up exercise, followed by "marching, jumping, double timing, gymnastic contests, and concluding or restorative exercises." Rifle exercises were recommended to increase "handiness with the piece" and to increase muscular strength. Recruits were cautioned to take frequent rests during rifle drills lest they become "muscle bound" at the expense of agility. Lastly, games were recommended as a means of restoring interest when men become bored with formal calisthenics. The objective of the camps was to develop "a physical hardihood far beyond the demands of the most vigorous civil life...."[21]

The military training camps were conceived as an "officer training" program and initially catered to college students on summer break. As the "preparedness movement" progressed and the potential for a "world war" grew, the camps began to target businessmen who could eventually serve as Officers if the US went to war. The businessman clientele prompted some to cast the military training camps as a social club. In an attempt to silence the critics, Major General Wood personally managed the strenuous military and physical training program that culminated with a 9-day "hike" with each man carrying a 42 pound load.[22] After the US declared war on Germany in the summer of 1917, Captain Herman Koehler assumed an integral role in the Army-wide physical training mission by conducting training sessions at the Plattsburg Training Camp on 25 June 1917 "for the purpose of conducting a course of physical training and bayonet fighting."[23] It has been estimated that over 40,000 men participate in military style training to include physical fitness, marching, and marksmanship at the Plattsburg Military Training Camp.

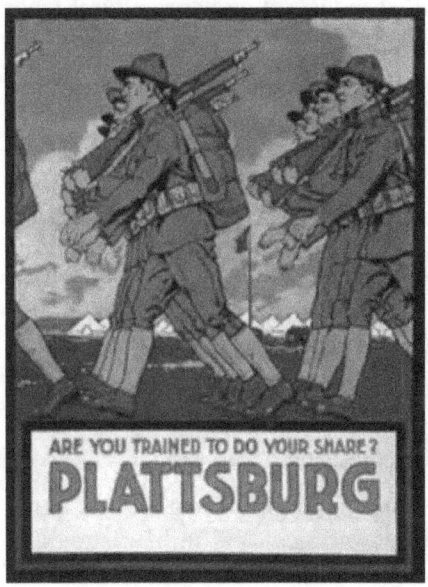 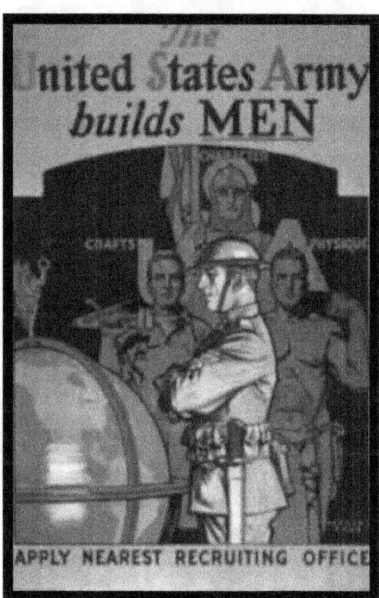

Figure 8. WWI Recruiting Posters for Plattsburg and the Army (1917).

In early 1917 when Germany declared its intent to sink all commercial shipping bound for Europe, Wilson's neutrality position became untenable. Following his speech to both houses of Congress on 2 April 1917, in which Wilson outlined his case for declaring war on Germany, the Congress passed a formal declaration of war on 6 April 1917. Although the provisions of the National Defense Act and the fervent wave of volunteerism following the declaration of war provided both the mechanism and the means to build the Army, Secretary of War Newton Baker and others argued that a voluntary enlistment process was an inefficient and ineffective way to build the military on the scale needed for a "world war." As early as 1916 Hugh Scott, former Chief of Staff, War Department, stated "The difficulty that is being now experience in obtaining recruits for the Regular Army and for the National Guard in service on the [Mexican] border and at their mobilization camps raises sharply the question of whether we will be able to recruit the troops authorized by Congress in the national-defense act...."[24] Baker's position on conscription was also diametrically opposed to Congress that favored a voluntary enlistment process. During two weeks of testimony before the House of Representatives Armed Services Committee, Baker outlined three advantages of a military draft: (1) it spreads the burden of military preparation both longitudinally and geographically, (2) it is "certain in its operation"—men will know "if and when" they are to be called to military service and this process can manage the force so as not to deplete the skilled industrial and agricultural labor needed to fight the war, and (3) the draft starts at the beginning of the "accumulation," and not as a penalty after a voluntary appeal has failed.[25] "We are now in the greatest war of all history. We are proposing to raise at the outset 500,000 men, because we think that is as many as can be presently trained.... Now, if that were a case of raising an army of 500,000 men, it might well be that some system of volunteers would be entirely adequate, although the best military opinion discredits that system as a means of raising armies...."[26] On 18 May 1917 the Congress finally passed the Selective Service Act and by the end of the year 516,212 soldiers had been drafted for military service. The Army end-strength had risen from 108,000 in 1916 to 421,000 by the end of 1917.[27] By the end of 1918 the number of conscripts would grow to 2.8 million and ultimately 72% of all soldiers who served during WWI were conscripted into service.[28]

Prior to the declaration of war, Soldiers were processed into the Army and sent directly to their units for basic physical and military training. There was no centralized basic combat training. Due to the number of Soldiers (size of the force) that were needed for World War I, it was readily obvious to Army leaders that deploying units could no longer continue to conduct basic combat training. The decision was made to establish more than 30 training camps throughout the US to manage basic combat training. Considering the lessons learned during the Mexican border campaign, Secretary of War Baker was legitimately concerned about the potentially immoral and destructive environment that seemed to develop in the communities surrounding Army training camps. "My experience with the Mexican mobilization was that our young soldiers had a good deal of time hanging rather heavily on their hands with two unfortunate results. 1. They became homesick. 2. They were easily led aside into unwholesome diversions and recreations, patronizing cheap picture shows, saloons, dance halls and houses of prostitution."[29] In a preemtive action, Baker created the Commission on Training Camp Activities, which was approved by President Wilson on 3 April 1917. "The Commission on Training Camp Activities represents the solicitude of the War Department in connection with the environment of the troops… the commission represents the method of attack by the War Department upon the evils which are traditionally associated with camps and training centers."[30] The commission's overarching objective was to create "a new kind of Soldier training camp…."[31] Because of his personal relationship with Secretary Baker and President Wilson, his experiences reviewing the Mexican border camps during the summer of 1916, and his familiarity with social issues in large organizations through his role on the Bureau of Social Hygiene (New York City) funded by J. D. Rockefeller, in March 1917 Secretary Baker selected Raymond Blaine Fosdick to "take charge of some voluntary work affecting recreation and leisure occupation in the Army…I regard the work as of great importance."[32] A short time later, Fosdick was formally appointed as the Chairman of the Commission on Training Camp Activities.

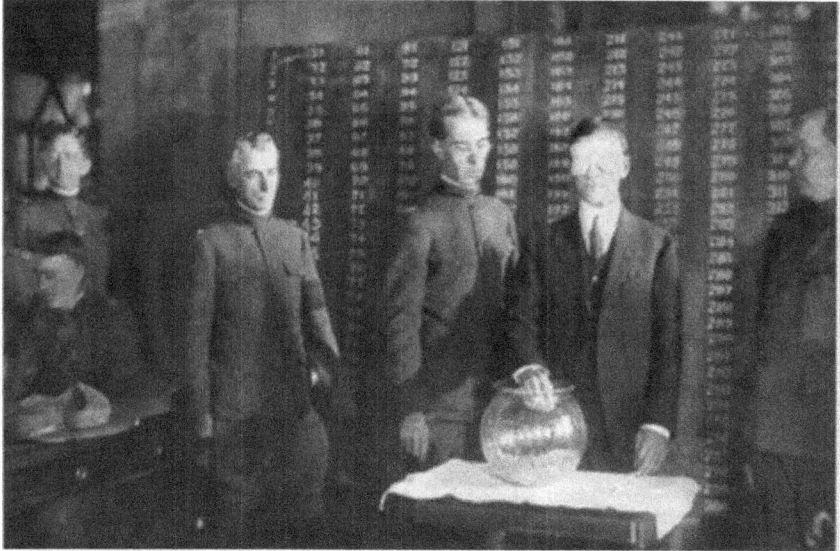

Figure 9. Secretary of War Newton Baker drawing the first Draft Number (1917).

Over concerns with prostitution and alcohol, the Commission's charter was clear: to supply the "normalities of life" and "keep the environs of those camps clean and wholesome."[33] "Secretary Baker is determined that the training camps shall be free from vice and drunkenness as is humanly possible to make them…The responsibility of the Government is doubly obvious in view of the measure of conscription."[34] Around the first of June 1917 Fosdick was dispatched to Canada to study their military training camps. However, it was Secretary Baker who framed the corp of the plan when he stated "that young men spontaneously prefer to be decent, and that opportunities for wholesome recreation are the best possible cure for irregularities in conduct which arise from idleness and the baser temptations."[35] One of the most pressing issues in the training camps was "free time." Most training programs allowed for seven hours of instruction/training per day.[36] In formulating the commission's action plan, Fosdick utilized lessons learned from his visits to Canadian and English training camps. Based upon the Canadian and British practices of utilizing athletics for recreation and moral, one of the Commission's most important tasks was the appointment of an athletic director in every training camp:

> The British understood the relaxing and therapeutic effect of vigorous games…they had had their men playing football almost before the battlefield was cleared. I had, myself, in the early days of the war, seen the invigorating effect of a baseball game on an exhausted squad of raw recruits returning to camp after a long hike. We came to the conclusion, therefore, not only that athletic supplies in quantity were necessary for the new army, but also that the administration of a carefully planned program should be in the hands of competent experts in each camp.[37]

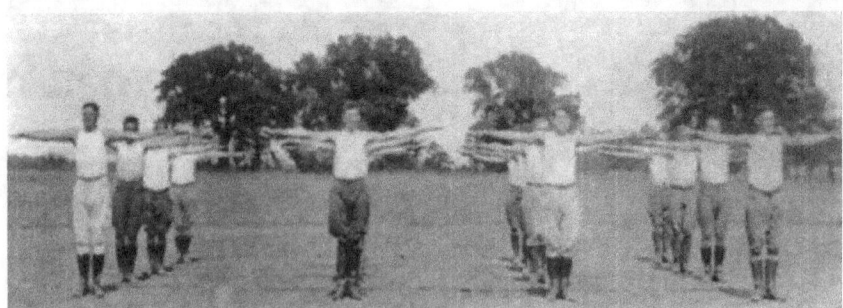

Figure 10. WWI Army Physical Training Formation.

In an attempt to remedy the "idle hands" issue and provide measured leadership for the athletic program, Fosdick turned to his Princeton

University affiliations and selected Dr. Joseph E. Raycroft as chairman of the Athletic Division of the Commission on Training Camp Activities from 1917 to 1919. At the time Raycroft had been serving as the Chairman/Professor of Hygiene and Physical Education at Princeton University since 1911. He was heavily influenced by early 20th Century physical educators such as James McCurdy, W.G. Anderson, Dudley Sergeant, and Mabel Lee, who proposed a change in focus of physical exercise from health, movement, strength and agility to athletic/sport performance. Many educators argued that focusing on sport as an outcome objective carried with it all the benefits of Turnen exercises with the added benefit of leadership development and the enhancement of social skills and moral-ethical behaviors.

Raycroft was well known for introducing the "mass athletics" model (intramural sports) into the physical education curriculum at Princeton. As chairman of the Athletic Division he quickly implemented the athletics model in the Army basic training camps in order to improve health, fitness, and morale. Raycroft introduced boxing and a variety of competitive sports to mitigate the drudgery of free time and the tedium of military drill, calisthenics, and gymnastics.[38] "Never before in the history of this country," wrote a newspaper sports editor, 'have so large a number of men engaged in athletics. Every kind of sport is involved—football, baseball, basket ball, volley ball, push ball, medicine ball, soccer, track and field athletics, and particularly boxing. Everybody's boxing, even the mountaineers and the boys from the farm who never saw a pair of boxing gloves in their lives. Men are learning to get bumped and not mind it. They eat it up.' That was the spirit and the kind of army we wanted."[39] As the war loomed, many physical education and sports professionals provided training input. Walter Camp (well known sports writer and football coach) developed his "daily dozen set-up" exercises, which were adopted by the Navy in 1918.[40]

Fosdick incorporated a myriad of traditional games like football, baseball, soccer, and boxing—running, tennis, fencing, swimming, and "laughter-provoking" games of swat tag, prisoner's base, and duck-on-the rock into Army mass athletics to help with self-control, agility, mental alertness, and initiative. Organizations like the Y.M.C.A., Knights of Columbus, and the Jewish Welfare Board were utilized to provide additional recreational experiences during basic training. Fosdick later concluded that "athletics offers a legitimate expression for the healthy animal spirit which, when put up, will invariably assert itself in some form of lawlessness. Important as this is, the greatest function of athletics is to educate the men into better fighters:"[41]

I have seen a boxing instructor stand up before a group of two thousand men and put them through a series of evolutions that would later be tried out in no man's land, for there is a close relationship between boxing and bayonet fighting. I have seen games of soccer in which four hundred players took part, and soccer, too, is one of the forms of sport which has a close parallel to fighting. While playing it, a man must be ready constantly to strike the ball with either foot. In this way he naturally acquires the short gait and balance that will serve him in good stead when he comes to crossing furrowed and shell-torn stretches of devastated land. It is a highly exhilarating game combining the maximum of exercise and recreation with valuable training.[42]

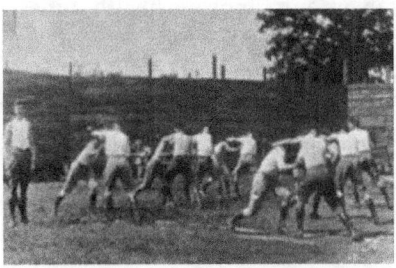

Boxing Instruction During Basic Training.

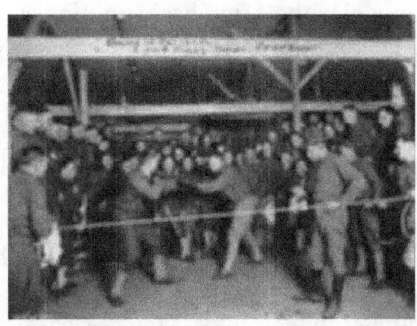

Boxing Barracks, 311th Supply Trains, Camp Grant (1918).

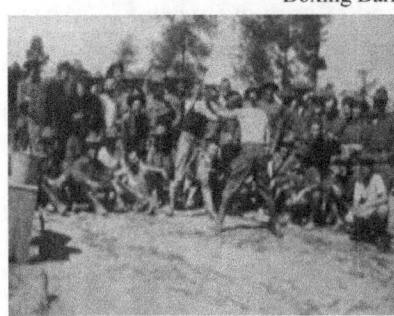

Boxing at Camp Greene, Charlotte, NC (1918).

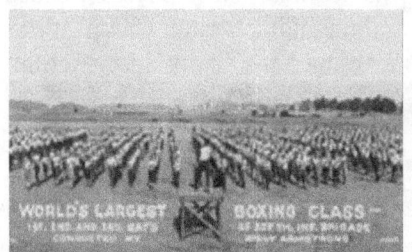

World's Largest Boxing Class, 337th Inf. Brigade, 27 June 1918.

Figure 11. Boxing Instruction and Contests—WWI Training Camps.

Photo 3 Source: Courtesy of the Robbins-Spangler Carolina Room -CharlotteMeclenburg Library.

Clearly for Fosdick the solution to the "tendency to mental and moral disintegration" that surfaced during basic recruit training was the introduction of recreational and educational programs. From his perspective the programs Raycroft introduced in the basic training camps constituted the largest social program ever undertaken. "It was the first time a government had ever combined educational and ethical elements with disciplinary forces, in the production of a fighting organism."[43]

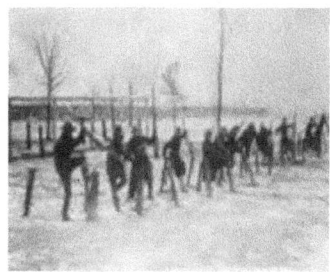

Wire Entanglement Negotiation Drills.

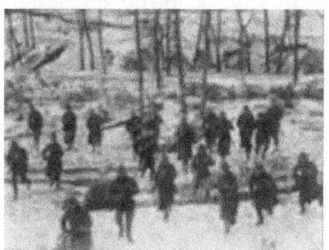

Trench Negotiation Drills.

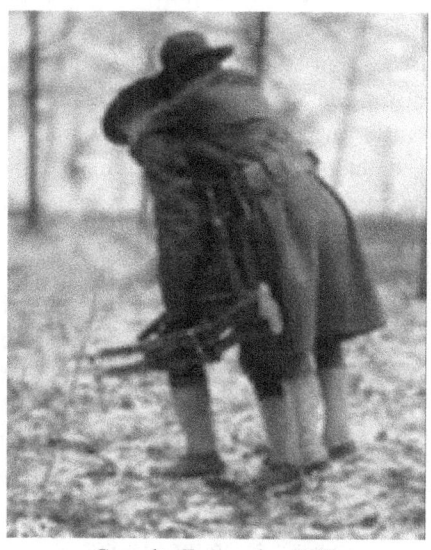

Casualty Evacuation Drills.

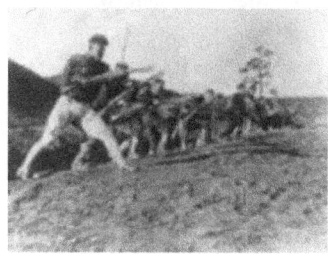

Bayonet Charge from Trench.

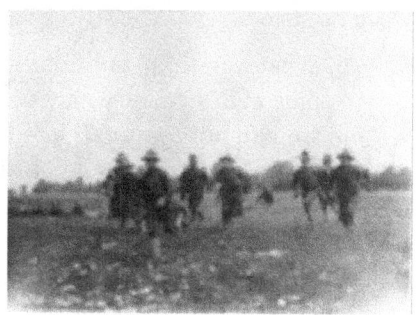

Rush Drills with Rifle.

Figure 12. WWI Combat Readiness Training.

By early 1917 Raycroft was introducing the athletic sport model into Army basic training, however, Koehler's gymnastics model remained the foundation of physical readiness training for the Army. Major Koehler continued to develop West Point officers and from May 1917 to September 1918 when he was detached on temporary duty to train physical fitness instructors and Soldiers at basic training camps throughout the US. He personally trained over 200,000 soldiers during WWI.[44] In 1917 Koehler published Special Regulations, No. 23—*Field Physical Training of the Soldier* to supplement his training program. This manual and Koehler's personal leadership and supervision at numerous basic training camps formed the foundation of physical conditioning during World War I.

With the cessation of hostilities in November 1918, World War I came to a rapid conclusion. During the post war after action reviews two competing physical training philosophies emerged: the Koehler disciplinary gymnastics model and the Raycroft athletic sport model. The battle for control of Army physical training came to a head in late 1919. Lieutenant Colonel Herman Koehler published *Koehler's West Point Manual of Disciplinary Physical Training*. In the "introduction" Koehler wrote: "in general, the manual is a revision of Special Regulations, No. 23, *Field Training of the Soldier*, a syllabus prepared by the author, and published by the War Department, by the direction of the Secretary of War, making it mandatory upon all to carry out this work in the service in accordance with these special regulations."[45] On a casual read, one might construe this publication to be Army doctrine; however Secretary of War Newton Baker stated in the "foreward" that "the appearance of Colonel Koehler's manual will...make available to a larger number of people the principle inclination of a system...which has stood the test under critical conditions."[46] Secretary Baker went on to address the historical propensity of the US Army to support physical fitness training only in times of crisis when he stated:

> Whatever form our future training of boys and young men in this country may take it is greatly to be hoped that we will not again fall into the habit of slighting the body as we were on the point of doing when the war forced us to realize its importance as the basis of our national strength.[47]

Approximately six months later, the Army War Plans Division under the direction of Major General William G. Haan approved the publication of the manual, *Mass Physical Training for Use in the Army and Reserve Officers' Training Corps* (1920) written by Dr. Joseph Raycroft.[48] In the forward Haan made it clear that this manual was the officially approved doctrine for Army training:

> This book was submitted to the War Department for publication as an official document; but in view of the delays that would probably be involved under this plan, it was decided that Dr. Raycroft should be requested to publish the book privately under his own name, so that it might

be available at the earliest possible moment for use in the army. To this end, this book has the approval of the War Plans Division of the General Staff. Its contents will form the basis for the training and instruction of the military service of the United States in the subjects included. (22 December 1919).[49]

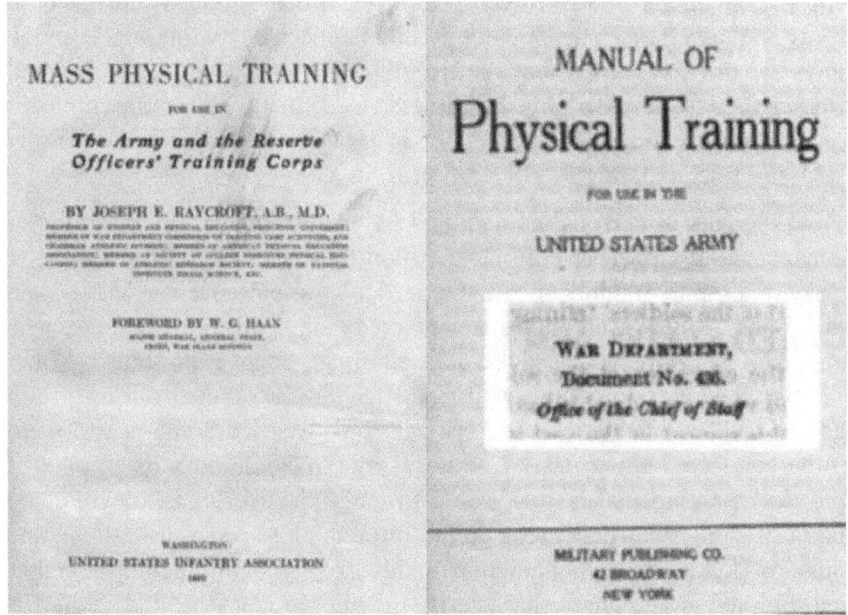

Figure 13. Post WWI PRT Manuals (Raycroft-Koehler).

Raycroft brought two notable biases to the 1920 *Mass Physical Training* manual. The Army of WWI was still a rather low tech, high maintenance organization. Most of the daily training involved significant manual labor on the part of the Soldier. "The daily program of the soldier, comprising as it does seven or eight hours of active outdoor work, provides all the physical exercise that is required to make and keep him physically fit."[50] The second bias was the pre-WWI training camp experience where a large number of soldiers experienced a significant amount of "free time" following the duty day. The Fosdick Commission's solution to these problems was to introduce the mass athletics model Raycroft had developed at Princeton University:

> To send a man out to dig a trench and to set him up in drill day after day, does not necessarily evolve a well-devel-

oped physical man. For the sake of such development, we have placed in every training camp in the United States an athletic director responsible to the commanding officer as his civilian aid.[51]

Following these central themes Raycroft identified six basic training domains: (1) physical drill, (2) group games, (3) drills in personal contact, (4) individual efficiency test, (5) mass athletics and competitive games, and (6) bayonet training. Raycroft's physical drill model varied in both form and function from Koehler's callisthenic and "setting-up" model. Physical drill was designed for disciplinary training and body control. Rather than to develop physical fitness, these drills placed an emphasis on "securing good posture, freedom of movement and accurate snappy response to commands."[52]

The drills in personal contact and bayonet training were designed to enhance aggressiveness, confidence, fighting spirit, and a "willingness to carry on in spite of punishment." Of particular importance was instruction in boxing. "Special emphasis is laid on boxing, not only because it is an excellent sport, but because of its intimate connection with bayonet fighting."[53] The competitive spirit and team work leaned during group games and mass athletics were critical objectives for Soldiers and were to be conducted every day. "In other words, this comprehensive plan of physical training makes it possible to carry the recruit far beyond the point of soldierly efficiency acquired through close order drill alone, and develops in him those fundamental qualities of resourcefulness, leadership and fighting spirit, which characterize the high-grade, seasoned soldier."[54]

Raycroft recommended two physical training periods per day. In the morning, not less than 1½ hours after the morning meal, Soldiers were to participate in a 1-hour lesson that concentrated on personal conditioning and combatives. The 1-hour afternoon session should concentrate on mass athletics/competitive sports and preparation for the Physical Efficiency Test. Raycroft stated that instructors should be junior officers or NCOs who were specifically trained, familiar and proficient in all phases of work, and capable of demonstrating and taking part in the performance of the work.[55] Lastly, following his natural disposition as an educator, Raycroft instruction in physical training should be part of the basic training of every officer, and that a "central school" (to include advanced courses) should be developed to "train and qualify experts who will serve as inspecting instructors and thus keep the work on a high plane of efficiency."[56]

Even taking into account the fact that Raycroft was a civilian educator, who had never served in the military, there were significant differences between the Raycroft and Koehler manuals. First, Raycroft's manual was obviously a consortial effort as he cited the contributions of a significant number of military and civilian physical training experts in the preparation of the manual (to include a liberal adaptation of the "setting up" exercises taken from Koehler's 1917 manual). In the preface, he acknowledged the assistance and input from 15:

> Athletic Directors, Special Instructors, and Physical Training Officers who contributed so generously of their technical training and experience and whose work in the Camps made it possible to organize this system and put it into operation during the war...The training material in this manual has been collected from many sources, both native and foreign, and no hesitation has been shown in adopting or adapting methods that have been found useful in the armies of our allies, nor in trying out any procedure that seemed to have merit and promised results.[57]

Second, Raycroft's manual was better designed, more comprehensive, and better written, with significantly more technical information about the science of exercise. It was clearly written/edited by a senior educator with the student/instructor in mind.

Third, over 50% of the manual (pages 149-280) pertained to the use of athletic sports and games for physical training. "The physical training officer should constantly keep in mind that the prime purpose of the supervised athletic period is to give the soldier the educational value of participating in different types of athletic contests."[58] Raycroft proposed using athletic sports and games in daily physical training as a means of improving mental and physical alertness and providing variety and interest to the regular work schedule. "It was demonstrated during the war that nothing was so valuable as competitive games in keeping alive the interest of the men and in preventing discontent and homesickness during a long training period or after a protracted tour of duty in the front lines."[59]

Fourth, and most importantly, the Raycroft manual was the first Army manual to identify quantitative physical outcome objectives for Soldiers, which were selected to measure "all-round physical efficiency." Although Koehler had used physical assessments to measure individual cadet development and program success since his arrival at West Point in 1885, Raycroft created a five-item battery (the Individual Efficiency Test—IET) to measure combat physical readiness (i.e., running, jumping, climbing, and throwing). The Individual Efficiency Test was composed of: 100 yd run (14 sec); running broad jump (12 feet); wall climb (8 ft unassisted);

hand grenade throw (30 yards into a 10' diameter circle); and obstacle course run. The Obstacle Course Run (OCR) presented in Raycroft's *Mass Physical Training* manual was the first recorded use of an obstacle course to obtain a quantitative assessment of functional fitness. The OCR utilized five obstacles spread over a 100-yard linear course. Soldiers were required to sprint 10 yards and vault a three-foot hurdle; sprint 15 yards and negotiate a wire entanglement; sprint 15 yards and climb a 5-foot high ramp/platform; leap from the platform over a 10-foot wide trench; sprint 15 yards and negotiate a 1-foot wide, 20 feet long plank bridge; sprint 15 yards and climb over an 8-foot smooth-faced fence; sprint to finish. The "passing" mark for the OCR was 30 seconds. The Individual Efficiency Test was designed to "stimulate the soldier to make the effort to attain a certain fixed standard, and serve also to call the attention of the Commanding Officer to those weak and inefficient men who need special attention and work to enable them to overcome their deficiencies."[60]

Raycroft further proposed that the Individual Efficiency Test contain a progressive component. He recommended that every recruit be tested as soon as they entered initial military training (Grade 3: test in service uniform without blouse and without equipment); if they fail, test again in 30 days; if they fail a second time they should receive remedial training. Once a soldier passed in "Grade 3," he should be tested in Grade 2: test the IET in service uniform without blouse and carrying a rifle. Once passing in Grade 2, he should be tested in Grade 1: test the IET in light marching equipment without blouse carrying a rifle. Raycroft was also the first to propose a "physical certificate" for each "grade" of the IET a soldier passed.[61] The last physical standard Raycroft proposed was to come at the end of three months of training. Each soldier was to demonstrate proficiency in hand-to-hand combat, knowledge of bayonet drill, and the ability to "acquit himself credibly in a three-round bout of boxing." Raycroft found that even a comprehensive program of physical training could "bring the recruit very much closer to the seasoned soldier as regards mental and physical preparedness" than previous training methods.[62] Finally Raycroft concluded:

> One of the most important of the many lessons which have come from the war is the demonstration of the fact that other types of physical activities besides calisthenics are not only extremely useful in the contribution which they make in the development of important soldierly qualities, but that they are capable of being used as an integral part of the formal program of training. Group games, wrestling, boxing, hand-to-hand fighting and other personal

contact drills give the soldier a kind of training which he can get in no other way short of battle experience. The inclusion of such activities in the regular training gives to the recruit, in a very effective way and in a relatively short space of time, an invaluable mental and physical experience and contributes greatly to the development of confidence and effectiveness in combat. In other words, activities of this type are an essential supplement to the disciplinary training received from the close order drill.[63]

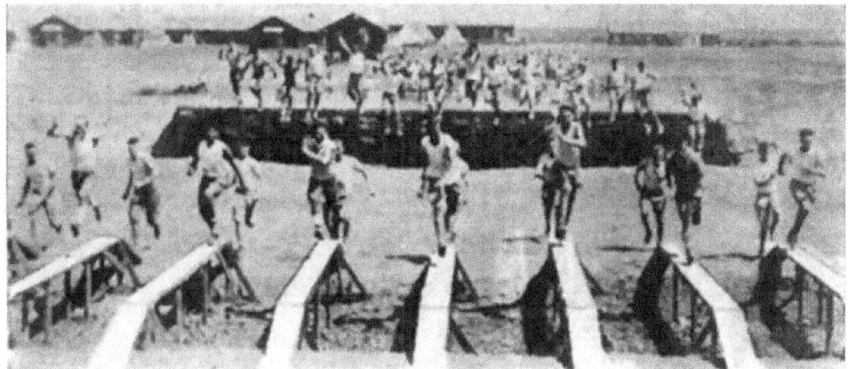

Figure 14. Obstacle Course Run. [64]

Soon after WWI Koehler's disciplinary gymnastics model went into rapid decline. There were several key factors that caused the Army to abandon Koehler's physical training model as Army doctrine. First, Koehler was retired from the Army in 1923. Second, and perhaps more significant, was the prevalence of anti-German sentiment in the US immediately following WWI. Although Koehler's physical training model was generally accepted as a viable training model, his program clearly epitomized the German Turnverein model. Having such inextricably links to an enemy that caused over 200,000 casualties was impossible to overcome in the short term. Even with the significant anti-German backlash following WWI, there was still some post-WWI allegiance to Koehler's PRT model among military leaders. Koehler's broad base of support was evidenced by the Secretary of War, Newton Baker, writing the "Foreward" for Koehler's 1919 training manual (which was never sanctioned by the Army). Although Raycroft's sport model was never fully implemented following WWI, it did serve as a template for physical readiness training and assessment models that would emerge shortly after the initiation of hostilities in WWII.

Post War Consideration of Army Physical Readiness Training

During the interwar years (1919-1939) three significant events hastened the evolution of Army physical fitness training: (1) comprehensive after action reviews from WWI, (2) discovery and utilization of antibiotics to reduce battlefield casualties, and (3) significant advancements in warfighting technology. From its inception the civilian leaders of the United States made the strategic decision to maintain a relatively small Regular Army in times of peace. In times of crisis the intent was to reinforce Regular Army forces "by such additional citizen forces as the particular emergency may require."[65] "If we intend to avoid a standing Army, (that bane of a republic, and engine of oppression in the hands of despots), our militia must be patronized and improved, and military information must be disseminated amongst the great mass of the people."[66] Although conscripted Soldiers were somewhat problematic from a fitness perspective during the Civil War, based upon results obtained by physical examinations during WWI approximately "one third of this enormous sample of the young men of the country were found to be [physically] unfit for duty with the fighting units of the Army."[67] Millions of men were drafted, but then rejected as physically unfit before being sworn into service. Medical examinations by local draft boards revealed the impact of poor nutrition and excessive and unsafe work conditions.[68] While studying bacteriology at Camp Funston, Kansas, Major George Draper noted "it is quite apparent that the physical condition of the men…is poor….their pale skins and flabby tissues bespeak lack of tone, and indicate the absence of any kind of exercise."[69] "Had the general public profited by the knowledge and experience of the Army in physical training it would not have been necessary, when the call for service in the Great War came, to discard one-third of the potential manpower because of physical disability."[70]

The "unfit for duty" problem was exacerbated by the sheer number of soldiers drafted. Basic training camps throughout the United States trained millions of men from mid 1917—1918. During the troop surge in late 1917, the Army found itself with large numbers of conscripts who were brought on active duty to meet growing manpower quotas; these men were unfit for duty. Some soldiers had such significant physical deficiencies that they were of little use to their unit. Whenever possible, commanders transferred these men to other units to "purify their organizations of poor soldiers, and men of deficient intelligence and physical stamina."[71] Finally the War Department created "convalescent units" in depot brigades where unfit men could rehabilitate and developed a limited service" category for these somplete non-combatant work. Due to generally poor fitness levels of these conscripted Soldiers, the entire country refocused on the physical fitness aspects of military training.

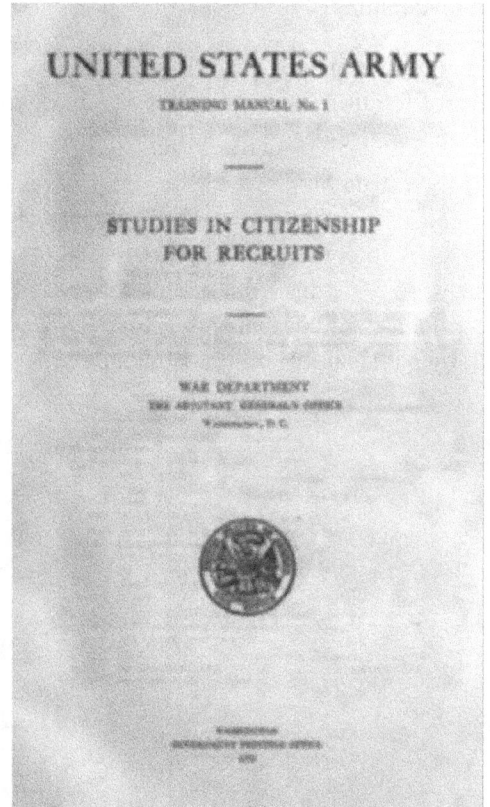

Figure 15. Studies in Citizenship for Recruits.

The growing emphasis on physical fitness was manifest in the four preparatory documents developed at the Citizens' Military Training Camp at Plattsburg during the summer of 1922. On 31 October 1922 the War Department published Training Manual No. 1—No. 4 entitled *Studies in Citizenship for Citizens Military Training Camps*, which were issued to all recruits upon entering the Army. Chapter 4, Training Manual No. 2, outlined the components and expectations of "military training" and provided a global view of the role of physical training in war:

> Fitness for survival, in time of war is the first and primary requisite for any preparedness program. No nation has ever survived, and no nation ever will survive, whose people are not physically, mentally, and morally fit for survival. Military training is not designed to enhance the

militaristic spirit. It builds men up physically. It gives them the discipline of self-control and inculcates obedience as the first step toward effective service and competence in leadership.[72]

The second significant event during the interwar years was the discovery and proliferation of antibiotics to treat combat casualties, specifically sulfa-based drugs and penicillin:[73]

> War is truly a struggle between life and death and, in war, death is caused equally as frequently by sickness and incapacity as by the bullets of the enemy…in few wars has the percentage of deaths from wounds exceeded that from disease…the loss of combat and of march are occasioned as much by physical disability as by bullets.[74]

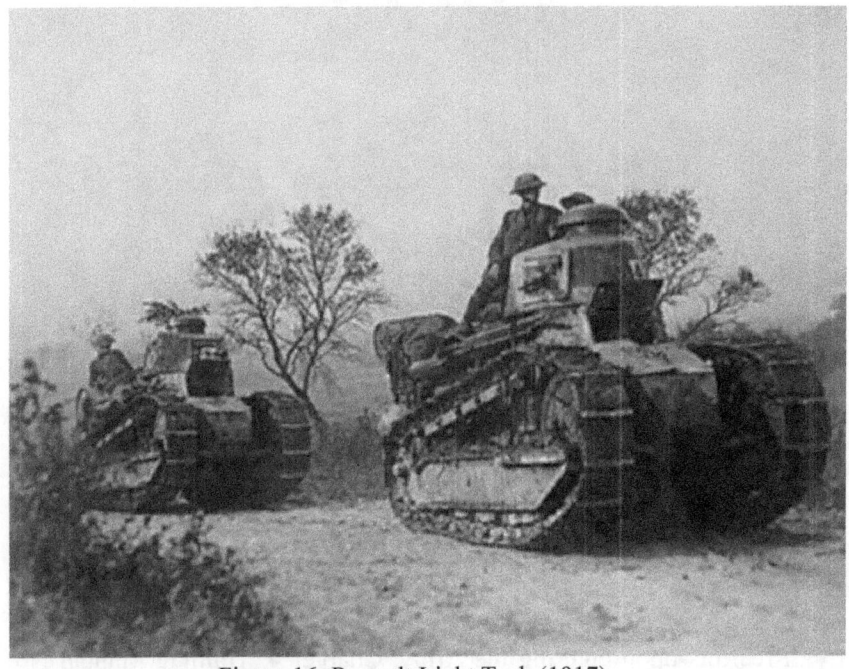

Figure 16. Renault Light Tank (1917).

The threat of conflict brought about great concerns for combat casualties. The greatest threat during these early years came from communicable and infectious diseases. From the Mexican War (1846) to WWI the percentage of war-time deaths attributable to non-combat injury/ illness was 64.36%.[75] In 1918 alone, the total number of American sailors and soldiers who died of influenza and pneumonia was over 43,000—about

80% of all Soldier deaths that year.[76] As a result of the non-combat threat to all cause mortality and morbidity the primary objective of virtually every military training program prior to 1941 was to improve the "organic vigor" (health) of the soldier.[77] Raycroft went so far as to state that "for the first time [soldiers were taught] how to combine health-giving exercise with play in the form of athletic games and sports."[78]

By comparison to the 64.36% non-combat casualty rate from 1846-1920, the non-combat casualty rate from WWII to Vietnam was 34.18%. This percentage represented a 100+% reduction in non-combat casualties. Along with improved emergency medical procedures and better combat casualty triage and evacuation, antibiotics significantly decreased the number of combat deaths. As a result, the historically salient outcome objectives of health and organic vigor virtually disappeared from Army physical training manuals after the publication of FM 21-20 in 1941, as the Army turned its attention from basic health-related fitness to functional fitness and combat readiness.

The third major event during the interwar years was the significant advancement in mechanized armor and rate of fire for personal and crew-served weapons.[79] With widespread use of machine guns during WWI, based upon the Hiram Maxim design, commanders became painfully aware of the need for strategies to mitigate casualties by enhancing mobility and improving personal protection. In the Battle of the Somme (1916), it has been estimated that the British Expeditionary Force suffered over 420,000 casualties in a span of five months and almost 58,000 casualties on the first day of the Battle.[80] In an attempt to break the trench-war stalemate, the French, working from the British model of the Little Willie (1915), developed the Renault Light Tank in 1917. "A solution for alleviating the casualties incurred in assaulting massed machine guns lay not in increasing the number of men exposed to the fire but in a technological advancement, the tank."[81] This light armored tank had a top speed of 4.8 mph on flat terrain with an operating range of 25-30 miles, which increased maneuver mobility by allowing soldiers to assault enemy positions from a protected position.[82] However, when used during penetration maneuvers, these light weight tanks became vulnerable when separated from infantry support. The increased need for mobility created by the first mechanized "tanks," coupled with the need for infantry support during combat maneuvers, translated directly to the need for Soldiers to develop greater speed, agility, and stamina.[83] Army leaders were aware that technological advancements in military weapons made the positional warfare of WWI obsolete; "… professional soldiers recognized that some change was necessary if they were to perform better the battlefield functions of penetration and exploitation that had proved so difficult during World War I."[84]

In reviewing the issues with the troop surge of 1917, Army leaders concluded that the civilian population would never maintain an adequate level of physical fitness required to meet minimum thresholds for combat readiness. After the Armistice, the leaders in the Training Camp Commission recommended to the War Planning Division that a permanent "course" be developed to maintain the current momentum in physical readiness training for Soldiers and instructors. In August 1919, F.E. Lacy, Colonel, Acting Director, War Plans Division staffed a memorandum through General Peyton March, Army Chief of Staff to establish a Physical and Bayonet Training course designed to train "instructors" (subject matter experts) to be taught at the Infantry School of Arms at Camp Benning, GA.[85] Lacy proposed that Dr. Joseph Raycroft use his "mass of data" to write the program of instruction in: (1) physical drill, (2) boxing and hand-to-hand fighting, (3) group games and mass athletics, including competitive games, and (4) bayonet fighting and that former Training Camp instructors serve as cadre for the physical and bayonet training course.[86] Dr. Raycroft developed a 21-day course (the first iteration to be conducted from September 5-30, 1919) and recommended that four officers be selected from each of the five branches of the service (Infantry, Calvary, Field Artillery, Coast Artillery Corps, and Engineers) to attend the first iteration. "In many ways the Benning school is the beginning of the largest physical education program ever attempted."[87]

As has been the pattern throughout the history of the US Army, the peacetime years of the 1920's and 1930's bought about a decade of complacency and diminishing expectations for physical readiness training.[88] On 10 September 1928 Adjutant General Lutz Wahl, by direction of the Chief of Staff C.P. Summerall, published Physical Training (Training Regulations, No. 115-5), which superseded Koehler's 1914 *Manual of Physical Training*.[89] TR 115-5 was prepared under the direction of the Lieutenant General Merch B. Stewart, Superintendent—United States Military Academy. Stewart was an 1896 graduate of the United States Military Academy and fought in the Spanish-American War and WWI. Although he graduated in the bottom half of his class, Stewart performed well in the physical program lead by Lieutenant Herman Koehler. Stewart authored several Army manuals to include *Physical Development of the Infantry Soldier* prior to his supervision of the publication of TR 115-5 as Superintendent. In the preface of his 1913 training manual, Stewart revealed his physical training philosophy for the infantry soldier: "every muscle, every organ, every faculty should be capable of working to the extreme human limit, then, if necessary, beyond.....The burden of combat is the expenditure of strength and energy required in moving from one position to another in battle, running at top speed, creeping, crawling, in crouching or lying behind cover, all in the while delivering a steady and accurate fire, in charging over long distances, and engaging in hand-to-hand fighting with butt and bayonet, and in the mental strain of facing injury or death."[90] Although Koehler had been retired from the Army for almost five years when TR 115-5 was published, the 1928 manual was basically an amalgam of his 1914 and 1919 manuals of physical training in two Parts. Part I contained all formations, setting-up drills, and calisthenics. Part II contained exercises with dumbbells and Indian clubs, gymnastic exercises with ropes, ladders, and apparatus, swimming, and combatives. All of the work by Raycroft, et al. and the Commission on Training Camp Activities following WWI was abandoned. The most conspicuous loss was the use of physical fitness testing to measure of combat readiness.

On 26 March, 1936 the War Department rescinded Training Regulation, No. 115-5 and established a new approach to disseminating training information with the publication of the *Basic Field Manual—Field Service Pocketbook*. The 1936 *Basic Field Manual* (BFM) was produced under the direction of General Malin Craig, Chief of Staff (USMA Class of 1898) and was the Army's first comprehensive basic field training manual. The BFM was published in two volumes and eight chapters. Chapter 4 (Volume 1) was dedicated to physical readiness training. As stated in the manual, Army physical training should be designed to achieve five objectives: (1) general health and vigor, (2) muscular strength, coordination, and endurance, (3) discipline and teamwork, (4) self-reliance, confidence, and courage, and (5) enthusiasm, pride, and morale.[91] Soldiers were directed to participate in physical training for two hours each day, divided into two 60-minute periods. The morning period should be scheduled at least 30 minutes after breakfast and should consist primarily of individual exercise and gymnastics.[92] In the afternoon session 30 minutes should be devoted to bayonet training and 30 minutes should be devoted to mass athletics and games. The manual identified 11 areas of physical development for soldiers including: setting-up exercises, marching, rifle exercises, gymnastics, jumping, mass athletics and combatives/ bayonet training.[93]

For the first time in a US Army manual the exercise running was accorded significant consideration. In his 1919 manual, Koehler stated "there is no exercise that will develop condition, vigor and endurance, lung and leg power in general as double timing at a moderate rate of speed."[94] He did however, caution instructors that "on account of its severity and tendency to permanent injury to the heart, instructors are cautioned to proceed carefully, especially when handling green men."[95] Koehler recommend that soldiers should conduct double-time runs fully equipped. In the 1936 BFM, running for long periods or a high rate of speed was described as "invaluable in the development of endurance and organic vigor."[96] The 1936 BFM would ultimately be given the numerical designator 21-20, which would guide Army physical training for the next 70+ years.

Notes

1. Wilson was a relatively talented baseball player and played one year of varsity baseball at Davidson College during his freshman year.

2. Leonard Wood was a trained medical doctor (Harvard) and avid athlete who aspired to be a combat line officer. He was a tireless champion of military preparedness and training and was the principle sponsor of the Plattsburg training camps, which gave young men their first orientation to military life. He was also a major player in the "preparedness movement" just prior to World War I; www.wood.army.mil/mgleonard wood.htm (accessed 6 June 2011). Herman J. Koehler, *Manual for Physical Training for use in the United States Army* (New York: Military Publishing Company, 1914), 3.

3. C. Thomas Lowman, "Does Current Army Physical Training Doctrine Adequately Prepare Soldiers For War?" Master of Military Art and Science thesis, Fort Leavenworth: Command and General Staff College, 2010, 13; The table of contents of the 1914 *Manual of Physical Training* could likely have been taken directly from Friedrich Jahn's "A Treatise on Gymnastics" (1828). The classic German gymnastics model served as the context for this manual as it did for other Koehler manuals. Of historical interest, it should be noted that Luietenant Colonel Sladen and Lieutenant Philips were USMA graduates (Fred W. Sladen (Class of 1890) and Philip Mathews (Class of 1906)). Luietenant Colonel Sladen was a Plebe during Koehler's first year on the faculty in the Department of Tactics at West Point. Cadet Sladen ranked 5/53 in "tactics," which included his physical education instruction from the Master of the Sword, Herman Koehler. In 1911 Captain Sladen returned to USMA as the Commandant of Cadets and was Koehler's immediate supervisor. Major General Sladen served as the 32nd Superintendent of the United States Military Academy from 1922-1925 and presided over Koehler's retirement ceremony.

4. Michael J. Reagor, "Herman J. Koehler: The Father of West Point Physical Education, 1985–1923." *Assembly*:3 (January 1993): 4; David J. Yebra, "Colonel Herman J. Koehler: The Father of Physical Education at West Point," (Paper written for LD 720: American Military History, United States Military Academy, 1998), 13.

5. Major General Leonard Wood was replaced as Chief of Staff of the Army on 22 April, 1914.

6. During the summer of 1915 and 1916 Major Herman Koehler was dispatched from West Point to the Plattsburg Military Training Camp to direct the disciplinary physical training "The Retirement of Colonel Herman Koehler," *The Pointer* (22 October 1923): 4. Penelope D. Clute, "The Plattsburg Idea," *New York Archives*:2 (Fall 2005): 11-12; *The Plattsburger* (New York: Wynkoop, Hallenbeck, Crawford Co., 1917), 13; Major General Wood established camps in Pennsylvania, California, Michigan, Vermont, and North Carolina.

7. Theodore Roosevelt, *America and the First World War* (New York: Charles Scribner's Sons, 1915), 209.

8. *The Plattsburger,* 13.

9. Arthur S. Link, *Woodrow Wilson and the Progressive Era, 1910-1917* (New York: Harper and Row, 1954), 200.

10. Raymond B. Fosdick, *Chronicle of a Generation: An Autobiography* (New York: Harper, 1958), 135; As a result of Mexican conflict a young Michigan high school student named Ted Bank joined the Army and was immediately deployed to the Mexican border—the future Colonel Bank would have a significant impact on Army PRT during and after World War II.

11. Fosdick, *Chronicle of a Generation*, 135.

12. "Army Heads Answer Militia Complaints." *New York Times*, 20 July, 1916.

13. Fosdick, *Chronicle of a Generation*, 136.

14. Raymond B. Fosdick, "The War and Navy Departments Commission on Training Camp Activities," *Annals of the American Society of Political and Social Science 79* (September 1918): 130.

15. Fosdick, *Chronicle of a Generation*, 140.

16. "Wants Mexico Cleaned Up—Senator Falls Fears Conflict with European Army There," *New York Times*, 22 March 1916.

17. In 1916 the regular Army at this time consisted of only about 100,000 Soldiers.

18. *The Plattsburger*, 14.

19. O.O. Ellis, and E.B. Garey, *The Plattsburg Manual – A Handbook for Military Training* (New York: The Century Co.): 21; A footnote to Chapter II read "These exercises are selected from those commonly given by Major H. J. Koehler, United States Army."

20. James Cole, and Oliver Schoomaker, *Military Instructors Manual* (New York: Edwin N. Appleton, 1917), 109.

21. *The Plattsburger*, 15.

22. Clute, "The Plattsburg Idea," 13.

23. "Bayonet Practice Again," *New York Times*, 25 June 1917; L. L. Little, "There is No Limit to Human Endurance," *Outing* November (1918): 113.

24. Hugh Scott, "Comments on Compulsory Military Service," *War Department Annual Reports, 1916*. Washington, DC: Government Printing Office, 1917), Volume I, 155-162, Reprint in *The Military Draft: Selected Readings on Conscription*, edited by Martin Anderson, 515-25, Stanford: Hoover Institution Press, 1982: 517.

25. *Selective-Service Act: Hearings before the Committee on Military Affairs, House of Representative, Sixty-fifth Congress, The Bill Authorizing the President to Increase Temporarily the Military Establishment of the United States* (April 7, 14, and 17, 1917), Washington: Government Printing Office, 1918: 273.

26. *Selective-Service Act: Hearings*, 14.

27. Online at www.sss.gov/induct.htm (accessed 14 July, 2010).

28. Jennifer Keene, *The United States and the First World War* (New York: Longman Press; 2000), 29.

29. Newton D. Baker, "Letter to President Woodrow Wilson – Mr. Fosdick and Army Recreation," in *The Papers of Woodrow Wilson, Vol. 4, January 24-April 6, 1917*, ed. Arthur S. Link (Princeton: Princeton University Press, 1983), 527.

30. Raymond B. Fosdick, "The Commission on Training Camp Activities," *Proceedings of the Academy of Political Science in the City of New York*:4 (February, 1918): 163.

31. "Making Vice Unattractive in Soldier's Camps," *New York Times*, 20 May 1917.

32. Newton D. Baker, "Letter to President Woodrow Wilson v. Raymond Fosdick," in *The Papers of Woodrow Wilson, Vol. 4, January 24-April 6, 1917*, ed. Arthur S. Link (Princeton: Princeton University Press, 1983), 506

33. The War Department, *Commission on Training Camp Activities, 1917.*

34. "Making Vice Unattractive in Soldier's Camps," *New York Times*, 20 May 1917; quoting Raymond Fosdick.

35. Fosdick, *Chronicle of a Generation*, 143.

36. Keene, *The United States and the First World War*, 29.

37. Fosdick, *Chronicle of a Generation*, 154.

38. Http://diglib.princeton.edu/ead/getEad?eadid=AC146&kw (accessed 24 June, 2010).

39. Fosdick, Chronicle of a Generation, 153-154.

40. Walter Camp, "A Daily Dozen Set-up," *Outing*:2 (1918): 98.

41. Fosdick, "The War and Navy Departments Commission on Training Camp Activities," 138-139.

42. Fosdick, "The War and Navy Departments Commission on Training Camp Activities," 139.

43. Fosdick, "The War and Navy Departments Commission on Training Camp Activities," 131.

44. Robert Degen, "The Evolution of Physical Education at the United States Military Academy," Master thesis, University of Wisconsin, 1967, 54; Herman Koehler, *Koehler's West Point Manual of Physical Disciplinary Training* (New York: E. P. Dutton & Company, 1919), v; Yebra, "Colonel Herman J. Koehler," 11.

45. Koehler, *Koehler's West Point Manual of Physical Disciplinary Training*, v.

46. Koehler, *Koehler's West Point Manual of Physical Disciplinary Training*, xiii.

47. Koehler, *Koehler's West Point Manual of Physical Disciplinary Training*, xiii.

48. A 2nd edition, which appears to be an exact reproduction of the 1st edition was published in 1924; the only addition is a preface by Briadire General H.A. Drum.

49. Joseph Raycroft, *Mass Physical Training for use in the Army and Reserve Officer Training Corps* (Washington:US Infantry Association, 1920), iv. In 1919 Colonel William H. Waldron published a secularized edition of Koehler's 1914 *Manual of Physical Training* entitled *Army Physical Training*. Waldron appears to have plagiarized much of his text directly from Koehler's manual. Waldron did change Koehler's photos to line drawings of a soldier in uniform.

50. Raycroft, *Mass Physical Training*, vii.

51. Fosdick, "The Commission on Training Camp Activities," 167.
52. Raycroft, Mass Physical Training, vii.
53. War Department, *Commission on Training Camps* (Washington: Government Printing Office, 1917), 13; Note: this section of the publication was attributed to Dr. Joseph Raycroft.
54. Raycroft, *Mass Physical Training*, vii.
55. Raycroft, *Mass Physical Training*, 3.
56. Raycroft, *Mass Physical Training*, viii.
57. Raycroft, *Mass Physical Training*, vi.
58. Raycroft, *Mass Physical Training*, 149.
59. Raycroft, *Mass Physical Training*, 34.
60. Raycroft, *Mass Physical Training*, viii.
61. Raycroft, *Mass Physical Training*, 143.
62. Raycroft, *Mass Physical Training*, vi.
63. Raycroft, *Mass Physical Training*, v.
64. Raycroft, *Mass Physical Training*, 147. The Obstacle Course Test run was published in *Mass Physical Training* Manual.
65. *Studies in Citizenship for the Recruit, US Army Training Manual No. 2* (Washington: Government Printing Office, 1922), 7.
66. Alden Partridge, "Lecture on Education," in *The Art of Epistolary Composition and Discourse on Education*, ed. Francois Peyre-Ferry's (Middletown, Conn.: E & H. Clark, 1826), 271.
67. James C. Magee, "Relationship of the Health of Civilians to the Efficiency of the Army," *American Journal of Public Health* 30 (November 1940): 1285.
68. Jennifer Keene, *World War I* (Westport, CT: Greenwood Press, 2006), 26.
69. George Draper, 1918, NA; as quoted in Keene, *World War I*, 26. George Draper was an Army Officer and physician and epidemiologist for the City of New York.
70. *Studies in Citizenship for the Recruit, Manual No. 2*, 33.
71. Jennifer Keene, Doughboys, *The Great War and The Remaking of America* (Baltimore: Johns Hopkins University Press, 2003), 27.
72. *Studies in Citizenship for the Recruit, Manual No. 2*, 7 & 33.
73. Sulfa drugs and penicillin were actually discovered in 1928, but were in limited production and availability until about 1945 when they were mass produced.
74. M.B. Stewart, *The Physical Development of the Infantry Soldier* (Menasha, WI: George Banta Press, 1913), 2, 4.
75. These percentages were calculated by averaging officialUS census statistics on combat and non-combat casualties for the given time periods.
76. Alfred Crosby, *Epidemic and Peace*, 1918 (Westport, CT: Greenwood Press, 1976) 260; *Annual Reports of the War Department* (Washington: Government Printing Office, 1:2, 1919), 1437, 2012.
77. Partridge, 1826, p. 265: "exercise for the preservation of health and confirming and rendering vigorous the constitution"; Koehler, *Manual for Physical Training*, 5: "general health and bodily vigor"; Raycroft, *Mass Physical Training*, iii: "to maintain him in a sound, healthful condition."

78. Joseph Raycroft, *Mass Physical Training*, iii.

79. Kenneth Finlayson, *An Uncertain Trumpet: The Evolution of US Army Infantry Doctrine, 1919-1941* (Westport, CT: Greenwood Press, 2001), 84.

80. Online at www.historylearningsite.com.uk/somme.htm; www.history-world.org/somme.htm (accessed 20 June, 2011). It has been estimated that over 1 million combatants died at Somme from July to November, 1916.

81. Finlayson, *An Uncertain Trumpet*, 80.

82. Richard M. Ogorkiewicz, *Armor: A History of Mechanized Forces* (New York: Frederick A. Praeger, Publisher, 1960), 170.

83. Jonathan House, *Toward Combined Arms Warfare: A Survey of 20th-Century Tactics, Doctrine, and Organization* (Fort Leavenworth, US Army Command and General Staff College, 1984), 29-31.

84. Bernard Brodie, and Fawn Brodie, *From Cross Bow to H-bomb* (Bloomington: Indiana University Press, 1973), 43.

85. Lacy, F.E., "War Department: Memorandum for the Chief of Staff; Subject: Physical and Bayonet Training, August, 1919," (Printed in "News Notes," *American Physical Education Review* 24, (October 1919): 419. There are few references to the "physical training and bayonet school"; one reference came from the biography of Brigadier General Jesmond Balmer when he became the Commandant of the Field Artillery School: LT Balmer returned to the United States in October, 1919, and was assigned to Camp Bragg, North Carolina, where he served with the 21st Field Artillery until March, 1920. He then went to Camp Benning, Georgia, to attend the Physical and Bayonet Training School until April 1920, when he went to Camp Jackson, South Carolina, as an Instructor in bayonet training. From June 1920, until August 1920, he served as an Instructor of the Army Olympic Games entries and in August returned to the 21st Field Artillery at Camp Bragg. He transferred to the 17th Field Artillery there in September, 1921. He became Provost Marshal at Fort Bragg in June 1923. (see "New Commandant, F.A.S." *The Field Artillery Journal* 32, (August 1942): 578).

86. Four individuals were recommended as instructors at the Physical and Bayonet Training program: Major John L. Griffith, Captain Carlton L. Brosius, Mr. George Blake, and Luietenant B.W Leman; Captain Brosius was the grandson of George Brosius, Director of the Milwaukee Normal School and Herman Koehler's teacher and mentor; all four instructors worked for Raycroft (Chairman of the Athletic Division, Commission on Training Camp Activities) during WWI; the Physical and Bayonet Training program of instruction was published by Raycroft in his manual—*Mass Physical Training* (1920).

87. On 5 October 1919 a wire service article concerning the new Physical Training and Bayonet School at Fort Benning was picked up by no less than three major newspapers *(Pittsburg Times, New York Evening Post, Miami News)*. The "article" described the formation of the school, the program of instruction, instructors, and overarching objectives.

88. Finlayson, *An Uncertain Trumpet*, 69.

89. Raycroft's manual of *Mass Physical Training,* which was identified by the War Plans Division as the standard for Army-wide PRT doctrine was summarily dismissed.

90. Stewart, *The Physical Development of the Infantry Soldier*, 4, 5.

91. Department of the Army, *Basic Field Manual, Vol. I, Chapter 4*, FM 21-20 Physical Readiness Training (Washington, DC: US Government Printing Office, 1936), 1-2.

92. "Men should not be required to indulge in strenuous exercise before breakfast," *Basic Field Manual* (1936), 4.

93. *Basic Field Manual* (1936), 2-5.

94. Koehler, *Koehler's West Point Manual of Physical Disciplinary Training*, 18.

95. Koehler, *Koehler's West Point Manual of Physical Disciplinary Training*, 18.

96. *Basic Field Manual* (1936), 2.

Chapter 5
World War II—A Return to Combat Readiness

Factors Influencing Army PRT Prior to World War II

Prior to the attack at Pearl Harbor on 7 December 1941, most Americans enjoyed an unrivaled quality of life due to an expanding array of consumer durables available for the home. The demand for "labor saving" devices spiked dramatically during the late 1930's due to technological innovations and significant increases in federal spending in preparation for war.[1] Mesmerized by the "World of Tomorrow," which was theme of the 1939 New York World's Fair, Americans began to envision an all-electric world. Electrical appliances transformed the landscape at home and in the workplace and significantly reduced much of the burden of manual labor required in last century.[2] "The first wave of innovations to home production came from the diffusion of electricity and piped water…For the country as a whole, in 1940, 83% of the total number of dwellings had electrical lights and 74% had running water."[3] By 1940, 61% of the wired households had a washing machine, and there was significant penetration of the electric iron, vacuum cleaner, dishwasher, and refrigerators. Although 43% of Americans were employed in "blue collar" jobs, improving technology reduced the amount of hard labor.[4] "Modern machines have to a great extent emancipated our muscles from work...and...have resulted in a lack of physical fitness in the youth of America, which seriously handicapped our war effort."[5] Unfortunately, the hard manual labor that remained in the US workplace was often more debilitating than constructive. In general Americans moved steadily away from a physically active industrial/agrarian society to a sedentary urban society, which further deteriorated personal health and fitness. Since the thought of another "world war" was inconceivable for most Americans, the need to maintain physical vigilance for national security was marginalized. During the interregnum from 1919 to 1939 the US and the Army lost focus of the painful lessons learned during combat in WWI. "Lack of physical fitness prevailed among the youth of the county because the nation failed to recognize its importance."[6]

As war beckoned, the United States found itself faced with a "perfect storm" created by 20 years of peace and emerging prosperity. The nexus of the "storm" was: (1) the need to rapidly mobilize a large number of combat soldiers, (2) measurable declines in personal health and fitness, which exacerbated the mobilization and training process, and (3) improvements in warfighting technology and mechanization.[7] The problems created by the cumulative effects of these issues were obscured by the perceived successes in mobilizing and training large numbers of civilians during

WWI. However, soon after the declaration of war, declining levels of personal health and fitness, exacerbated by increased needs for stamina and mobility, created near desperation in the mobilization and training of soldiers. It became readily apparent to most civil and military leaders that significant changes in secular physical fitness and Army physical training and assessment doctrine would have to occur to successfully resource the war effort:

> Fifty percent of inductees cannot swim well enough to save their lives, and lack the strength to jump ditches, scale walls, throw missiles and survive forced marches. Colonel Bank…conducted physical tests with 400 troops at Fort Knox and 11 other camps… The results proved that 20-25% are in very good shape, 40% in fair shape, but not good enough for combat and 35% are in miserable shape.[8]

Over a four-year period (1940-1944) civil and military leaders developed three joint initiatives to mitigate the systemic physical fitness and manpower issues facing the Army: (1) a national public relations and youth fitness campaign, (2) passage of the Selective Service and Training Act and establishment of the Women's Army Auxiliary Corps, and (3) revisions in Army physical readiness training doctrine. In October 1940, President Franklin Roosevelt named John Kelly, the 3-time Olympic gold medal rower, as the National Director of Physical Fitness. This position was generally acknowledged to be a public relations post where Kelly could use his notoriety to promote physical fitness during the War.[9] In late 1940, when Army leaders realized that the public relations campaign alone would not resolve the manpower demands for the armed services, the War Department restructured several federal agencies to attack the medical/fitness issue. The newly established Federal Security Agency (FSA) was given broader authority to promote/develop/sustain the physical fitness of US citizens. Under the leadership of Paul V. McNutt, the FSA established several "committees" designed to enhance physical fitness. Key players on these committees were C. Ward Crampton, Colonel Leonard Rowntree (MD), Arthur H. Steinhaus (MD), and Colonel Theodore Bank.

With the national public relations campaign underway, on 14 September 1940 Congress moved to resolve the evolving military manpower issue by passing the Burke-Wadsworth Act (better known as the Selective Training and Service Act). This Act mandated the first peace-time conscription in the history of the United States. Between November 1940 and October 1946 over 10,000,000 men entered military service through the Selective

Service system.¹⁰ By early 1941, the two historical nemeses of "military conscription" again emerged: (1) "draft boards" were identifying an alarmingly high number of candidates who were physically/medically unfit for service, and (2) basic training programs were ineffective in transforming sedentary recruits into "hardened" soldiers. In 1941 only about one half of high school men participated in a regular physical education/fitness program. "This generation of draftees as a whole is considerably softer and weaker than its fathers were in 1917."¹¹ "Many young men are entering the Army today totally unprepared for military life. It takes weeks to bring them into the physical conditioning necessary for military training."¹² During congressional hearing on youth fitness Commissioner of Education John W. Studebaker stated:

> I wonder if you understand what the usual program of physical fitness training in this country in the ordinary high school has been! It has consisted of about two periods per week. The program we recommend includes five periods per week. The recommended program was prepared by Army and Navy experts in physical fitness and others representing the schools and colleges.¹³

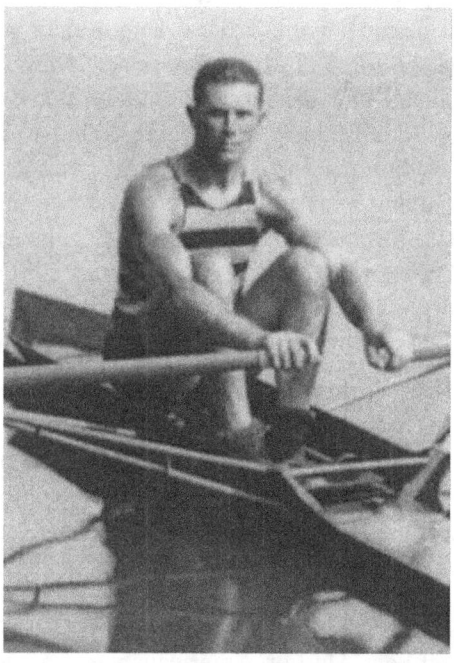

Figure 17. John B. Kelly, Chair—National Physical Fitness Council.

In subsequent testimony Colonel Rowntree, medical director for the Selective Service, stated that:

> We are accustomed to regard ourselves, as a Nation, as healthy and rugged...but when we look at the facts as they are revealed by the statistics on rejection, a very large proportion of our manhood is far below par.[14]

Bank agreed:

> Our young men are being sent into our Armed Services without the ability to swim, without the leg strength to jump combat obstacles such as ditches and fences; without the arm and shoulder strength which would enable them to pull themselves up over ledges, or save their lives by climbing up or down ropes and rope ladders, and without the agilities, developed by athletics, that would increase their chances of staying alive in various combat situations.[15]

By most estimates Selective Service rejections averaged about 30%; however Colonel Rowntree testified that out of the first 2,000,000 men examined, 1,000,000 were rejected and about 90% were rejected for physical fitness and medical issues.[16] Based upon data collected during WWII for the Army Air Force physical fitness test, Karpovich and Weiss concluded that "enlisted and aircrew personnel entered the Army Air Forces in fairly poor condition."[17] Men were found to be deficient in running speed and endurance and abdominal endurance; however they were most deficient in arm and shoulder strength as measured by the pull-up. As the United States progressed towards war, it again became clear that many of the men who reported to the Military Entrance Processing Station (MEPS) were not physically fit for military duty. By 1943 the number of unqualified men would rise to 2.5-3 million:[18]

> Of the first two million men examined under Selective Service, fully half were found unfit for military combat service! Of these, 500,000...could finally be accepted for limited service. But the rest were rejected completely! Of those rejected, 400,000 men were physically unfit... they weren't healthy enough to meet Army physical standards![19]

After the attack at Pearl Harbor, Americans were infused with a sense of national purpose to defeat the Axis powers; however in 1941 when the

US declared war on Japan and Germany, the armed services faced critical manpower shortages:

> In the beginning, the Selective Training and Service Act of 1940 was designed to provide the authority for the leisurely procurement of an army for national defense. This was most fortunate because it afforded Selective Service an opportunity for orientation...prior to the great pressure for manpower that followed the declaration of war.[20]

Although the Selective Service boards increased rates of induction, many of the recruits were physically unfit. "...many of the registrants were found to be pampered, soft, flabby, and in need of conditioning. Special training in physical fitness was necessary, after induction, which represented weeks of wasted time and effort which could have been avoided if every young man prior to induction had made himself physically fit."[21] In an attempt to remediate physical fitness deficiencies, which existed prior to service, Army Chief of Staff - George C. Marshall directed a major revision of the 1936 *Basic Field Manual*, Volume I, Chapter 4. On March 6, 1941 FM 21-20 *Basic Field Manual, Physical Training* was published under the direction of Brigadier General Robert Eichelberger, Superintendent, United States Military Academy. FM 21-20 superseded Ch. 4, Vol. I, BFM (1936) and TR 115-5, Part II (1928). The stated purpose of the 1941 revision was to produce a state of health and general fitness that would enhance physical efficiency and allow soldiers to perform arduous duties, which were essential to military effectiveness.[22] Although FM 21-20 (1941) was the primary physical training doctrine for the first two years of WW II, it represented only modest improvements in the evolution of physical training and assessment of the combat Soldier.

The 1941 *Basic Field Manual* (BFM) partitioned physical training into eight domains: disciplinary exercises; setting-up exercises; marching and exercises while marching; running, jumping, and climbing; personal contests; mass athletics and group games; rifle exercises; and swimming.[23] Unit commanders were directed to conduct two physical training sessions per day: 30-minute session in the morning for personal fitness and conditioning and a 60-minute session in the afternoon for testing, mass athletics, and games.[24] FM 21-20 stressed the need for a balanced in the training program, which would allow the Soldier to develop "discipline, endurance, agility, good posture, body control, and health."[25] "Model schedules," designed to help the instructor develop a proper daily exercise program, were provided for the trained and untrained Soldier in Chapter 3.[26]

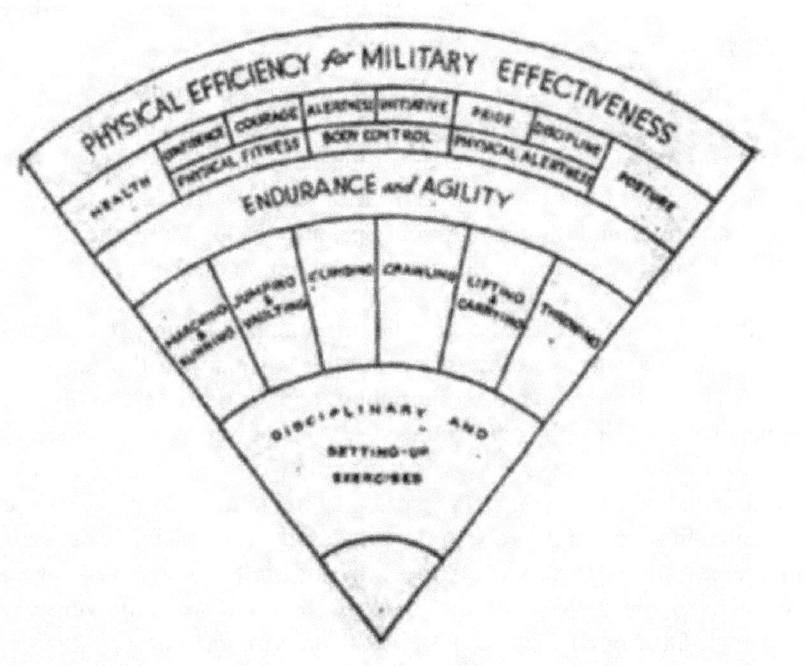

Figure 18. Physical Efficiency Matrix.

There were three unique aspects to the 1941 manual. First, the authors developed a hierarchical "model" to define "physical efficiency for military effectiveness."[28] Three levels of physical training were used to achieve physical efficiency: Level 1: "disciplinary and setting-up exercises"—which consisted of military drill (facing movements), general calisthenics, and stretching exercises designed to develop military discipline, general muscular development, and prepare the body for skill and endurance exercises; Level 2: basic movement pattern/skill exercises—throwing, jumping, crawling, climbing, lifting, etc.; and Level 3: endurance and agility training. If physical training was conducted properly the soldier would achieve total physical efficiency as expressed by the acquisition of the physical fitness, body control, posture, and health:

> Setting-up exercises should be conducted so that they impart the physiological, as well as the disciplinary, benefit of which they are capable. Accuracy and precision of performance will be insisted upon whenever they are possible of attainment.... But this insistence upon accuracy and precision of performance should be with the aim in

mind of insuring that the men get the maximum physical benefit from the exercises and should not be employed for purely disciplinary motives.²⁹

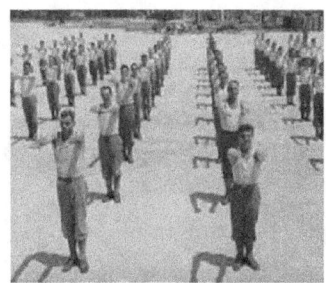
Air Service Command PT Formation (1943).

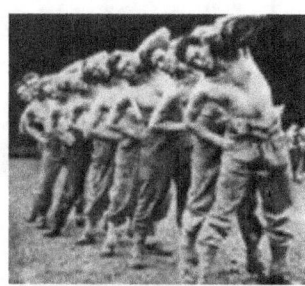
Darby's Rangers Training (1942).

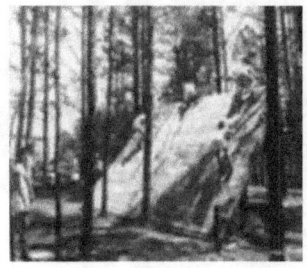
Obstacle Course Training, Fort Jackson, SC (1943).

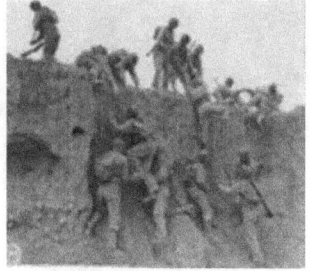
Commando Training, Camp Carson, CO (1943).

Figure 19. WWII Physical Readiness Training.³⁰

FM 21-20 (1941) was the first manual to establish basic principles of exercise to guide physical training. The two principles were: (1) progression: "a course progressively arranged will so condition the men and increase their aptitude that they will reach the standard required…," and (2) balance: "…the work [should be] organized so as to include as many as possible of the basic skills required of the soldier."³¹

The second unique aspect of FM 21-20 was the inclusion of various fitness assessments and the acknowledgement of their value in physical readiness training.³² "The physical training program should be based upon the condition and aptitude of the men to be trained. The best method of determining this condition and aptitude of the group is by comparison with known standards."³³ Four "primary" assessments (with associated criterion-referenced standards—pass/fail) were recommended for commanders to use in assessing the physical readiness of their Soldiers. A significant number of secondary assessments was also identified.

The most combat-specific assessment proposed in the 1941 manual was the "obstacle" course test—OCT (Figure 20). The OCT allowed the commander to evaluate functional fitness by measuring a soldier's speed, strength, coordination, and agility; skills that were specified for "field service."

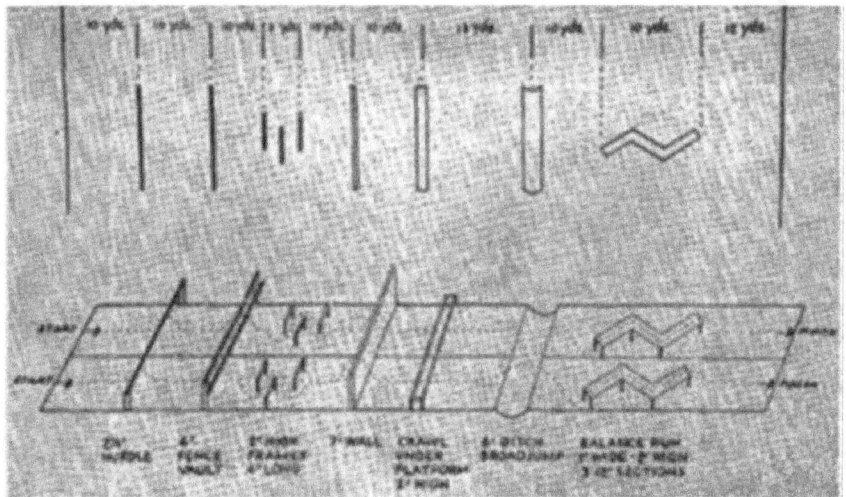

Figure 20. Obstacle Course Test (1941). [34]

Raycroft's Obstacle Course Run, which consisting of five obstacles, and the FM 21-20 Obstacle Course Test, which consisting of seven obstacles, were remarkably similar. Both tests were 100-yard linear courses that used a low hurdle (3' v. 2½'), a wall (fence) climb (8' v. 7'), a running jump (6' ditch v. 10' trench from a platform), and balance test (24' v. 20'). Raycroft's test used a "wire entanglement" to assess agility as opposed to the 2' high frames in the 1941 OCT. The 1941 OCT added two obstacles; a 4' fence vault and a 2' high low crawl. The minimum time specified for Raycroft's OCR was 30 seconds, while the minimum time for 1941 OCT was at the commander's discretion. The authors concluded that "tests can be conducted with little, if any, interference with the scheduled program, and require nothing more than a little planning on the part of the instructor. Their value to the program is so great that they should be held at regular intervals."[35]

The third unique aspect of the 1941 physical training basic field manual was the inclusion of a detailed chapter on swimming, lifesaving, and water safety. Since ancient Greece, armies have valued the tactical advantages and safety benefits of survival swimming and basically all Army manuals from Clias to MacLaren to Koehler ascribed significant value to survival swimming. Although the 1928 *Physical Training Manual* (TR 115-5) included some aquatic information, BFM (1936) Vol. 1, Chapter 4 Physical Training included no information on swimming or lifesaving. "All soldiers should receive instruction and training in swimming, both without and with equipment…Soldiers who have been properly instructed should be able to ford streams, participate in landing operations, and take care of themselves in the water in emergencies."[36] This swimming section was eerily prophetic for the soldiers who assaulted the beaches of Normandy, 6 June 1944. Although many soldiers died from plunging fire, "Even the lightly wounded die by drowning, doomed by the waterlogging of their overloaded packs. From Boat No. 1, all hands jump off in water over their heads. Most of them are carried down. Ten or so survivors get around the boat and clutch at its sides in an attempt to stay afloat. The same thing happens to the section in Boat No. 4. Half of its people are lost to the fire or tide before anyone gets ashore."[37] It is believed that a significant number of the 4,000+ soldiers killed in action during the D-day assault actually drown as they abandoned their landing crafts or were "put ashore" in water that was 10-15 feet deep.[38]

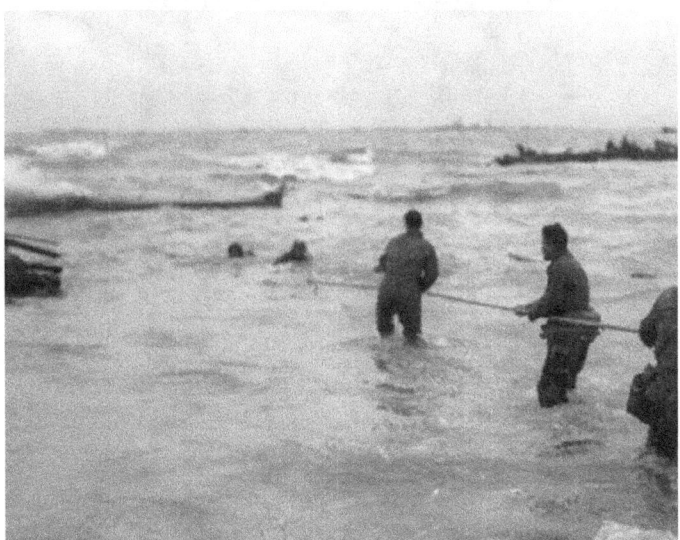

Figure 21. Rescuing Soldiers during the Normandy Invasion (1944).

Meeting the Combat Readiness Needs of World War II

Colonel Theodore Paul "Ted" Bank would become the central figure in the continuing evolution of Army physical readiness training during WWII. As a decorated Soldier with significant combat experience in France during WWI as a member of the American Expeditionary Force, Bank understood the physical needs of combat.[39] After the war he enrolled at the University of Michigan, joined the football team, and ultimately became the starting quarterback for several successful seasons (1920-1921) under Coach Fielding Yost. After college Bank enjoyed a successful football coaching career at the high school and college level where he nurtured his interests in physical fitness and sport. Bank had remained in the Army Reserves since 1919 and in February 1941 he was ordered back to active duty at the rank of Captain. Bank was quickly advanced to the rank of Colonel and ultimately appointed as the Chief – Athletic and Recreation Branch and worked for Major General Joseph Byron, head of the Army's special services division.[40]

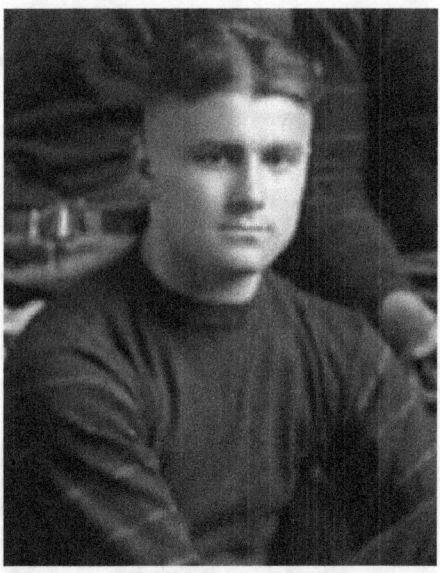

Figure 22. Colonel Theodore Paul "Ted" Bank.

Even with a well coordinated national public relations campaign and the extensive revision of the Army physical training manual, there were still critical manpower issues by 1942. Based upon the dramatic rejection rates of greater than 50% of the registrants, more direct action was required to ensure adequate manpower for the armed services. In October 1941

President Roosevelt initiated a plan to "rehabilitate" 200,000 recruits. The Army selected the most promising dental and orthopedic cases for rehabilitation; however the entire program was soon terminated because of meager positive results. Instead the Manpower Commission chose to initiate a "prehabilitation" program to address the greater physical fitness problem. Local doctors, dentist, and school health professionals were directed to conduct a "pre-examination" to assess and provide corrective programs for adult males who failed to meet the standards required for military service.[41]

Since the mid 1930s the science of exercise and fitness assessment had developed at a torrid pace in US universities and colleges. The "prehabilitation" efforts of 1941 leveraged these advancements to prepare young adult men for military service. Subject matter experts like Charles McCloy (University of Iowa), Thomas Cureton (University of Illinois), A. A. Esslinger (Stanford University), Karl Bookwalter (Indiana University), and Peter Karpovich (Springfield College) served as excellent resources for the research needs of the armed services. Through his coaching experiences at Tulane University and the University of Idaho, Ted Bank became familiar with these physical education professionals and their innovative approaches to fitness assessment and program design. In late 1941 and early 1942 Colonel Bank (Chief of the Athletic and Recreation Branch) enlisted the services of Charles McCloy and A.A. Esslinger to develop a new physical training and assessment program for the Army.[42] They began by administering 25 different physical fitness assessments to over 400 soldiers to determine which fitness assessments best measured combat readiness. Upon analysis, McCloy and Esslinger determined that ten fitness items best discriminated between fit and unfit soldiers: pull-ups, 20 sec. burpee, 3 successive broad jumps—riple bound, shot put, push-ups, 75-yd pick-a-back run, dodging run, 6-sec run, sit-ups, and 300-yd run.

During the summer of 1942 a newly designed PRT program was assessed in a series of training studies conducted throughout the Army by Esslinger, Bank, and McCloy. In the first 6-week training study significant improvements in total physical conditioning were observed: 30% in pull-up strength, 50% in push-up and abdominal strength, 8% in cardio-respiratory endurance, and 11% in muscular endurance.[43] During the autumn Colonel Hallenbeck, Commander of the 125th Infantry Regiment stationed at Camp Page Mill (California), requested that these tests be given to all personnel in the camp. Esslinger conducted a 5-week training study utilizing two experimental and two control companies. Soldiers in the control and experimental companies were assessed with the 10-item physical fitness battery at the end of the 5-week training period. The control company reported a 3.5% increase in physical fitness, while the experiential group reported a 23.5% increase in total physical conditioning.[44]

In March 1942, as Esslinger, Bank, and McCloy were working to develop a new scientifically based PRT doctrine for the Army, the War Department initiated a major reorganization of the force. The Army Ground Forces was tasked to provide ground force troops that were properly equipped and trained for combat operations. The AGF preempted Bank's new PRT doctrine by issuing a Training Directive (Letter) on 19 October 1942 that reduced the time allotted to individual (basic) training from 17 weeks to 13 weeks and outlined the requirements for a new physical fitness test—the Army Ground Forces Test (AGFT). The AFGT was primarily designed to assess unit effectiveness on mission essential tasks. It was recommended that commanders administer the test every 8-12 weeks. The test items were push-ups, 300 yard shuttle run, 20-sec. burpees, 70 yard pig-a-back run (carrying a man of equal weight), 70 yard zigzag run (involving creeping, crawling, jumping, and running on seven legs of ten yards each), and a four mile march (50 minutes).[45] Although the administration of the AGFT was encouraged, it was not mandatory.

Only a month after the Army Ground Forces Directive was published, the Army published Bank, et al.'s new physical training guidance in the form of Training Circular 87 (TC 87).[46] Based upon their findings at Fort Knox and other Army camps, "Colonel Banks and his board came up with 15 Calisthenic exercises that use every muscle in the body if given and taken properly. This Training Circular 87 was accepted by the government 17 November 1942."[47] The publication of Training Circular No. 87 once again represented the Army's historical propensity for being behind the physical training curve and playing catch-up with the start of hostilities. Although FM 21-20 had just been published on 6 March 1941 and the AGF Directive in March, 1942, they were already outdated. TC 87 stated, "The exercises listed below differ from those now in general practice [i.e., published in FM 21-20] in that they are more strenuous and varied in nature. They are presented for the purpose of placing greater emphasis on the physical conditioning of troops."[48] While FM 21-20 (1941) was more process based, TC 87 was more outcomes based. TC 87 contained specific distances/times for ruck marching and more specific guidance for calisthenics, grass and guerilla drills, and running exercises. Special emphasis was given to mobility runs and "double exercises." In order to increase the leg and shoulder strength and endurance, soldiers were directed to lift a partner (via the Army, Fireman's, Cross, Single shoulder lift) and carry him some specified distance (i.e. effectively "doubling" the training load). These exercises utilized the overload principle to enhance strength and power, as well as improving casualty evacuation skills. They also served as the impetus for the 75-yard pick-a-back test item, which was included a year later in the Physical Efficiency Test Battery. Based upon the research by Bank, McCloy, and Esslinger, for the first time the Army had empirical data to support a physical training program and assessment battery.

In the April 1943 issue of the *Journal of Health and Physical Education,* Colonel Bank presented a detailed review of "The Army Physical Conditioning Program." He outlined the developmental process and the basic "program of instruction" (POI), attributing much of the physical training program development to McCloy and Esslinger. He provided a basic outline of Training Circular 87, which involved marching, calisthenics, guerrilla exercises, grass drills, combative events, and running exercises to enhance soldier fitness. Although Colonel Bank was an advocate for Soldiers fitness relative to combat readiness, he also subscribed to the "Raycroft" mass athletics model. In the final section of this article Bank described the genesis of the Special Service Corps (Officer) and its impact on soldiers through athletic participation. "Every company that goes overseas carries with it two athletics kits. It has boxing equipment, footballs, basketballs, and soccer balls…In addition we have activated the Special services units comprised of five officers and 118 enlisted men, all of whom are specialists" in music, athletics, and theater.[49]

Since 1940 the United States had instituted a military draft, launched a massive public awareness campaign on physically fitness, registered approximately 10,000,000 men for armed service, revised FM 21-20 (1941), developed the AGF combat readiness test, and issued new PRT guidance in the form of TC 87. However, by the beginning of 1943 it was becoming apparent that these efforts were not sufficient to provide enough recruits who were physically prepared for initial military training or combat. During the Senate subcommittee hearings on HR1975 (March 1943), Colonel Leonard G. Rowntree Chief of the Medical Division, Selective Service System and Vice Chairman, National Committee on Physical Fitness testified that "In the beginning we were selecting for a peacetime Army…Now we are at the bottom of the barrel, and we are not only lowering our standards, but we are going back through our rejected list…trying to determine what can be salvaged and made available for military service."[50] Following the historical pattern exhibited by every Army with manpower shortages, the Selective Service Board made two changes to increase inductions: (1) they lower the physical standards required for selection and (2) they changed the age range of eligible draftees from 21-36 to 18-45.⁵¹ Although these changes provided some relief to the acute manpower shortages, with no end to the war in sight national leaders remained concerned about chronic manpower shortages. With a growing sense of unease, the Office of Education was directed to formulate a plan to change the public high schools curriculum. Under Commissioner John W. Studebaker's leadership, the Federal Security Agency developed a plan to prepare high school youth for war and for the war-time labor market by developing the "Victory Corps" program.⁵²

The Office of Education produced a series of six "pamphlets" designed to proscribe and coordinate a voluntary "Victory Corps" curriculum for junior and senior high schools. In the overview (Pamphlet No. 1) Secretary of War Henry L. Stimson wrote "The Victory Corps, with its emphasis on a thorough mastery of fundamental subjects—physical training, special studies, and other activities that can properly be a part of any school's program—will enable the boys and girls to serve more usefully after graduation, both in the war effort directly and indirectly in other related pursuits."⁵³ Pamphlet No. 2: *Physical Fitness through Physical Education* was designed to "make secondary school pupils physically fit to undertake the unusually heavy tasks they will probably be called upon to assume in the near future."⁵⁴ In the preface to Pamphlet No. 2, Victory Corps Chairman Eddie Rickenbacker wrote "there are many data and reports of observations by competent persons which indicate that American youth are deficient in the physical characteristics needed by soldiers, sailors, and airman."⁵⁵ "No part of the secondary school program is affected more in this war period than that which pertains to health and physical education… complete adaptation of the physical education program to wartime needs is essential."⁵⁶ During the 1943 Senate hearings on the Victory Corps program Lieutenant Colonel Harley West testified that "The Army has a tremendous task. We are fighting a war all over the world, we are training men by the millions. We feel that we have the right to ask for inductees who have a sound high school [physical] education on which we may build."⁵⁷

The Victory Corps physical education program was designed to develop: (1) strength, endurance, stamina, and bodily coordination, and (2) physical skills of direct value to the armed forces and war work. On the title page of *Youth Goes to War*, Lieutenant General Brehon B. Somervell, Commanding General, Army Services Forces stated:

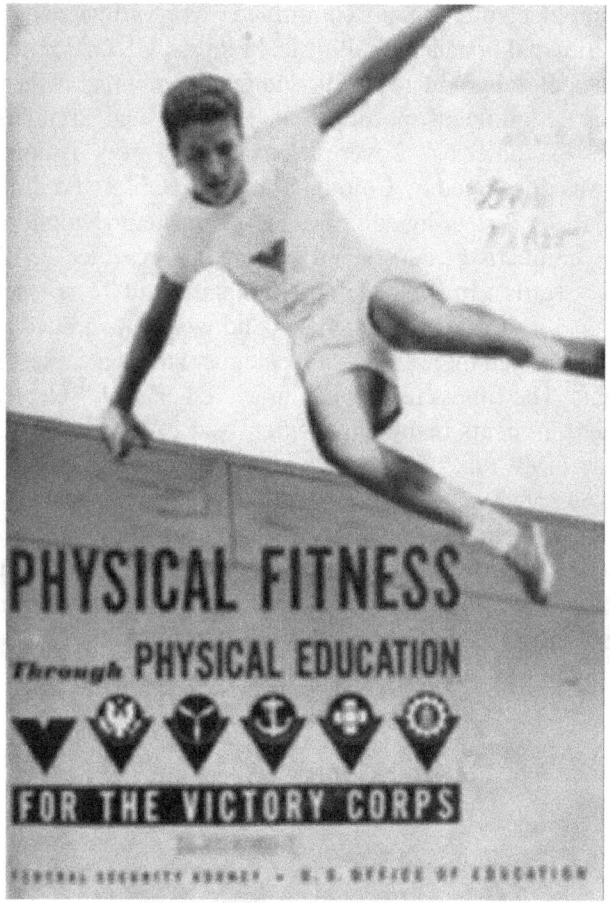

Figure 23. Victory through Fitness—The Victory Corps.

Let us be realistic. Every able-bodied boy is destined at the appointed age for the armed services…Those who do not or cannot go to college must begin now…to prepare themselves for the tasks which are for them inevitable and unavoidable. Young people in high school must be trained specifically to become better warriors…a selectee who is rejected from military service because of physical disability is no good to the Army…Far too many young people are unable to serve their country because they are not in tip-top physical shape.[58]

By July 1943 more than 70% of high schools in the United States had tried and 52.2% had adopted the Victory Corps program.[59]

The Pamphlet No. 2 steering committee was coordinated by Jackson R. Sharman, Principal Specialist in Physical Fitness, US Office of Education, a Columbia doctoral graduate (1929) and faculty member at the University of Alabama. Significant portions of the physical training program presented in Pamphlet No. 2 were taken directly from Training Circular 87, which was developed by Colonel Theodore Bank (who also served on the Pamphlet No. 2 steering committee). A robust curriculum of aquatics, gymnastics, combatives, games and sports was presented in Chapters IV (boys) and V (girls). In Chapter VI—Standards and Tests teachers, were provided a menu of fitness assessments and were encouraged to select 10 events (no more than three from each category) to create a test battery for their students. The fitness testing events were generally selected from the test and measurements textbooks written by Bovard and Cozens (1938) and McCloy (1939) and from drills proposed in TC 87. The suggested test events by category were: arm/shoulder—pull-ups, pushups, dips, 15' rope climb, bar vault; abdomen/back—sit-ups, hanging half lever, leg lift, forward bend, bank twist; legs—potato race, jump and reach, standing long jump, running long jump, running high jump, 100-yd dash, 440-yd run, 880-yd run. A fairly complex military obstacle course was also presented in the Appendix.[60]

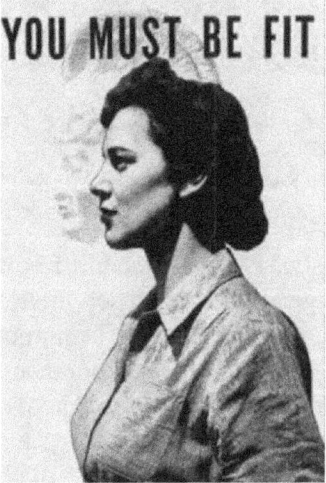

Figure 24. Women's Army Corps Fitness (1943).[61]

With an ever increasing need for combat forces and an ever expanding role for women in the armed services, the Honorable Edith Nourse Rogers, Congresswoman from Massachusetts introduced the Army Women's

Auxiliary bill in May, 1941. The objective of the bill was the development of an auxiliary corps to complement the Army Nurse Corps. "On 14, May 1942, Congress approved the creation of a Women's Army Auxiliary Corps (WAAC) and Oveta Culp Hoppy was appointed the first Director."[62] On 1 July 1943 the Women's Army Corps was signed into law and women were given military status as enlisted and officer personnel. Approximately 150,000 women served in the Army during WWII.[63]

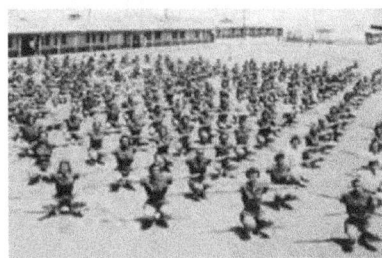

WASP Pilot Physical Training (1942).

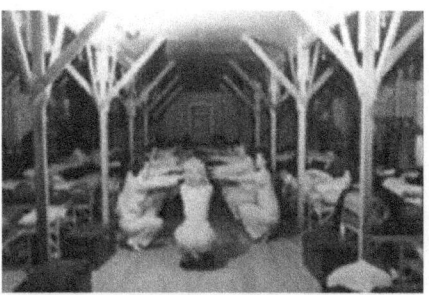

WACs Physical Training in Barracks.

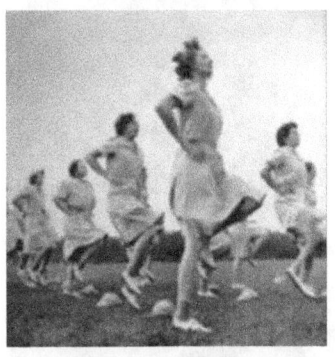

WACs Performing Calisthenics (1942).

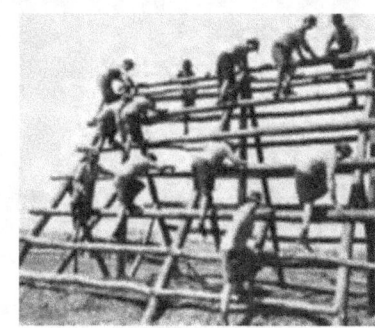

Obstacle Course Training to Increase Agility.

Figure 25. Women's Army Corps (WAC) Physical Training.

As the role of women in the Army expanded and they assumed more rigorous jobs, physical fitness became an increasing priority. On 15 July, 1943 the War Department published the *Women's Army Corps (WAC) Field Manual—Physical Training* (FM 35-20). The purpose of the manual was to establish a physical fitness program that would prepare women for their non-combat roles in the Army (i.e., to "take over" jobs that would allow men to fight). The preface succinctly stated the mission:

> The demands of war are varied, endless, and merciless. To satisfy these demands, you must be fit....Your task is to

do the things which, if you did not do them, would have to be done by men taken from the fighting ranks; men whose presence in the battle line may mean victory, whose absence might mean defeat. You must be able to do these.[64]

Various conditioning drills were described in the "daily exercise series," which when properly executed in a progressive manner would improve performance in each of the four WAC physical conditioning domains: strength, stamina, coordination, and stability. Although there was no required physical readiness assessment, FM 35-20 did present a battery of fitness "self test" items, which consisted of: full dips (push-ups), sit-ups (bent knee modified), wing lifts (prone trunk extensions—hands behind the head), endurance: squat thrusts or running in place or running for a distance at a "dog trot" pace, and balance: "stork stand."[65] There was also instruction in swimming, unarmed combatives, and recreational games.

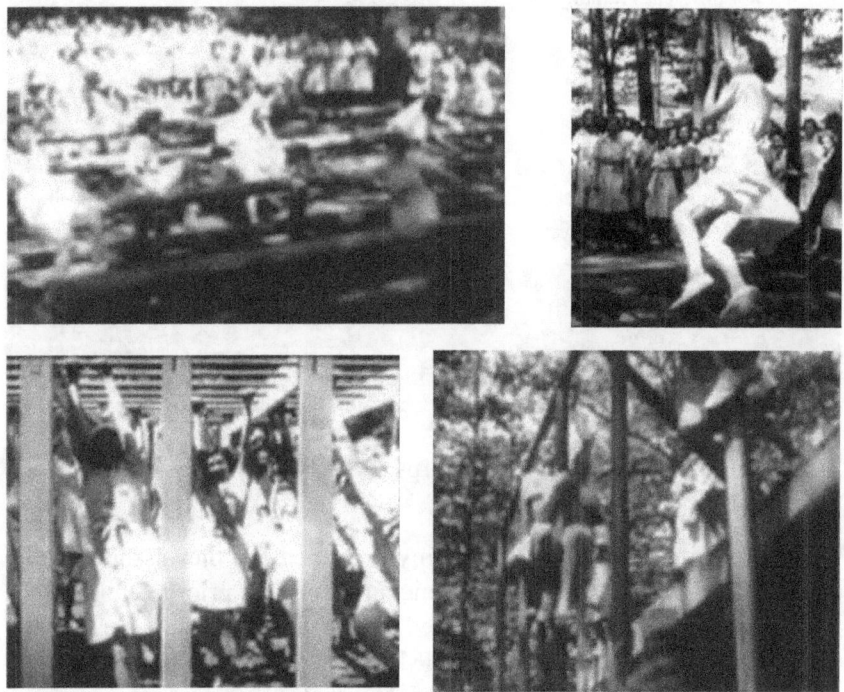

Figure 26. WAC Combat Readiness Training.

In late 1943, at the height of the United States' involvement in WWII, the national emphasis on physical fitness training reached its zenith. While the Selective Service Boards were in-processing thousands of soldiers per week, Colonel's Rowntree and Bank convinced civilian and Army leaders that individual Soldier fitness would be a the key determinate of a successful war effort.[66] Some of these efforts coalesced around the National Committee on Physical Fitness, which was commissioned by President Roosevelt in early 1943. The committee was chaired by the former Olympic champion John Kelly and co-chaired by Colonel Leonard Rowntree, Chief of the Medical Division for the Selective Service System. The National Committee on Physical Fitness was charged with developing and operating a program for improving physical fitness throughout the nation. "Such a program would include evaluation of the physical state of our young men and women and increase the activities and responsibilities of schools and colleges in physical education…and enlist the active support of industrial, social, religious, patriotic, professional and other groups."[67] Rowntree enlisted the support of various medical and physical education organizations (primarily the American Medical Association (AMA) and the American Association for Health, Physical Education, and Recreation (AAHPER) to actively support this national mission. In 1943 AAHPER dedicated the national association to the year of Army fitness. The theme of their annual convention (the National War Fitness Conference) was "Victory through Fitness." Each of the monthly issue of the *Journal of Health and Physical Education* were replete with articles like: "The Role of Exercise in Physical Fitness"—Steinhaus; "The Physical Fitness Program of the Army Air Forces"—Stansbury; "Psychological Factors in Total Fitness for War"—Bonney; "Military Physical Fitness and Physical Education"—McCloy, and "The Army Physical Conditioning Program"—Bank.[68] The National Committee on Physical Fitness designated 1944 as the "Physical Fitness Year" with an implementation date of 1 September 1944.[69]

In light of the rapid developments in the science of exercise and fitness from 1938 – 1943 and Colonel Bank's successes in influencing basic recruit fitness in 1942, the Army Ground Forces initiated an aggressive program to study fitness assessment as a means of shaping physical training and ensuring combat readiness. Over the next several years numerous physical fitness tests were developed and research studies conducted by military and civilian personnel in an attempt to predict combat physical readiness. These assessments were designed to accomplish three objectives: (1) to screen soldiers into and out of the military, (2) to identify soldiers who needed remedial training, and (3) as performance criterion for certain military jobs (i.e., for pilot or parachute training).[70]

One example of these efforts was the creation of the Army Ground Forces Medical Research Laboratory (AGFMRL) at Fort Knox, KY. In response to growing issues with "aircrew fatigue," from 24 September, 1942 to 10 March 1944 the AGFMRL analyzed a variety of physical fitness tests that might be used to predict fatigue. As a foundation for these studies Eichna, Bean, and Ash defined the physically fit man as one who possessed: (1) the capacity to do multiple types of "high energy" work, (2) the ability to endure and continue to do work for long periods of time, (3) significant muscular and cardio-respiratory reserves to minimize the disturbance of "physiologic functions," and (4) the capacity to do meaningful work following the exercise bout.[71] They compared Soldier performance on four different physical fitness tests: Army Ground Forces test (AGF), Army Air Forces test, Navy step test, and Harvard step test. For purposes of analysis, performance on the four tests was classified into three categories: poor, average, and good. Based upon a "mean" performance on the four tests, the 7-item AGF test was found to over predict physical fitness (resulted in the most soldiers classified as "good"), while the AAF test was found to under predict physical fitness (resulted in the most soldiers classified as "poor"). Ultimately the researchers concluded that fitness tests did not possess a high degree of predictive validity and should therefore only be used as one aspect of assessing physical fitness/readiness.

During this two-year period, many of the research projects coalesced around Colonel Bank's efforts to continuously update and improve Army physical fitness training and assessment. On 1 May 1944 the War Department published Pamphlet No. 21-9 (PAM 21-9): *Physical Conditioning* under the signatures of Major General J.A. Ulio, Adjutant General and General George C. Marshall, Chief of Staff.[72] As stated in the Introduction, Training Circular 87 was fielded in the summer of 1942 in response to the need for more strenuous training.[73] The function of PAM 21-9 was to provide an entirely new approach to physical conditioning in the Army. PAM 21-9 proposed that Army physical conditioning should focus on "total military fitness," which was composed of three domains: (1) technical fitness—knowledge, (2) mental and emotional fitness—habits, sense of mission, and willingness to win, and (3) physical fitness—developing the body to function effectively under physical stress. The "constituents" of physical fitness were defined as: freedom from disease and injury, strength, endurance, agility, and coordination. PAM 21-9 identified eight components of physical conditioning: marching, calisthenics, guerrilla exercises, grass drills, combatives, running exercises, swimming, and relays.[74] A separate section devoted to the use of "athletics" in the physical training program as some of Raycroft's work from WWI was again reemerged.

PAM 21-9 recommended a minimum of 1½ hours of physical training per day. Exercise prior to breakfast was approved as long as there was an adequate warm-up period prior to strenuous exercise.[75] PAM 21-9 suggested that the average man could be "put in good physical condition " in about 12 weeks (approximately the length of basic combat training), if the program was balanced and progressive. Training programs were to begin at a moderate intensity and progress gradually and steadily. For the first time in an Army training manual the authors identified the concepts of "overload" and "intensity" as key principles of physical development. "As physiologists have discovered, the nearer an exercise approaches the limits of one's ability [overload] the greater the development…development depends not upon the amount of work done, but the amount of work done per second [intensity]."[76] In the first week of a new physical training program, instructors were directed to concentrate on calisthenic exercises for 40-45 minutes each day, since they provided the greatest benefit for the general body. Although a myriad of exercises were described; "Running is the best single conditioning activity and should be used every day."[77] Again for the first time in any Army training manual, three stages of conditioning were defined. Stage one was the "Toughening Phase," which should last one to two weeks and is where the Soldier concentrated on mastering good form; calisthenics and running were the most favored activities.[78] Stage two was the "Slow Improvement Phase," which should last 6-8 weeks and constituted the period of most rapid development. Stage three was the "Sustaining Phase," in which the Soldier reached peak performance and strives to maintain this high level.[79] PAM 21-9 was quite sophisticated relative to the science of exercise and provided greater clarity on preparing Soldiers for the physical rigors of combat.

PAM 21-9 also introduced a new physical readiness test titled the Physical Efficiency Test Battery (PETB). The PETB was designed to replace the Army Ground Forces Test. "This test battery was developed after a tremendous amount of testing experience in the Army. It represents the 7 best tests out of an original group of 25."[80] The test items selected for the PETB were: pull-ups, 20-sec. burpee, squat jumps, pushups, 100-yard pig-a-back run (which was increased from 75 yards from the AGF); sit-ups, and the 300-yard shuttle run.[81] The 70-yard zigzag run and the four mile road march from the Army Ground Forces Test were eliminated.[82] As fitness testing evolved the importance of standards of performance, uniforms, and testing environments emerged. The manual also provided guidance concerning the importance of testing order, uniformity of judging/scoring, and the condition of the test areas and facilities.[83] The most radical addition to PAM 21-9 was the inclusion of normative scales for each of the seven test items. The normative scales provided Commanders with a "man's total score," which was a powerful motivation to excel. "By using these tables, the competitive spirit of the men is aroused because they want to make the highest total score and beat their friends."[84] Raw scores were converted to scale scores that ranged from 0 – 100 (making the highest total score = 700). A Soldier's performance could be classified as Very Poor, Poor, Average, Good, or Excellent for each of the seven test items. "Every company commander should have a physical fitness profile for every man in his organization," which can be used to identify and remediate weak performers.[85]

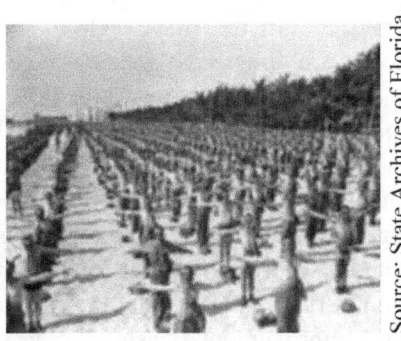

Figure 27. Army Air Corps Physical Training (Miami Beach, c.1943).

At approximately the same time Bank was completing PAM 21-9 and the Physical Efficiency Test Battery, the Army Air Force (AAF) began to diverge from traditional Army PRT doctrine. Captain Edgar B. Stansbury, Chief, Physical Fitness Branch, Special Services Division summarized the AAF's program in Physical Fitness Program of the Army Air Forces (AAF).[86] From the outset the fledgling AAF acknowledged the need for "physical training specialists," and due to the force size/structure set about to "procure specialists who were qualified in physical education to aid commanding officers in maintaining superior physical condition of AAF personnel."[87] The effort to provide trained fitness instructors contradicted the staffing plan for Army PRT. Only six months prior, Colonel Bank stated that "Physical training specialists as such, do not exist in the Army…the very size of the ground forces prohibits the use of such specialists…it is doubtful that as many as 10,000 would suffice to handle the task of conditioning the troops."[88] The AAF also took a slightly different approach to physical training by adopting the "whole man" unitary philosophy, which focused on physical fitness, social fitness and mental fitness. In reality the "whole man" concept was an extension of the "mens sana in corpore sano" philosophy (prayer) published in *Satire X* by the Roman poet Decimus Juvenalis in the mid 1st Century AD, and was secularized into the "mind, body, spirit" triad proposed in 1891 by Luther Gulick as the central dictum for the YMCA.[89]

The AFF developed a two part physical training program consisting of "required" and "voluntary" activities. There were two components to the "required program" and each component accounted for 50% of the Soldier's physical program. Fifty percent of the "required program" mandated the completion of the activities specified in TC 87, while the other 50% could be selected from TC 87 or any other "pertinent publication." For the "required program" each Soldier was to exercise between three to six hours per week distributed over a minimum of three days. The voluntary program was designed to supplement the required program and followed the Raycroft's mass athletics model utilized by the basic training camps in WWI. Since PAM 21-9 did not require units to use the Army's Physical Efficiency Test Battery, the AAF developed their own Physical Fitness Test (PFT), which was published in Regulation No. 50-10 (28 April, 1943). Stansbury alluded to an empirical study where the 3-item PFT was developed; the three test items were: sit-ups, chinning, and 300-yd shuttle run, which were a subset of the 7-item Physical Efficiency Test battery.[90] The PFT was designed to determine individual fitness status and program effectiveness. Lastly the AAF established a Physical Fitness Rating (PFR) system (excellent, very good, good, poor, very poor) to evaluate an Officer/NCO's progress in the physical program. These rating cards became a permanent part of the Officer/NCO's records and followed them from station to station.[91]

The Effects of World War II on Army PRT

> *War places a great premium upon the strength, stamina, agility, and coordination of the soldier because victory and his life are so often dependent upon them.*[92]

From a physical readiness program and assessment perspective the first and most important PRT changes during WWII was the growth in the use of empirical, scientific approaches to program development. In 1942 McCloy, Esslinger, and Bank developed an alternative PRT program for the Army.[93] Over the summer they utilized an empirical research design to test the hypothesis that their training POI was better (i.e., produced greater gains in physical fitness) in a controlled environment. The results demonstrated that their PRT program was quantitatively better that the existing 1941 FM 21-20 training POI, which ultimately resulted in the publication of TC 87 and PAM 21-9 and preciptated numerous changes in the 1946 revision of FM 21-20.

As with every war, WWII confirmed the universal axiom that physical fitness is a key and essential combat skill.[94] "A man who is more clever, agile, and mentally alert than his opponent will be defeated by that less skillful and less imaginative individual if the latter has greater strength and endurance and knows no rules of fairness except one—to win at any cost."[95] "Success in battle goes to the troops who can take one more step and fire one more shot than the enemy."[96] "The generals…realize that the military wizard but physical moron should be relegated to the same classification as the Samson who is a military dud."[97] The fitness issues during WWII were again exacerbated by the conscription of men into the Army who were physically unprepared to fight. "Had we had proper physical fitness programs in America for the 23 years prior to Pearl Harbor, many of our boys that made the supreme sacrifice would be alive today."[98] "Approximately a million men have been returned from overseas physically unfit."[99]

One application of the progress in physical readiness training during WWII came from General Lucian Truscott. The "Truscott Trot" was legendary during World War II and stemmed from Truscott's belief that the ordinary infantryman was no different from elite forces that were made to endure strenuous physical training.[100] "You can't lead your men from a command post."[101] Instead of the old infantry marching rate of 2 1/2 miles per hour, Truscott required his division to march five miles the first hour, four miles in each of the next two hours, and 3 1/2 miles per hour for the remainder of a march lasting 30 miles.[102] Truscott also prepared his soldiers to operate in mountainous terrain by exposing them to mountain walking and running techniques, night and day operations in the mountains, and numerous rope climbing skills. "This pre-invasion mountain training paid off in Italy where in five days, after fierce fighting in Agrigento, the 3d Infantry Division marched 100 miles to Palermo…a classic for its speed and success."[103]

WWII again confirmed that the Army needed to commitment greater energy and resources to the development of physically fit Soldiers.[104] Army leaders like Colonel Leonard Rowntree worked to define combat related fitness: "Physical fitness is the bodily state which combines maximum power and efficiency, with the minimum time for recovery after exhaustion" and the physical attributes needed to succeed in combat: "strength, endurance, stamina, special agilities, leadership, initiative, emotional stability and the indomitable 'will to win.'"[105] While Rowntree worked to define physical fitness, Colonel Theodore Bank worked to apply his concepts to physical development programs for the Army and society in general: "Physical fitness should be based on a continuing and graded progression, and is especially important while our youth are in formative years, long before they arrive at 'military age.'"[106]

We can learn a valuable lesson from the dramatic changes in attitude relative to the importance of physical training that occurred in many combat units shortly after the United States entered WWII. Historical records from the 2nd Army provide a cogent example. In a 1941 training memoranda from the 2nd Army Commander, Lieutenant General Benjamin Lear directed subordinate commanders to provide minimal emphasis on physical training and cautioned that excessive fatigue and exhaustion were to be avoided. Physical exercises should consist of mass calisthenics for general physical develop and competitive contests for the "physical benefit…and to develop team spirit."[107] In a subsequent memorandum Lear stated "It is not intended to have physical conditioning unduly stressed."[108] By mid 1942, the complexion of physical training in the 2nd Army had changed significantly. In subsequent training memoranda Lear directed that "physical hardening was to be brought to such a state that infantry units could "make a continuous foot march of 25 miles with full field equipment…we must do all in our power to train…all units [so] they are physically and emotionally prepared for the realities of the war."[109] In training directive No. 40, Lear directed his subordinate commanders to develop a physical training program that was more extensive than directed by Army Ground Forces. Lieutenant General Lear's replacement, Lieutenant General Lloyd Fredendall, had recently returned from commanding II Corps in northern Africa where he saw significant combat action.[110] Fredendall placed a heavy emphasis on physical training and stated "if all soldiers were physically hardened to the extent of being 'tough guys'…military operations would be a success…All troops should undergo a course of training paralleling that of our Ranger Battalion. It would involve maximum physical hardening, training for personal physical combat…[and] training in all weapons."[111] The lessons learned in combat quickly filtered back to the training bases in the US and significantly influenced the pace and intensity of Army PRT.

The extensive after action reviews following WWII were predictably similar to those that followed WWI relative to recruit/soldier fitness, physical training, and remediation. All three issues were identified as serious impediments in prosecuting the war. With the memories of combat still vivid in their minds, Army leaders acknowledged the shortcomings in the physical readiness program and set about to rectify these problems. Following nearly the identical course of action that led to the development of the Physical and Bayonet Training 'course' at Camp Benning (1919) and Raycroft's 1920 revision of physical training doctrine, the Army formally established the Physical Training School (PTS) in late 1945 and tasked them with the revision of FM 21-20. Originally the School was to be located at Camp Lee, VA, but it was ultimately activated at Camp Bragg, NC.[112] Upon inception the Physical Training School was assigned two primary tasks. The first task was to develop and implemented two educational courses: the Physical Education Supervisors Course and the Physical Training Instructors Course. Both courses were designed to provide knowledge and skills on how to design and implement a scientifically based physical training program. The supervisor's course lasted seven weeks and the instructor's course lasted three weeks. The ability for graduates to implement the practical lessons learned at the PRT School varied by command.[113]

Again similar to the task list developed for the Physical Training and Bayonet School (1919), the second task assigned to the PTS was to rewrite FM 21-20 *Physical Training*, which was revised for the second time and published in January, 1946.[114] FM 21-20 (1946) superseded FM 21-20 (1941), TC 87 (1942), and PAM 21-9 (1944). The general focus of the 1946 revision was the application of the "total military fitness" concept to combat effectiveness; "without physical fitness [the soldier] lacks the strength and stamina to fight."[115] Since WWII saw great advances in mechanized warfare, the authors were careful to caution against the perception that enhanced mechanization reduced the need for physically fit Soldiers. "The fact that warfare has become mechanized has accentuated rather than minimized the importance of physical fitness."[116]

FM 21-20 (1946) focused in much more detail on the "planning and development of physical training" (Chapter 3), rather than the execution of physical training that was so dominant in previous Army PT field manuals. Predictably, after the issues with the fitness levels of conscripted Soldiers, the 1946 manual went into great detail concerning the pace of training sedentary recruits and the hazards of over training. There was an in-depth discussion on exercise progression and the manual even presented a crude periodized training model. Due to the number of troops deployed during WWII and the time requirements to transport large numbers of soldiers to Europe, there were extensive discussions about maintaining fitness levels while in transport aboard ship and while in combat. On several occasions throughout the manual the authors acknowledged the need for and benefit of "variety" in physical training as a preventative for overuse injuries and to reduce boredom and improve motivation. With West Point no longer actively directing the physical training program of instruction for the Army, the 1946 revision moved away from the traditional Turner gymnastics terminology of setting-up and disciplinary exercises and employed a more secular construct-based approach to physical training. Gone also was the overarching philosophical model of "physical efficiency for military effectiveness" and any significant mention of health and vigor as an outcome objective of physical training.

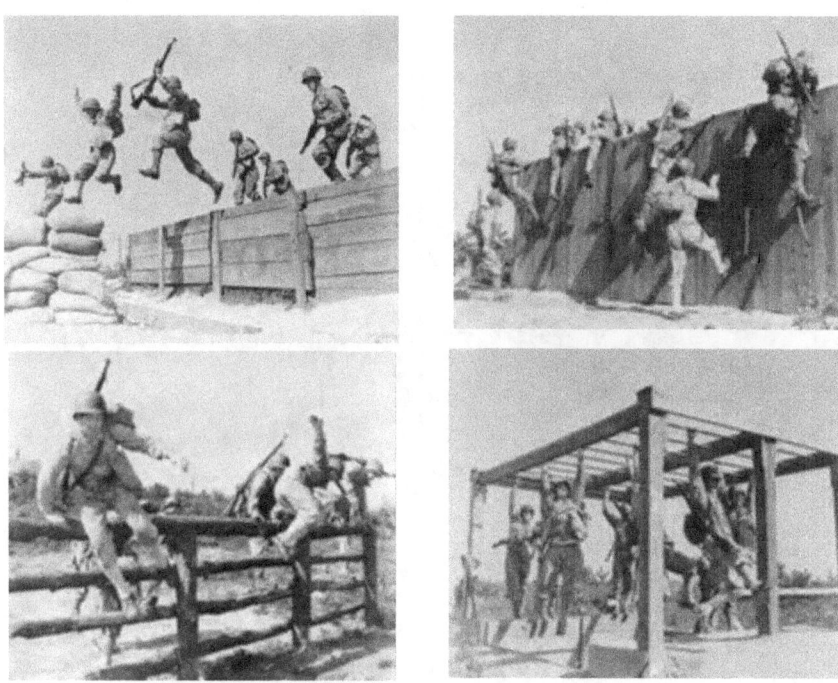

Figure 28. WWII Combat Readiness Training.

The exercise focus of the 1946 revision was on the integration of strenuous physical activity into all aspects of military training "in order to produce a soldier with the staying power and mental confidence to win."[117] A variety of calisthenic exercises were introduced: conditioning, rifle, log, and guerilla; cardio-respiratory exercises: marching, running, grass drills; combatives; swimming; athletic and games; and posture training. In Chapter 3.36 there was a significant increase in specificity when describing the "model" or purpose of exercise activities like guerrilla drills, running, and combatives.[118] The 1946 manual reaffirmed that "running is the best single conditioning activity for developing endurance and should be used every day."[119] Three new chapters were added to the 1946 revision of FM 21-20: Chapter 7—The Strength Course, Chapter 13—Combative

Activities, and Chapter 14—Tumbling. The "strength course" combined content on how to train both muscular endurance (pull-ups, decline sit-ups, war-club—similar to a kettle bell, squat jumps, etc.) and muscular strength (dead lift, snatch, curls, military press).

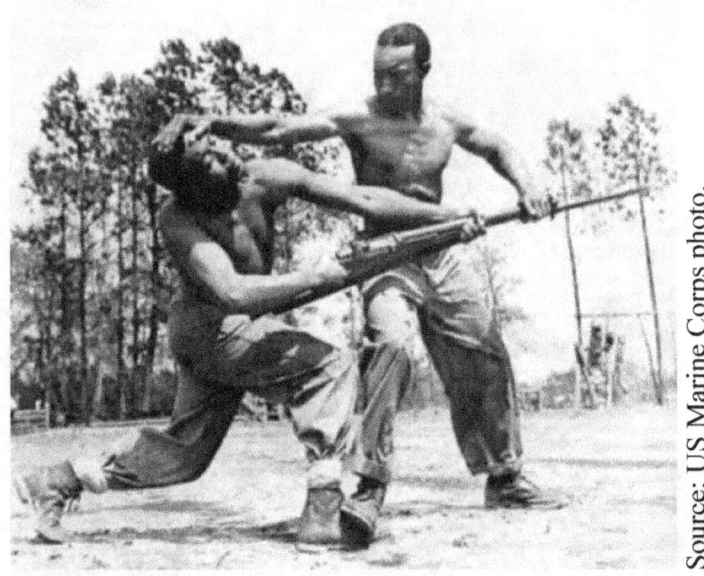

Figure 29. Bayonet and Unarmed Combat Instruction.

Since there were extensive discussions about boxing, wrestling, and gymnastics in previous Army PT field manuals, the most conspicuous new materials in the 1946 manual pertained to combative training. The combative activity chapter contained the usual "personal contests" like Indian wrestling, cock fighting, and grappling. However, for the first time in any Army field manual, Chapter 13 presented 20 pages of material on "hand to hand fighting" (the forerunner to modern Army close quarters combat training). The "hand to hand fighting" skills included strikes, chops, kicks, gouges, stomps, chokes, etc.[120] Following the combatives chapter was Chapter 14—Tumbling. Considering the focus on combat applications throughout the 1946 manual, it was interesting to find a chapter on tumbling that included 33 pages of stunts and tumbles to include rolls, vaults, and somersaults and a number of "partner" stunts like the knee hand spring, the shoulder balance, and the groin pitch. The tumbling chapter contained the first "military gymnastic" materials since Koehler's 1914 *Manual of Physical Training* and seemed decidedly out of context. Although FM 21-20 (1946) was authorized by the Secretary of War—Dwight D. Eisenhower and approved by the Acting Adjutant General—Edward F. Witsell, there is no indication or record of who actually authored the 1946 revision. The chapters on combatives, boxing, wrestling, tumbling, and swimming, however, seem to closely emulate the 4th Class Physical Education curriculum at the United States Military Academy in the 1940's; therefore the Academy's influence on this manual seems undeniable.

In the 1946 manual an entire chapter (Chapter 17) was dedicated to the discussion of "physical fitness testing." The fitness assessments were designed to achieve five objectives: measure current status, track progress, identify deficiencies, motivate soldiers to train, and drive training. Conspicuously gone from the manual was a "title" for the fitness test. Neither the Ground Forces Test nor the Physical Efficiency Test Battery was included in this revision. The 1946 FM 21-20 described an outdoor and indoor "test battery."[121] The outdoor battery consisted of pull-ups, squat jumps, push-ups sit-ups, and 300 yard shuttle run; gone were the 20 sec. burpee and the 100 yd pig-a-back run from Bank's 1944 Physical Efficiency Test Battery. The indoor battery substituted a shuttle run (25 yards x 10 laps = 250 yards) or 60 sec. squat thrusts test for the 300-yd shuttle run. The purpose of the indoor/outdoor tests was to "find out the condition of the troops and then to do something about the deficiencies revealed."[122] Commanders were encouraged to develop individual performance profiles, using the updated normative 100-point scales. The average score per test item was expected to be 50 points (out of 100 points), which allowed for a total of 500 points. Performance on the test items was categorized from Very Poor to Excellent and the "average" category was changed to "fair." Although all combat troops were encouraged "to achieve a high standard of physical fitness regardless of age—for military combat takes no cognizance of age," scales scores were adjusted for men over the age of 30.[123] Men were to be tested about every 8-12 weeks. Interestingly, the last line of Chapter 17 (printed in "bold" print) stated "Whether or not to employ these test is, of course, a command responsibility."[124]

On 31 May, 1946 the Army Medical Research Laboratory, Fort Knox (formerly the Army Ground Forces MRL) was approved to conduct a second study to critique various physical fitness tests. Bean, et al. stated that the purpose of physical fitness tests was to logically employ pre-selection, measure the effects of training, and determine the stages of convalescence.[125] This study was an extension of the 1944 study by Eichna, et al. Although generally the results were similar to those of the 1944 study, the analysis of some specific test items produced interesting results: (1) the 300-yd shuttle run exhibited a poor correlation with the

Harvard Step Test and therefore should not considered a good measure of aerobic capacity, (2) the change in performance on the pull-up test following 57 days of training was 7 to 9 pull-ups, leading the researchers to conclude that pull-up score distributions would always be fairly skewed and somewhat leptokurtic; and (3) the 4-mile march is not sufficiently rigorous to differentiate among levels of performance.

Notes

1. Sue Bowden, and Avner Offer, "Household Appliances and the Use of Time: The United States and Britain since the 1920s," *The Economic History Review* 47: (1994): 732; William Tuttle, "Part Two: The American Family on the Home Front," in *World War II and the American Home Front*. Marilyn M. Harper (Washington, DC: US Department of the Interior, October 2007), 51. "In January 1939, President Franklin D. Roosevelt submitted a $9 billion budget that contained $1.3 billion for national defense. Just a week later, he asked Congress for an additional $525 million for building a "two-ocean" navy, strengthening the nation's seacoast defenses, and manufacturing military aircraft."

2. David Ney, *Electrifying America: Social Meanings of a New Technology, 1880-1940* (Cambridge, Mass: MIT Press, 1990), 16, 368.

3. Emanuela Cardia, "Household Technology: Was It the Engine of Liberation?" Unpublished manuscript, University of Montreal, April 2010, 3.

4. Emanuela Cardia, "Household Technology," 3; Bowden and Offer, "Household Appliances and the Use of Time" Table 1, 729; William Tuttle, "Part Two: The American Family on the Home Front," 88.

5. Theodore Bank, "Trends Toward Separate Commission on Fitness," *Aim for Industrial Sports and Recreation—A Sports World Digest (AIM)* 4: (1945): 22.

6. Leonard Rowntree, "National Program for Physical Fitness," *The Journal of the American Medical Association* 125: (22 July 1944): 825.

7. For example, by 1938 the United States had developed the M36 tank with a top speed of 28 mph; the M36 tank significantly increasing mobility requirements during combined arms maneuvers

8. Ardmore Army Air Field (1942-1946): *Chronological Reminders of the Past* (reference: November 27, 1943), www.oklahomahistory.net/airbase/1jogger.html (accessed 21 June 2011).

9. Robert France, *Introduction to Physical Education and Sports Science* (Clifton Park, NY: Delmar, Cengage Learning, 2009), 18.

10. *Induction Statistics*, www.sss.gov/induct.htm (accessed 24 September, 2010); Marcus Goldstein, "Physical Status of Men Examined through Selective Service in World War II," *Public Health Reports* 66: (11 May, 1951): 592.

11. Bank, "Trends Toward Separate Commission on Fitness," 22.

12. High School Victory Corps, *Hearings before the Committee on Education and Labor, United States Senate on S.875* (Washington: Government Printing Office, 14 April, 1943), 37 (testimony of Colonel Theodore Bank).

13. High School Victory Corps, *Hearings on Senate Bill S.875*, 16 (testimony of Commissioner Studebaker, PhD).

14. High School Victory Corps, *Hearings on Senate Bill S.875*, 32.

15. Bank, "Trends Toward Separate Commission on Fitness," 23.

16. High School Victory Corps, *Hearings on Senate Bill S.875*, 32.

17. Peter Karpovich, and R. A. Weiss, "Physical Fitness of Men Entering the Army Air Forces," *Research Quarterly* 17: (1946): 192.

18. High School Victory Corps, *Hearings on Senate Bill S.875*, 33 (testimony of Colonel Rowntree).

19. Lyle M. Spencer, and Robert K. Burns, *Youth Goes to War* (Chicago: Science Research Associates, 1943), 165.

20. Rowntree, *National Program for Physical Fitness*, 821.

21. Rowntree, *National Program for Physical Fitness*, 825.

22. Department of the Army, FM 21-20 *Physical Readiness Training* (Washington, DC: US Government Printing Office, 1941), 1.

23. FM 21-20 *Physical Readiness Training* (1941), 3.

24. From FM 21-20, *Physical Readiness Training* (1941): "Exercises before breakfast are not recommended; if indulged in at all, they should be confined to a few arm stretchings and relaxed trunk-bending exercises—just exertion enough to accelerate circulation mildly. To exercise strenuously before breakfast is likely to affect the digestive operation seriously, and is more apt to weaken than to strengthen the body, which is at a very low state of physical efficiency immediately after arising, when its resistance is low," 7

25. FM 21-20 *Physical Readiness Training* (1941), 12.

26. FM 21-20 *Physical Readiness Training* (1941), 56.

27. There is no clear evidence who actually developed FM 21-20; if the process followed the pattern established for TR 115-5 and BFM Vol. 1, Chapter 4, it was likely developed at West Point under the direction of Colonel John W. Harmony, FM 21-20 Master of the Sword. Physical Readiness Training (1941), 2.

28. FM 21-20 *Physical Readiness Training* (1941), 2.

29. FM 21-20 *Physical Readiness Training* (1941), 37.

30. FM 21-20 *Physical Readiness Training* (1941), 12.

31. The second photo on the right, "Darby's Rangers" was taken in England in 1942 where US Rangers trained with battle-hardened British Commandos; the first man in line was Mr. Warren "Bing" E. Evans, "Evans helped spearhead four invasions—North Africa, Sicily, Salerno and Anzio—and was a POW for more than 14 months. His third escape attempt was successful, shortly before he was scheduled to be shot on April 22, 1945. "I was overseas for three years and seven months," said Evans, "and probably had more combat experience and time behind enemy lines than anyone." Darby's Rangers, who underwent rigorous training by the famed British Commandos, were pioneers in night operations and fighting— in mountains, fields and on water. They specialized in surprise night attacks from unlikely and difficult directions, often the backside of an enemy-occupied mountain. They were skilled in hand-to-hand fighting, often using knives and bayonets when they didn't want to be discovered at night." (Eckerle, 2008); Evans began the war as an NCO, but received two battlefield promotions to Captain; he was awarded the Purple Heart and the Silver Star.

32. Physical fitness tests/assessments had not been included in an Army training manuals since Raycroft's *Mass Physical Training* (1920); although FM 21-20 *Physical Readiness Training* (1941) included a menu of physical fitness assessments, it stopped short of establishing a standardized physical readiness battery/test.

33. FM 21-20 *Physical Readiness Training* (1941), 5.

34. FM 21-20 *Physical Readiness Training* (1941), 6.

35. FM 21-20 *Physical Readiness Training* (1941), 43.

36. FM 21-20 *Physical Readiness Training* (1941), 96.

37. S.L.A. Marshall, "First Wave at Omaha Beach," *The Atlantic Magazine* (November, 1960) online at http://www.theatlantic.com/ magazine /archive /1960/11/first-wave-at-omaha-beach/3365/ (accessed 2 March 2012).

38. Michael D. Krause, "History of US Army Soldier Physical Fitness," in *National Conference on Military Physical Fitness-Proceedings Report*, ed. Lois A. Hale (Washington, DC: National Defense University, 1990), 22. Statistics were provided by The National D-day Memorial-www.dday.org (accessed 20 June 2011); S.L.A. Marshall, *The Soldier's Load and the Mobility of a Nation* (Quantico: The Marine Corps Association, 1980), 35; Reports from the Pacific Theater during World War II suggested that more soldiers died in the island campaigns from drowning than from Japanese bullets. Whether fact or anecdote, the drowning, on D-Day drove the inclusion and assessment of the "bob and travel" in the USMA aquatic curriculum for the last 60 years; Marshall, S.L.A. "First Wave at Omaha," *The Atlantic Magazine*, November 1960, "At one thousand yards, Boat No. 5 is hit dead on and foundered. Six men drown before help arrives. The other six boats ride unscathed to within one hundred yards of the shore, where a shell into Boat No. 3 kills two men. Another dozen drown, taking to the water as the boat sinks."

39. Ted Bank enlisted in the Army in 1916 at age 18 (immediately upon graduating from high school in Clint, Michigan). He saw considerable combat during the Mexican Border dispute and in France with the American Expeditionary Force during WWI. He was wounded in combat and received the French Croix de Guerre for gallantry in battle, "Former Michigan Quarterback Considered for Texas Coach: Has Colorful, Fighting Career," *San Antonio Express*, 10 January 1934.

40. Bank, "Trends Toward Separate Commission on Fitness," 22. The football photo was cropped with permission from the *1919 Michigan Football Roster* photo, University of Michigan, Bentley Historical Library.

41. Rowntree, *National Program for Physical Fitness,* 822; Stanley J. Reiser, "The Emergence of the Concept of Screening for Disease." *The Milbank Memorial Fund Quarterly, Health and Society* 56. (1978): 409; Mary McElroy, "A Sociohistorical Analysis Of US Youth Physical Activity And Sedentary Behaviors," in *Physical Activity and Sedentary Behavior-Challenges and Solutions*, ed. Alan L. Smith and Stuart J.H. Biddle (Champaign, IL: Human Kinetics Inc., 2008), 65.

42. Dr. Charles H. McCloy was the noted professor of physical education at the State University of Iowa. Dr. A. A. Esslinger was an associate professor and Director–Division of Physical Education for Men at Stanford University and a major in the US Army Reserve.

43. Theodore Bank, "The Army Physical Conditioning Program," *Journal of Health and Physical Education* 14: (1943): 197.

44. "Annual Report of the President of Stanford University, 1943," 230; Bank, "The Army Physical Conditioning Program," 197; War Department, Pamphlet 21-9 *Physical Conditioning* (Washington: Government Printing Office, 1944), 6.

45. History.amedd.army.mil/booksdocs/wwii/medtrain/ch8.htm (accessed 8 September 2010). William B. Bean, Charles R. Park, David M. Bell, and Charles R. Henderson, *A Critique of Physical Fitness Tests* (Fort Knox, KY: *Army Medical Research Lab,* Report 56-1(07), 19 February 1947), 14; Ludwig Eichna, William Bean, and William Ashe, *Comparison of Tests of Physical Fitness* (Fort Knox: Army Ground Forces Medical Research Laboratory, 1944), 1; ; John P. Ladd, "US Army Physical Fitness Testing: Past, Present and Future." Student paper written for the Communicative Arts Program, March, 1971, 12. Based upon the fitness testing items selected for the Army Ground Forces test, its development was clearly influenced by the work of Bank, McCloy, and Esslinger.

46. *Army Training Circular 87* was developed by McCloy, Esslinger, and Bank.

47. *Ardmore Army Air Field (1942-1946)*, http://www.oklahomahistory.net/airbase/ 1jogger.html (accessed 10 September 2010).

48. *Army Training Circular No. 87*, 1942, 1.

49. Bank, "The Army Physical Conditioning Program," 196; Ward C. Crampton, *Fighting Fitness: A Preliminary Training Guide* (New York: McGraw-Hill Book Co, 1944), 10.

50. Subcommittee on the Committee on Appropriations, *US Senate Hearings on H.R. 1975,* 1943, 60 (testimony of Colonel L.G. Rowntree); Richard M. Ugland, "Education for Victory: The High School Victory Corps and Curricular Adaptation during World War II," *History of Education Quarterly 19*: (1979): 443.

51. High School Victory Corps, *Hearings on Senate Bill S.875*, 37 (testimony of Colonel L. G. Rowntree, Chief, Medical Division, Selective Service System). Subcommittee of the Committee on *Appropriations on HR1975,* 55. Testimony of Dr. J.W. Studebaker, 59. Testimony of Colonel L.G. Rowntree; Rowntree, "National Program for Physical Fitness," 824.

52. High School Victory Corps, *Hearings on Senate Bill S.875*, 1.

53. *Physical Fitness through Physical Education–Pamphlet No. 2*, iv.

54. *Physical Fitness through Physical Education–Pamphlet No. 2*, Victory Corps Series (Washington: Government Printing Office, 1942), 1-2.

55. *Physical Fitness through Physical Education—Pamphlet No. 2*, v.

56. D.A. Emerson, and Joy Hills, *The Victory Corps Program: A Wartime Program for High Schools* (Salem, OR: Superintendent of Public Instruction, 1943), 21.

57. High School Victory Corps, *Hearings on Senate Bill S.875,* 26 (testimony of Luietenant Colonel Harley B. West, General Staff Corps).

58. Spencer and Burns, *Youth Goes to War,* cover page. Spencer and Burns, *Youth Goes to War*, 5, 29, 129.

59. Ugland, "Education for Victory," 439.

60. *Physical Fitness through Physical Education—Pamphlet No. 2*, 1942, 26, 52, 91.

61. Online at www.armywomen.org/history.shtml (accessed 22 November, 2010).

62. Judith Bellafaire, *The Women's Army Corps: A Commemoration of World War II Service* (Fort McNair, DC: Center for Military History Publication 72-15, 17 February 2005), 2; online at http://www.history.army.mil/brochures/WAC/WAC.HTM).

63. War Department, FM 35-20 *W.A.C. Field Manual Physical Training*(Washington.: US Government Printing Office, 1943), 1a.

64. FM 35-20 *W.A.C. Field Manual Physical Training* (1943), 1, 4.

65. A successful repetition was one in which a woman lowered her body in a generally straight/rigid manner until the arm's reach a 90o angle and the chin touches the ground/floor.

66. Bank, "The Army Physical Conditioning Program," 197; Bank, "Trends Toward Separate Commission on Fitness," 22; Rowntree, "National Program for Physical Fitness," 821.

67. "Physical Fitness Program – Editorial," *The Journal of the American Medical Association* 125: (22 July 1944): 851; Note: the National Committee on Physical Fitness was the forerunner of the President's Council on Physical Fitness and Sport.

68. "Victory through Fitness-National War Fitness Conference." *Journal of Health and Physical Education* 14: (1942): 131.

69. Goldstein, "Physical Status of Men Examined," 608.

70. David E. Thomas, "Selection of the Parachutist," *Military Surgeon Magazine* 91 (1942) and *Military Review* 86 (1942): 64; In order to qualify for parachute training, candidates were "required to demonstrate good physical strength, stamina and coordination by his ability to do fifteen push-ups and perform coordination exercises with an acceptable degree of proficiency…a history of excellence in some competitive sport is desirable but not required."

71. Eichna, et al., *Comparison of Tests of Physical Fitness,* 1.

72. This document was clearly written or directed by Colonel Theodore Bank based upon the inclusion of research results from 1942 and also the "Bank twist" on page 35.

73. Pamphlet 21-9 *Physical Conditioning*, 5.

74. Pamphlet 21-9 *Physical Conditioning*, 2-8.

75. War Department Pamphlet 21-9 *Physical Conditioning*, 10; FM 21-20 *Physical Training* (1941) stated that in some hot climates exercise early in the morning may be preferable and the Surgeon General had determined that hot weather exercise was not harmful if Soldiers were give adequate time to acclimatize (S.G.O. Circular Letter No. 119, 3 July 1943, "Acclimatization, Including Water and Salt Requirements in Hot Climates.")

76. War Department Pamphlet 21-9 *Physical Conditioning*, 64; "The amount of work done per second" was the authors attempt to describe what we not call "work intensity".

77. War Department Pamphlet 21-9 *Physical Conditioning*, 64.

78. The concept of "toughening" grew from the poor condition of conscripted Soldiers during WWI and WWII as evidenced by the testimony of Colonel L. Rowntree: "These boys when they come up are soft and flabby. It is not their fault. It is the fault of civilization and these boys are not touch and the Army and Navy has set up within their organizations ways and means of toughening and conditioning these men" *Hearings on H.R. 1975-First Deficiency Appropriations Bill for 1943* (Washington, DC: US Government Printing Office, 1943), 60).

79. War Department Pamphlet 21-9 *Physical Conditioning*, 61.

80. War Department Pamphlet 21-9 *Physical Conditioning*, 71.

81. Pushups were to be completed continuously to exhaustion—no rest was allowed; the Soldier was required to keep his body in a generally straight line from head-toe and lower his body until his chest touched the ground; to facilitate rater reliability the rater would place his hand flat on the ground, about the center of the chest; the Soldier testing was required to lower his body until his chest touched the raters hand.

82. War Department Pamphlet 21-9 *Physical Conditioning*, 71; Ladd, *US Army Physical Fitness Testing*, 13.

83. Ladd, *US Army Physical Fitness Testing*, 14; War Department Pamphlet 21-9 *Physical Conditioning*, 76.

84. War Department Pamphlet 21-9 *Physical Conditioning*, 78.

85. War Department Pamphlet 21-9 *Physical Conditioning*, 81.

86. Edgar B. Stansbury, "The Physical Fitness Program of the Army Air Forces," *The Journal of Health and Physical Education* 14: (1943): 463; War Department Pamphlet 21-9 *Physical Conditioning*, 82.

87. Stansbury, "The Physical Fitness Program of the Army Air Forces," 463.

88. Bank, "The Army Physical Conditioning Program," 195.

89. Martti Muukkonen, "Orandum Est Ut Sit Mens Sana In Corpore Sano- Formation of the Triangle Principle of the YMCA," presentation to the TUHTI Seminar of the Finnish Youth Research Society. Helsinki, 20 September 2001, 6; Note: Luther Gulick was a gymnastics instructor at the YMCA Springfield Training College and a close personal friend and professional colleague of Major General Leonard Wood.

90. Stansbury, "The Physical Fitness Program of the Army Air Forces," 503.

91. "The Physical Fitness Program of the Army Air Forces," 503.

92. Department of the Army, FM 21-20 *Physical Readiness Training* (Washington: US Government Printing Office, 1946), 1.

93. Bank, "The Army Physical Conditioning Program," 196; Hagen, 1996, 85-86.

94. D'Eliscu, 1943, 3; Perhaps one of the more definitive lessons on the benefits of physical and mental toughness came from the Third Army's maneuver to relieve the 101st Airborne at Bastogne during the Battle of the Bulge. Following the meeting at Verdun with General Eisenhower, late on 19 December 1944 General George S. Patton broke contact with the Germans near Saarbrucken almost 100 miles from Bastogne. In approximately 72 hours Patton marched elements of the

Third Army over 100 miles of rugged terrain in the dead of winter to interdict the Germans at Bastogne. With little or no rest "his forces still had the stamina and discipline in engaging the German forces and succeed in breaking through them." (http://threeo.ca/outstandingpmsgengeorgespattonc 758.php - accessed 21 December 2011); Agostino Von Hassell, and Ed Breslin, *Patton: The Pursuit of Destiny* (Nashville: Nelson, 2010), 157; Don Fox, *Patton's Vanguard: The United States Army Fourth Armored Division* (Jefferson, NC: McFarland & Company, Inc., Publishers; 2003), 304; Tim McNeese, *The Battle of the Bulge* (Philadelphia: Chelsea House Publishers, 2004), 77-79.

95. Francois D'Eliscu, *How to Prepare for Military Fitness* (New York: W. W. Norton & Company, 1943), 3.

96. Gerald Astor, *Battling Buzzards: The Odyssey of the 517th Parachute Regimental Combat Team* (New York: Dell Publishing, 1993), 97. This statement was attributed to Colonel Lewis A. "Lou" Walsh, Commander, 517 parachute Regimental Combat Team, October, 1943.

97. C.L. Brownell, "We Learned About Fitness from Them," *Journal of Health and Physical Education* 15: (April 1944): 183.

98. Bank, "Trends toward Separate Commission on Fitness," 23.

99. Bank, "Trends toward Separate Commission on Fitness," 23.

100. Lucian Truscott, *Command Missions, A Personal Story* (New York: Dutton, 1954), 180: "I was confident then that an average infantry battalion could approximate Ranger and Commando standards for marching, but I realized that I would have to approach the objective gradually. Officers and men would have to be imbued with the importance of such preparation and with confidence in their ability to attain it. It would be some time before each battalion could be required to attain a marching speed of five miles in one hour, four miles an hour for twenty miles, and three and a half miles an hour for distances up to thirty miles. But each battalion would attain it."

101. Will Lang, "Lucian Truscott," *Life* (2 October 1944): 106.

102. Lang, "Lucian Truscott," 106; Truscott, *Command Missions*, 185; Truscott went as far as establishing the proper stride length (30"-36") and stride rate (104-146 steps per minute) to achieve a 3, 4, 5 mph pace. Truscott's training schedule required each Officer and Enlisted person to march five miles in one hour twice each week and eight miles in two hours once each week. The purpose was to develop physical condition and stamina and determine combat readiness and capabilities.

103. Mark Hertling, "Physical Training and the Modern Battlefield: Are We Tough Enough?" Monograph, School of Advanced Military Studies, Fort Leavenworth: US Army Command and General Staff College, 1987, 20; Lang, *Lucian Truscott*, 106; "Palermo was a hundred miles to the northwest. Our first forty or so miles led through rugged mountains which rose to a height of more than 4,000 feet...Our three tortuous roads northward had steep grades, numerous hairpin turns, and many bridges...I told them I expected them to be in Palermo in five days and be the first to arrive." (Truscott, *Command Missions*, 224).

104. Major A.A. Esslinger, Chief, Physical Training, Army Service Forces, 10 October 1945; in a personal letter to the Master of the Sword, Department of Physical Education, United States Military Academy he wrote: "My conviction that the Army has failed miserably in conditioning our troops makes me disappointed that more is not being done at the Academy to bring about an improvement in this situation....While the physical condition of a regimental or divisional commander is important it is far more important that regimental or divisional commander have the proper attitude and knowledge in relation to the physical condition of his troops."

105. Rowntree, "National Program for Physical Fitness," 825.

106. Bank, "Trends toward Separate Commission on Fitness," 24.

107. Bell L. Wiley, and William P. Govan, *History of the Second Army* (Study No. 16) (Washington: Historical Section, Army Ground Forces, 1946), 53.

108. Wiley and Govan, *History of the Second Army*, 55.

109. Wiley and Govan, *History of the Second Army,* 108, 111.

110. Major General Fredendall was the commander of II Corps during the Tunisia Campaign and was defeated by Rommel and von Arnim at the Battle of Kasserine Pass. He was relieved by Eisenhower and returned stateside where he was ultimately given the command of 2nd Army on 1 June 1943.

111. Wiley and Govan, *History of the Second Army,* 122.

112. Richard W. Whitfield, *History of the US Army Artillery and Missile School, Volume 3: 1945-1957* (Fort Sill, OK: US Army Field Artillery School, 1957), 17; World War II (USAPFS Archived Historical Documents, 1987), 37, 40-41.

113. World War II (USAPFS Archived Historical Document, 1987), 40-41.

114. *Basic Field Manual-1:4* (1936) was never officially designated as *Field Manual 21-20*, therefore for chronological purposes FM 21-20 *Physical Readiness Training* (1941) will be identified as the originating document in the "FM 21-20 Field Manual" series. According to two sources (*Physical Fitness Symposium Report* (Fort Benning, GA: US Infantry Center, 12-14 October 1970), 9 and Krause, *History of US Army Soldier Physical Fitness*, 22; the Physical Fitness School was "transferred to Fort Bragg in 1946 and was placed in charge of the revision of FM 21-20." The date given above (1946) for the Physical Training School's formation and its involvement in the revision of FM 21-20 are contradictory, since FM 21-20 *Physical Readiness Training* (1946) was published in January, 1946. Generally the revision of this type of manual took about six-eight months. There are three possible explanations for this contradiction: (1) the PTS was operational at Fort Bragg prior to 1946 and was tasked to revise FM 21-20 *Physical Readiness Training* (1941) beginning in 1945-with a January 1946 publication date; (2) the 1946 revision was written by individuals who were later assigned to the Physical Training School at Fort Bragg in 1946; or (3) the FM 21-20 *Physical Readiness Training* revision alluded to in the Physical Fitness Symposium report and by Krause was actually the 1950 revision.

115. FM 21-20 *Physical Readiness Training* (1946), 1.

116. FM 21-20 *Physical Readiness Training* (1946), 1.

117. Krause, "History of US Army Soldier Physical Fitness," 22.
118. FM 21-20 *Physical Readiness Training* (1946), 34 (see Table 1, p. 36).
119. FM 21-20 *Physical Readiness Training* (1946), 35.
120. FM 21-20 *Physical Readiness Training* (1946), 217.
121. FM 21-20 *Physical Readiness Training* (1946), 333.
122. FM 21-20 *Physical Readiness Training* (1946, 349.
123. FM 21-20 *Physical Readiness Training* (1946), 345.
124. FM 21-20 *Physical Readiness Training* (1946), 349.
125. Bean, et al., *A Critique of Physical Fitness Tests,* 1.

Chapter 6
The Cold War Era—Fomenting a National Fitness Policy

As America settled into a post war routine and lives returned to their normal peace-time pace, the Army again grew complacent about physical readiness training. American occupational soldiers in Japan enjoyed the easy life of an occupational army.[1] Families joined their husbands and life took on a very social atmosphere. An eight-hour duty day, parties and social functions for the married Officers and NCOs was a way of life. The younger, single soldiers found recreation in the form of drinking and dating Japanese women. Ultimately, American soldiers in Japan became soft.[2] "When World War II ended in 1945, the American Army was the most capable in the world…Five years later, by June 1950, the Army was a shadow of its former strength…the Army had lost its warfighting edge…"[3] The Army's peacetime rhythm relegated tactical and physical training to a low and under resourced priority, which resulted in an Army that was ill prepared physically, mentally, or emotionally for combat in Korea.[4]

On 25 June, 1950 the North Korean Army (NKA) invaded South Korea.[5] Several days later a US Army task force under the command of Lieutenant Colonel Charles Smith was committed to the battle to stop the advancing NKA somewhere north of Osan. Outnumbered and out resourced the US forces made contact at 0816 on 5 July 1950.[6] By 1430 the NKA had overrun or flanked the US positions and Lieutenant Colonel Smith gave the order to disengage.[7] Although US forces were confronted with a larger, better equipped, and better trained NKA, many analysts attribute the poor combat performance of Task Force Smith to a lack of preparation for war.[8] "By failing to train properly, by failing to develop esprit, and by failing to develop the physical and mental conditioning required to fight, the companies and battalions of the Eighth US Army set themselves up for failure long before the first airplane or ship landed in Korea."[9] The advantages of the NKA's superior forces were enhanced by the extremely poor physical conditioning of US troops: "The first indications of a decline in the physical strength and ability of young Americans became apparent among United States soldiers in the early stages of the Korean War."[10] "Dismounted soldiers who bypassed the roadblock by moving cross-country over the steep Korean hills realized in no uncertain terms what a lack of physical preparation for the rigors of combat actually meant."[11]

As part of the on-going after action review for the Korean War, several faculty members of the Department of Physical Education at West Point surveyed recent graduates that had seen combat in Korea.[12] Of those who completed the survey: 35% responded that American troops were inferior to other UN troops in physical conditioning; 93% responded that a vigorous physical conditioning program prepared soldiers for combat; 68% responded that combat fitness could not adequately be developed through routine field training; and 50% responded that adequate physical training programs were provided for their unit prior to combat.[13] These results are supported by the reflective statement published in the historical summary of FM 21-20 (1957): "as the reports came back from Korea, an alarming number of casualties were attributed to the inability of the US soldiers to physically withstand the rigors of combat."[14]

On 30 November 1950 the Army revised FM 21-20 for the third time, which was one year ahead of the previous 5-year revision cycle and only five months after the Task Force Smith debacle. Interestingly there were only minor changes in the physical training doctrine: (1) the principles of exercise were identified as—progression and overload; and (2) the phases of physical development were identified as—toughening, slow improvement, and sustaining. From an exercise prescription perspective there were no significant changes to the training program. Chapter 14—"Tumbling" was removed and replaced with "Mass Games and Contests." Most of mass games materials were taken from Chapter 7—"Personal Contests and Games" (FM 21-20, 1941). The most significant content revision was the deletion of all "hand to hand" fighting activities that had been incorporated for the first time in the post-WWII FM 21-20 (1946). There were no significant changes to Chapter 17—"Physical Fitness Testing" and the approved physical fitness test was the 5-item Physical Fitness Test Battery (Outdoor): pull-ups, squat jumps, pushups, sit-ups, 300-yard shuttle run or the alternative fitness test battery (indoor), which allowed for the substitution of an indoor shuttle run (250-yards at 25 yards per link) or 60-sec. squat thrust test for the 300-yard shuttle run. The normative scoring scales remained unchanged.[15]

Only strength can cooperate. Weakness can only beg.
—Dwight D. Eisenhower

The post Korean War period was a particularly contentious time in theUS, especially relative to the doctrine of communism. Senator Joseph McCarthy's "red scare" created an ideological schism between America and much of the world. Virtually every facet of American life became a competition with the Soviet block; industrial productivity, technology, space exploration, and ultimately physical fitness.[16] The tensions that arose from this competitive environment ultimately had a dramatic effect on secular and Army physical readiness training. In 1953 the former German physiotherapist Dr. Hans Kraus and his colleague Dr. Sonja

Webber developed the Kraus-Weber Test of Minimum Muscular Fitness (see graphic below). In 1954 Kraus and his assistant Ruth Hirshland conducted clinical trials assessing minimum muscular fitness of American and European children.[17] Later that year, at the height of the "red scare," Kraus and Hirshland published their findings in several seminal articles.[18] Kraus and Hirshland reported that 57.9% of American children failed the 6-item fitness battery as opposed to 8.7% of European children. Following a White House luncheon on 11 July 1955, Kraus and Hirshland presented their data to 30 government leaders including President Eisenhower and Vice President Nixon. Shocked by the results, Eisenhower declared this to be a serious problem that was even more alarming than he had imagined. Kraus and Prudden attributed the cause of the problem to a range of factors "from the playpen to the school bus to television—in short, America's plush standard of living."[19] On 16 July 1956 President Eisenhower issued Executive Order 10673 to establish the President's Council on Youth Fitness, which started a 7-year national campaign to promote physical fitness.[20]

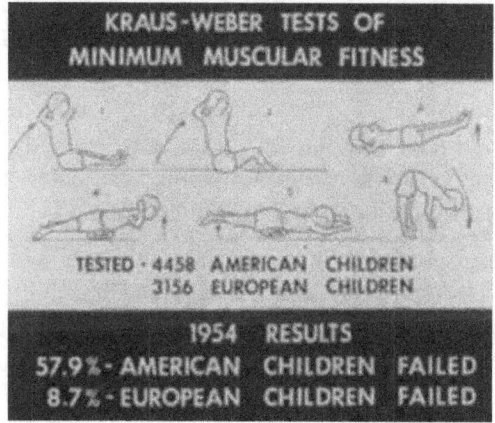

Figure 30. Exercises from the Kraus-Weber Test.

Contrary to the direction of the Nation, which was earnestly promoting a national commitment to physical fitness, the Army was losing ground on the physical readiness training problem. One of the victims of the Eisenhower budgetary reductions was the Physical Training School at Fort Bragg.[21] Over the protests of Representative Carl Durham—top minority member of the House Armed Services Committee (Chapel Hill, NC) the PTS was closed on 1 January, 1954 to save the Army $250,000.[22] The projected Army budget in FY1954 was $6.9 billion.[23] Both Durham and then Secretary of the Army Robert T. Stevens acknowledged that field commanders in Korea were calling for a greater emphasis on physical conditioning of troops. "It just doesn't make sense, Durham said, to save money by cutting out something…you admit you need urgently."[24] 1953 marked the second time the Army's physical readiness training school was eliminated.

On 25 January 1956 *Physical Training—Women's Army Corps* (FM 35-20) was revised and published for the second time. Although not as patronizing as the 1943 version, the 1956 revision still portrayed the physical character of women as "the weaker sex." FM 35-20 (1956) established a new format for Army field manuals and appears to be the precursor to the 1957 revision of FM 21-20 (TM 21-200). FM 35-20 (1956) presented chapters on planning/administering PRT; leadership and organization of physical training programs, general conditioning, posture training, body mechanics, and team sports, relays, and swimming. While the upcoming 1957 revision of FM 21-20 (for men) focused on combat readiness, FM 35-20 focused on personal and social wellness and included phrases like "the contents consist of…various types of physical training activities suitable for female personnel" and survival swimming is "one of the finest means of developing grace and coordination."[25] Although the swimming and sport chapters were relatively gender neutral, the conditioning exercises, body mechanics, group and relay games were generally devoid of any significant exercise intensity and rigor. Lastly, the limited discussion on fitness testing for women presented in the initial FM 35-20 (1943) was not included in the 1956 revision.

With the demise of the Physical Training School in January 1954, proponency for physical readiness doctrine and training was transferred to the Special Services Division (specifically the Ranger Department) at the US Army Infantry School at Fort Benning. From 1953 to 1957 various Army-wide physical fitness "conferences" were held to support physical fitness training and development. On 8 October 1957 *Physical Training* (FM 21-20) was revised and published for the fourth time and superseded Physical Training (FM 21-20,1950), Change No. 1 (26 October 1951), Change No. 2 (15 September 1952), and TC 21-3 (18 April 1957). During this revision Army leaders elected to segregate PRT "concepts" from "applications." The conceptual information relating to PRT development, planning and organization was published in FM 21-20-*Physical Training*. Applied information related to exercise prescription, physical conditioning, and exercise was published several months later in TM 21-200—Physical Conditioning. The revised FM 21-20 (1957) assumed a decidedly more scientific foundation with new chapters on the influence of exercise on body structure—muscle and skeletal systems, and body function—circulatory, respiratory, endocrine, and lymphatic systems. Chapter 6—Program Planning was significantly more dogmatic than the 1950 version. Approximately 50% of all physical training was dedicated to Drill 1—the enhanced Army Dozen.[26] In addition FM 21-20 (1957) prescribed that running, grass and guerrilla drills, combatives and games, relays, and sports were to be incorporated into the training schedule to enhance variety and balance.

On 31 December 1957, a little over two months after the revised FM 21-20 was released, the Army's applied physical training doctrine was published in *Physical Conditioning* (TM 21-200). The 588 page "hip-pocket" manual provided detailed descriptions of conditioning activities designed for Drill Sergeants and NCOs. The manual reiterated the five (5) components of physical fitness: muscular strength ("power of contracting is regularly challenged by maximum load"), muscular endurance ("performing continuous work over long periods"), circulo-respiratory endurance ("Wind—ability to use oxygen to do work over an extended period"), agility ("ability to change direction quickly"), and coordination ("Timing—"ability to move all body parts in a smooth, efficient, concerted effort"). It described the three overarching principles of physical conditioning: (1) moderate beginning (build a foundation), (2) gradual progression, and (3) overload; and the three stages of development: (1) The Toughening Stage—for untrained men, (2) The Slow Improvement Stage—slow, progressive, steady improvement, and (3) The Sustaining Stage—sustaining high levels of fitness with little improvement. TM 21-200 provided extensive instructions on developing each component of physical fitness, most of which was taken from the 1950 FM 21-20.[27]

Physical fitness/combat readiness testing and evaluation doctrine was also segregated by manual. FM 21-20 contained information related to the philosophy of physical readiness testing in Chapter 11—"The Evaluation of Physical Fitness" and TM 21-200 contained information related to the administration of physical readiness tests in Chapter 11—"Administration of Physical Fitness Tests." The 5-item Physical Fitness Test Battery (PFTB) remained the Army's approved fitness test. Although PFTB items remained the same, there were slight adjustments in the normative scales. At the 100 point level pull-ups decreased from 20 to 18, squat jumps increased from 75 to 95, push-ups increased from 54 to 60, sit-ups increased from 79 to 85, and the 300 yard shuttle run remained unchanged. Perhaps in response to "lessons learned" from combat experiences in Korea, the 1957 manuals also included a new test called the Physical Achievement Test (PAT), which was designed for "combat-type units" to assess combat-related skills. The 5-item PAT included: 5-second rope climb, 75-yard dash, standing triple broad jump, 150 yard man carry, and 1-mile run.[28] Although "distance runs" had been included in army training manuals since 1826 as an effective measure of stamina, the addition of a low intensity, aerobic capacity event (1-mile run) was a significant change for Army fitness testing. The administration and application of these fitness tests was still at the discretion of the commander and the emphasis continued to shift from program effectiveness (unit readiness) to individual readiness. For the first time the administration of both physical fitness tests became mandatory during basic combat training:

> The costly lessons learned from our past military experiences have led to...the ever increasing realization that our troops must be well conditioned.[29]

As a part of the national emphasis on physical fitness initiated by President Eisenhower, on 21-24 April, 1958 the US Army Infantry School (USAIS) hosted its first major Physical Fitness Seminar at Fort Benning, GA.[30] The myriad of military and civilian conferees were organized into five working committees: (1) the role of the Nation in the Army's progress towards fitness, (2) physical fitness and total military fitness, (3) the physical needs of the pentomic soldier, (4) the program for fitness, and (5) the evaluation of physical fitness.[31] The seminar was hosted by the Ranger Department, a subordinate unit of the USAIS, which was responsible for Army-wide physical training policy and doctrine and the resident instruction of students in physical training.[32] Over 65 civilian and military organizations were represented at the seminar. Some of the keynote speakers were Brigadire General Stanley Larsen (assistant commandant USA Infantry School), Dr. Ott Romney (President's Council on Youth Fitness), Dr. Ray Duncan (American Association for Health and Physical Education), and Lieutenant Colonel Frank Kobes (Director/Master of the Sword, Department of Physical Education, USMA). Brigadire General Larsen succinctly outlined the four key fitness question facing the Army and the Nation in his welcoming address: (1) how does civilian fitness affect us?, (2) what should we be fit for?, (3) how do we attain fitness?, and (4) how do we measure fitness?"[33]

As part of the seminar Lieutenant Colonel James Reilly (Chairman, Combat Conditioning Committee) outlined the Army physical training model, which consisted of three stages: (1) the toughening stage, where soldiers first experience a regular exercise program, mostly during initial entry training; (2) the slow improvement stage, where soldiers built upon their "toughening" foundation through progression and overload; and (3) the sustain stage, where soldiers use greater balance and variety of physical exercises and sport to maintain motivation and interest as long as troops are on active military duty. After two days of discussions, each of the five working committees reported their conclusions and recommendations:

Committee 1: What part can the Nation play in the Army's progress towards fitness? This committee reported eight conclusions and two recommendations, the most salient of which were:

Conclusions:
1. The nation must awaken to the necessity of physical fitness.
2. Communities with sound fitness programs send men to the Army in a better state of physical, mental, and technical fitness.
3. The American Soldier must be in good physical condition through participation in a variety of sports and other recreational skills.
4. The nation should maintain higher standards for youth fitness.

Recommendations:
1. Endorse physical education programs that contain a combination of body building, athletic, and recreational sport activities.
2. Oppose the substitution of ROTC for physical education.[34]

Committee 2: Is physical fitness necessary for total fitness? This committee reported four conclusions and four recommendations, the most salient of which were:

Conclusions:
1. Physical fitness is essential to total military fitness and should receive equal emphasis with the development of technical skills.
2. Benefits of physical fitness support emotional and mental fitness, physical aptitude is essential to military leadership.

Recommendations:
1. Ensure Command emphasis on physical fitness at all levels.

2. Establish a program of instruction to train military physical fitness supervisors.

3. Establish a Division/Post level physical training course to train unit instructors. [35]

Committee 3: Determine the degree of physical proficiency required of the pentomic Soldier. This committee reported 11 conclusions and seven recommendations, the most salient of which were:

Conclusions:

1. Current concepts and doctrine are adequate.

2. Personnel who are continuously engaged in physical training will be physically fit for their job assignment.

3. The physical fitness program is for all military regardless of duty assignment.

Recommendations:

1. Current doctrine (FM 21-20/TM21-200) should be sustained including current definitions relating to physical fitness.

2. Increased motivation methods to include awards programs for individuals and units.[36]

Committee 4: Determine the adequacy of the physical training program to include training aids and research. This committee reported 10 conclusions and three recommendations, the most salient of which were:

Conclusions:

1. The current fitness training program is adequate to meet the requirements of the present concept of warfare.

2. Current BCT/AIT programs do not allocate sufficient hours to physical conditioning.

3. Reduce time devoted to "Drill One" and increase time devoted to developing stamina.

4. There is a need for continuous research and evaluation of all aspects of the physical training program.

Recommendation:

Mandate one hour per day of physical conditioning for all personnel. [37]

Committee 5: The over-all evaluation of the physical fitness program. This committee reported seven conclusions and three recommendations, the most salient of which were:

Conclusions:

1. Physical fitness tests should assess endurance, stamina, strength, and activities that produce a combat effective soldier.
2. Physical assessments should be multidimensional, including individual achievement tests, road marches, obstacles courses and field training exercises.
3. Physical fitness type tests should be used by a superior when rating a subordinate.

Recommendations:

1. Additional emphasis be placed on the evaluation of the over-all physical fitness program by the commander.
2. Incorporate fitness assessment data in NCO evaluation reports.
3. DA Form 705 should be a permanent part of a Soldiers 201 file.[38]

During the decade of the 1960's the United States experienced the most prolific growth in secular physical fitness, which many attribute to the number of Soldiers that received physical fitness training during WWII and Korea and the fears aroused by the "Cold War." The President's Council for Youth Fitness provided significant programmatic and public relations support to the effort. The American Association for Health, Physical Education, and Recreation served as the dissemination network for thousands of public school students and their parents through physical educators and coaches. US colleges and universities provided extensive empirical research to support the development of the science of exercise. Our national leaders, specifically Presidents Eisenhower and Kennedy, provided cache for the "fitness movement" through their personal commitment and active involvement in fitness development. Kennedy leveraged his knowledge and experience as a combat naval officer to further our national emphasis on physical fitness. In a poignant article for *Sports Illustrated,* published in December 1960, president-elect John F. Kennedy argued:

> The physical vigor of our citizens is one of America's most precious resources... throughout our history we

have been challenged to armed conflict by nations which sought to destroy our independence or threatened our freedom…our growing softness, our increasing lack of physical fitness, is a menace to our security…the stamina and strength which the defense of liberty requires are not the product of a few weeks' basic training or a month's conditioning…[however, they] come from bodies which have been conditioned by a lifetime of participation in sports and interest in physical activity.[39]

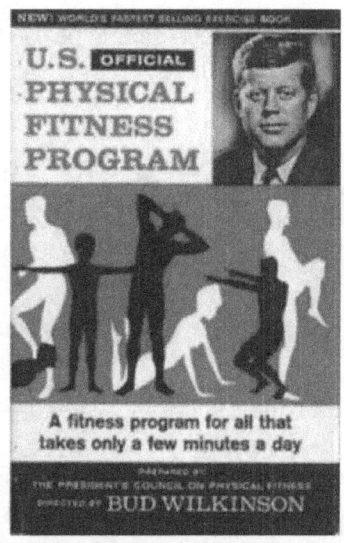

Figure 31. US Physical Fitness Training Program manual (1963).

On 2 October, 1959 the Army published Change 1 to TM 21-200. This rather innocuous change had one significant historical implication that would change Army physical readiness testing forever. Change 1, TM 21-200 established the Army Physical Fitness Test and Physical Achievement Test as a service requirement for all Soldiers with a minimum total score to pass each test of 200 points.[40] Passing thresholds for each individual test item were not established. On 25 July, 1961 the Army published Change 2 to TM 21-200, where the lessons learned in Korea finally caught up with PRT doctrine. Change 2 marked a return to "combat readiness" as the primary focus of Army fitness testing (as was the case in 1920 and again in 1946). As described in Change 2 (TM 21-200) the major emphasis of Army physical fitness testing was to assess those components of fitness and functional skills that were deemed necessary in combat. Essential military skills were defined as: running, jumping, dodging, climbing and traversing, vaulting, carrying, balancing, falling and swimming. Both the Physical Fitness Test and the Physical Achievement Test were discarded in favor of the Physical Combat Proficiency Test (PCPT). The PCPT became the required physical fitness test for the US Army and incorporated assessments of both individual fitness and unit readiness. The PCPT events were (including minimum performance time/score): 40-yard low crawl (36 sec.), horizontal ladder (number of rungs in one minute—36), dodge run and jump (agility run—26.5 sec.), grenade throw (15 pts), and a one mile run (8:30).[41] The PCPT was mandatory for basic combat training and generally used to assess combat readiness of most Soldiers. Each event was worth 100 points with a maximum score of 500 points. A minimum of 300 points was considered passing and a soldier must achieve a minimum of 60 points/event to be considered "combat qualified."[42]

> We find ourselves now in a rather serious predicament, one which is becoming more serious each year. Incoming cadets possess less physical ability than they did twenty or thirty years ago and the time allotted for developing physical ability in these cadets has gradually been reduced—31% since 1945. At the same time it is apparent that the officer of today and tomorrow will need more physical coordination, strength, and stamina than his predecessor.[43]

During the summer of 1962 the US Army Infantry Center developed a document entitled Your Individual Physical Fitness to help USAIS students better understand fitness development and aid them with the planning and execution of individual physical activity program.[44] The document was quite sophisticated relative to the discussion in Section IV – "Building Your Fitness Program." The manual presented the five elements (principles) of a sound physical training program: overload—a level of intensity greater than you are accustomed to doing; progression—regularly increasing your workload; balance—working all body parts/systems; variety—using a variety of exercise to prevent overuse and boredom; and regularity—exercising on a regular and predictable schedule.[45] In order to facilitate progression and recovery, the manual presented six Tables ("progression guides") that regulated frequency and intensity of physical work.

Once the Army made the PCPT a service requirement in 1959 with performance criteria of 200 points and 300 points (TM 21-200 Change 1 and Change 2 respectively), it became necessary to formalize this requirement. On 7 January 1963 *Army Physical Fitness Program* (Training Circular

21-1), outlined the regulations for administering/grading the PCPT. The PCPT was mandatory for:

> All personnel under forty years old in Active Army divisional and non-divisional combat and combat support TOE units, every six months; personnel attending service schools longer than twenty weeks, preferably about midway through the course; basic trainees, twice during basic combat training and once during advanced individual training; and all others on active duty with available facilities, semiannually.[46]

Those soldiers who did not have access to the physical testing facilities were required to take the Army Minimum Physical Fitness Test—Male twice each year. A soldiers' performance on the physical fitness test was to be included in his official file. On 26 July 1963 the Army published TC 21-1, Change 3, which mandated that the physical fitness test card become a permanent part of an individual's field 201 file for all Soldiers less than 40 years of age.[47]

On 7 January 1963 the Department of the Army also issued two additional physical training pamphlets, DA PAM 21-1—*Physical Fitness Training Program for Specialist* and *Staff Personnel and DA PAM 21-2*—Physical Training Program for Women. During the ramp-up to the Vietnam War there was a significant need for additional "non-combat" troops. The physical expectations for these "support" troops were generally lower than for combat-type troops.[48] These lower expectations necessitated the development of the Army Minimum Physical Fitness Test – Male (PAM 21-1), which was designed for personnel who were assigned to duties that "precluded" them from "training" for the PCPT. The Army Minimum—Male test consisted of six events, one for each focus area: flexibility, shoulder girdle, abdominal, back, leg, and circulo-respiratory. Each focus area had a primary and alternate test; the Soldier had the choice of which event he would take. The primary events included: squat bender, push-ups, sit-up, "legs over," squat thrust, and stationary run. The alternate events included: squat stretch, 8-count pushup, body twist, leg spreader, mountain climber, and one-half mile run. The test could be administered indoors or outdoors and there were no published standards of performance.[49]

PAM 21-2 established the Army Minimum Physical Fitness Test—Female to assess the five exercises that comprised the "5-10 Plan."[50] The five items in the AMPFT—Female were: arm circle (18 reps), twister (15 reps), bent-over airplane (15 reps), sit-up (15 reps), jumping jacks (16 reps). There was no time limitation and female Soldiers "passed" if they could execute the requisite number of repetitions. The AMPFT—Female was required for all WAC trainees during and upon completion of basic training.

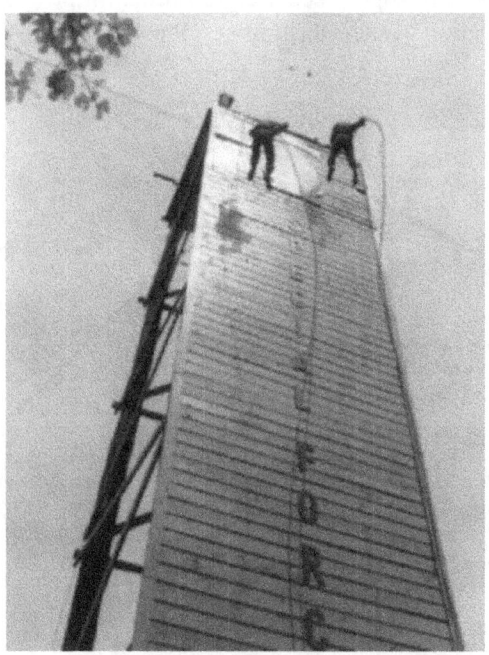

Figure 32. Army Special Forces Rappel Training (1963).

Between 1960 and 1964 US involvement in Vietnam and the concomitant increase in casualty rates were doubling each year; in 1965 the number of casualties jumped to 1,862. Prior to 1969 the majority of Soldiers voluntarily enlisted in the Army. With the increased need for Soldiers and increased risk of deployment to Vietnam, enlisted Soldiers were not always among the most physically fit. A part of the physical fitness problem was an ever increasing issue with body composition. On 25 October 1963 the Army institutionalized the policies and procedures of the Army weight control program with the publication of Weight Control (AR 600-7). This document superseded DA Circular 600-7, which was published on 10 September 1962. Army Regulation 600-7 applied to all active duty Soldiers and the AWCP was administered by the commander. Body weight standards by age and gender for enlistment, reenlistment, and extension of service for all Officer and Enlisted personnel were published in AR 40-501.[51] Since relatively little was known about the assessment of lean and fat body mass, obesity was defined in terms of body weight. DA Form 2738-R was established as the counseling form for body weight.

"Personnel whose weight exceeds the appropriate standard established in table I or II, appendix III, AR 40-501, and whose obesity has been determined by a physician to be attributable to nonmedical causes, will be placed on a medically supervised weight reduction program regardless of the date of expiration of their term of service."[52]

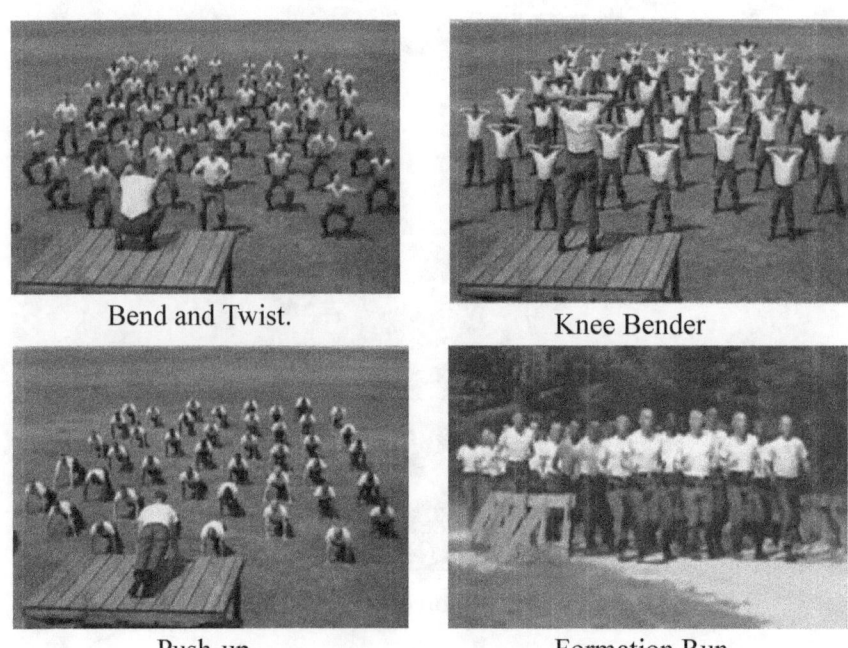

Figure 33. Physical Readiness Training (1967).

Although US advisors had been in Vietnam since 1955, combat troops were not used until after the Gulf of Tonkin incident on 2 August 1964. By the end of 1965, "President Johnson announced plans to deploy additional combat units and increase American military strength in South Vietnam to 175,000..."[53] As the Army prepared for combat in Vietnam, 5 January 1965 would become a seminal date in the history of physical readiness training and assessment for the US Army. Although TC 21-1 specified army-wide fitness assessment requirements, it was not until January, 1965 that the physical training and testing requirements were formally codified in Army regulations. Army Chief of Staff, Harold K. Johnson directed the publication the *Army Physical Fitness Program (*AR 600-9), which established the regulatory framework for Army physical readiness training and assessment. Physical fitness was identified as "an indispensable part of leadership" and individual commanders were given the authority and responsible for executing the Army physical fitness program. AR 600-9 did not provide specific PRT doctrine; "Detailed objectives for male personnel are as indicated in TM 21-200 and DA Pam 21-1; and for female personnel as indicated in FM 35-20 and in DA Pam 21-2."[54] AR 600-9 established Army-wide minimum physical fitness standards for all personnel and the implementation policy for the Army's physical fitness program. All personnel were required to take a fitness test "periodically." When tested on a semi-annual basis, tests were to occur about every six months. All male personnel were required to take the Physical Combat Proficiency Test or during inclement weather the Army Minimum Physical Fitness Test—Male. Female personnel were required to take the Army Minimum Physical Fitness Test—Female, which was to be administered twice to "WAC trainees" as proscribed in DA PAM 21-2 and "periodically" upon completion of basic training.

Throughout 1965 there were many additional changes to Army physical readiness training and doctrine. On 26 February 1965 Headquarters DA published the first revision of *Physical Fitness Program for Women in the Army* (DA PAM 21-2). While some of the materials overlapped *Physical Training—Women's Army Corps* (FM 35-20, 1956), PAM 21-2 provided the rationale for why women needed to exercise and build a strong physical fitness program. The unique feature in PAM 21-2 was the required basic exercises for women—the "5-10 Plan." The rather parochial 5-10 Plan outlined the "five basic exercises to be performed each day in just 10 minutes."[55]

On 26 May 1965, the Army issued Change 4 to TM 21-200 *Physical Conditioning*. Other than minor revisions to two exercise drills, the primary purpose of Change 4 was to supersede Change 2—Physical Fitness Testing and bring TM 21-200 (1957) into alignment with AR 600-9 (1965). Change 4 outlined the three authorized Army fitness tests: Physical Combat Proficiency Test, Army Minimum Physical Fitness Test—Male, and the Airborne Trainee Physical Fitness Test. The only scoring change to the PCPT was to lower the dodge run and jump time from 26.5 seconds to 25 seconds.

On 23 June 1965 Weight Control (AR600-7) was revised and published for the second time. There were no substantial changes; AR 600-7 provided regulatory control of body weight for active duty service members. "Maintenance of proper body weight is a prerequisite to achieving a satisfactory degree of physical fitness."[56] The weight control program was still command-driven. After determining an overweight condition was not due to a medical issue, the Soldier was counseled by completing DA Form 2738-R and began a program to reduce his/her body weight.

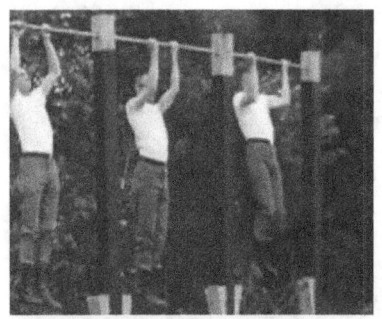 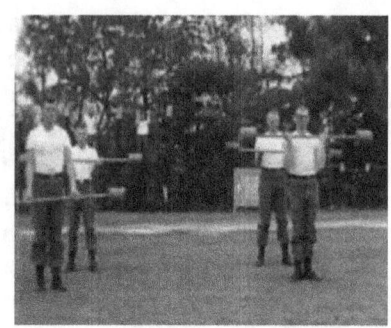
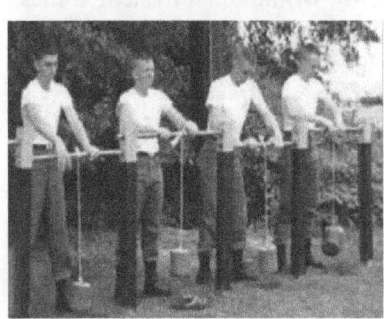 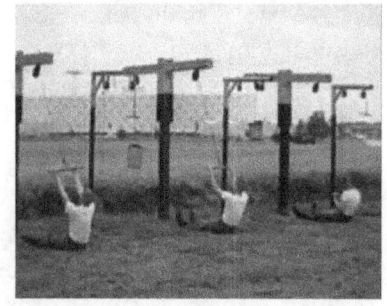

Figure 34. Strength Circuit in Basic Combat Training (1967).

On 2 September 1965 *Physical Training—Women's Army Corps* (FM 35-20) was revised and published for the third time. The 1965 revision signified a dramatic departure from previous parochial attitudes about women, exercise, and fitness and brought FM 35-20 into alignment with AR 600-9 (1965). As stated in the purpose "this manual provides guidance in the planning, execution, and evaluation of physical training" for women.[57] Like their male counterparts, the primary physical components were defined as: strength, stamina, coordination, flexibility, and sports-related skills. Exercises were divided into seven chapters: physical conditioning—mostly calisthenics; posture training; body mechanics—functions skills like lifting, pushing, etc.; group games; relay games; team and individual sports; and swimming. Interestingly, even though physical fitness testing requirements for women were specified in AR 600-9 (January, 1965), there was no mention of a physical fitness testing requirement for women in either revision of PAM 21-2 (February, 1965) or FM 35-20 (September, 1965).

In 1966 the number of Army physical fitness tests grew when the Inclement Weather Physical Fitness Test was introduced in the Continental Army Command Pamphlet 600-1.[58] The Inclement Weather Test was designed to insure there was no disruption to the training/testing schedule for Soldiers in basic, advanced individual or combat support training as a result of weather. Test events were selected to measure muscular strength and endurance and coordination of the five basic muscle groups. The test items were: push-ups, knee bender, sit-ups, side step (jumping jacks) and the squat thrust. Males older than 40 years of age were exempt from all physical fitness testing.

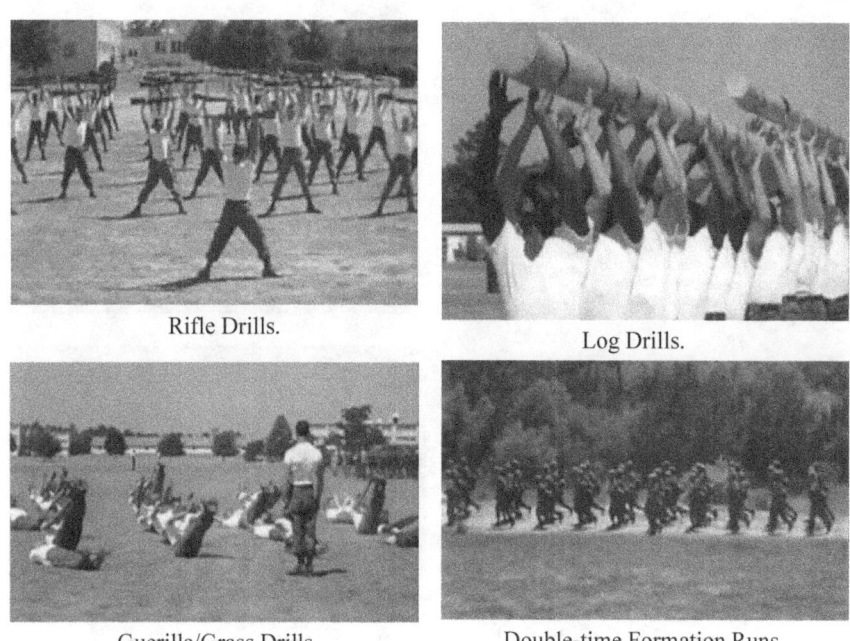

Rifle Drills. Log Drills.

Guerilla/Grass Drills. Double-time Formation Runs.

Figure 35. Combat Readiness Physical Training (1967).

With US troop levels peaking in Vietnam, *Physical Readiness Training* (FM 21-20) was revised and published for the sixth time on 31 January 1969.[59] Taking advantage of the exponential growth in the body of knowledge on exercise science, the 1969 revision made substantial changes to the 1957 physical training doctrine. The basic anatomy and physiology presented in Chapters 2 & 3 (1957) were enhanced and moved to Part Six—"The Human Body. Chapter 28—"The Body and Physical Fitness," a discussion of the applied science of exercise physiology, and Chapter 31—"Posture Training" were added. The 1969 revision previewed a new chapter entitled "Development of Physical Readiness."[60] This chapter provided a concise summary of the types, components, stages and principles of exercise. The terms isotonic and isometric were used for the first time in Army PRT doctrine. The five basic principles of exercise (overload, progression, balance, variety, and regularity) were operationally defined.[61] In an attempt to centralize Army doctrine and training, all conditioning drills and sport activities, which were published separately as TM 21-200 in 1957, were reintegrated into FM 21-20 (1969) in Chapters 10-23. *Physical Conditioning* (TM 21-200) was discontinued.

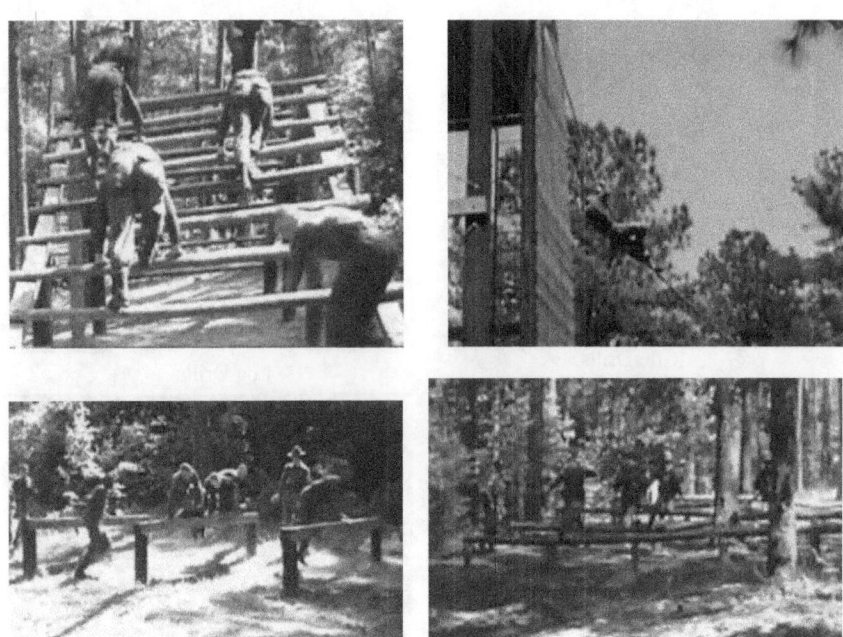

Figure 36. Combat Obstacle Course Training (1967).

In FM 21-20 (1969) commanders were allowed to choose from four physical fitness tests. These tests were designed to assess the essential components of fitness and combat-related skills. Essential combat skills were defined as: running, jumping, dodging, climbing and traversing, crawling, throwing, vaulting, carrying, balancing, falling and swimming.[62] The four fitness tests available to male soldiers were: Physical Combat Proficiency Test (PCPT), Army Minimum PFT—Male, Airborne Trainee PFT, and the Inclement Weather PFT. Tests were ostensibly selected to fit with the unit's mission. The revised PCPT included the 40-yard low crawl; horizontal ladder; run, dodge and jump; grenade throw (the 150-yard man-carry was substituted for the grenade throw in basic combat training, advanced individual training, and combat support training); and a one-mile run.[63] For the first time, a minimum standard was established for each PCPT event; all soldiers were required to achieve 300 total points, with a minimum of 60 points/event for combat soldiers and 45 points/event for combat support personnel. The Army Minimum PFT—Male (AMPFT-M) consisted of six events each with a specific focus; flexibility, shoulder girdle, abdominal, back, leg, and circulo-respiratory. Each functional area had a primary and alternate test event and the soldier had the choice of which event he would take. The primary events included: squat bender, push-ups, sit-up, legs over, squat thrust, and stationary run. The alternate events included: squat stretch, 8 count push-up, body twist, leg spreader, mountain climber, and one-half mile run. The Airborne Trainee Qualification Test was the only Army test with criterion-referenced standards for each event. This test required trainees to achieve minimum standards of: 6—chin-ups, 20—bent leg sit-ups, 22—pushups, 80—half knee bend (2 min.), 8:30—1-mile run.[64]

Birth of the Soldier Fitness Center

With the influence of Presidents Eisenhower and Kennedy and the President's Council on Youth Fitness, the secular fitness movement grew exponentially during to the decade of the 1970's primarily through the influences of two exercise professionals: Dr. Kenneth Cooper and Mr. Arthur Jones. In 1968 Cooper published his seminal work *Aerobics,* which started a generation of "baby boomers" on the aerobic path to fitness.[65] In early 1970 Arthur Jones produced his first strength training machines, which were marketed under the brand name "Nautilus." The Nautilus machines allowed the beginner to engage in varying intensities of strength training with a minimum level of instruction and supervision. Nautilus machines enhanced work capacity by reducing the rest interval between exercise sets.

As the Army entered into the turbulent 70s with a protracted conflict in Southeast Asia, the United States once again resorted to forced conscription to manage manpower requirements.[66] The concomitant poor initial entry fitness levels were exacerbated by two persistent human resource problems: (1) how to manage the expanding role of women in the Army, and (2) the growing physical fitness/weight management/body composition issue. Following the secular trends of women's emerging contributions to sport and the workplace from 1940 to 1970, society's perceptions of women's physical abilities were changing dramatically. Although it was generally believed women were physiologically incapable of successfully engaging certain strength and endurance events (e.g., running long distances), in December 1963 American Merry Lepper ran the first competitive marathon since 1926.[67] In 1966 Roberta Gibb unofficially ran the Boston Marathon and completed the 26+ mile race in 3:21:25.[68] The civil rights and affirmative action movements of the 1960s and 1970s further impacted women's roles in the Army. Although women had made some strides in athletics, this progress was not evidenced in the 1970 publication of the Army Training Program (PAM 21-114: male and PAM 21-121: female). There remained significant gender differences in the physical aspects of basic combat training that resulted from the divergent missions of men and women in the Army. Men were trained for combat-related tasks requiring muscular strength and stamina, while women were trained for administrative tasks that required only marginal levels of general fitness and conditioning. For the Army there were still questions about a woman's "inability to withstand arduous physical exercise."[69]

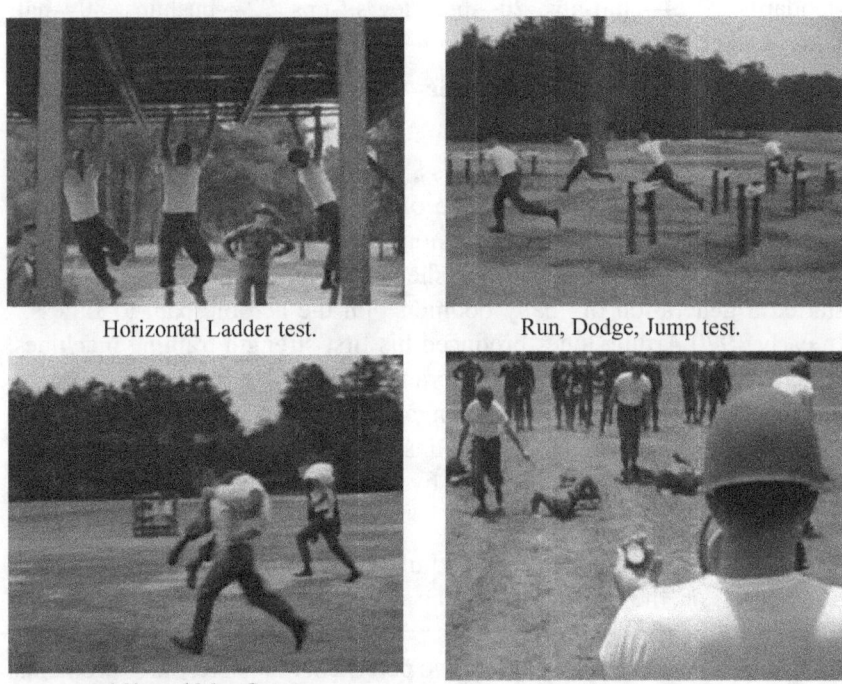

Horizontal Ladder test.   Run, Dodge, Jump test.

150-yard Man Carry.   40-yard Low Crawl.

Figure 37. Physical Combat Proficiency Test (1969).

On 12-14 October, 1970 the US Army Infantry School (USAIS) hosted its second Physical Fitness Symposium at Fort Benning, GA. There were seven objectives for the conference: (1) discuss new developments in fitness programming, (2) nurture liaisons between military and civilian fitness experts, (3) discuss recent PRT developments by the Infantry School, (4) evaluate Army PRT programs, (5) learn about civilian research and development, (6) determine the relationship between fitness and military job performance, and (7) evaluate the Army's physical fitness testing program.[70] The symposium was hosted by the Leadership Department and the Office of Doctrine, Development, Literature, and Plans (ODDLP), which was the USAIS's proponent agency for Army physical fitness programs.[71] Over 80 leading "civilian and military physiologists, medical specialists, physical fitness educators and military training specialists" gathered for the symposium.[72] Some of the keynote speakers were Brigadier General John Carley, Dr. Paul Ribisl (Kent State), Dr. Edwin Fleishman (American Institute for Research), Dr. George Cousins (Indiana University) and Colonel Frank Kobes (Department of Physical Education, USMA).

When the Physical Fitness Symposium concluded on 14 October 1970, participants had established fifteen (15) conclusions and nine (9) resolutions. The most noteworthy conclusions were: (1) physical fitness is essential to total military preparedness and should receive equal emphasis with the development of technical skills, (2) the application of "aerobics" is a required component for physical fitness training, (3) physical training programs should be implemented by qualified school-trained personnel, and (4) all soldiers, regardless of age, should meet minimum physical fitness standards. There were two noteworthy resolutions; the Army should develop: (1) a national research and documentation center that would serve as the focal point for research in physical fitness, and (2) an "Army Physical Fitness Institute" to teach selected officers and enlisted men the skills and expertise to properly implement approved fitness programs.[73] This was the fourth time since 1885 that an Army planning and operations committee recommended that the Army develop and resource a school to train Army Officers and NCOs about physical fitness.

On 12 November 1971 the *Army Physical Fitness Program* (AR 600-9) was revised and published for the second time. In a consolidation of authority and responsibility, proponency for the Army Physical Fitness Program was given to the Assistant Chief of Staff for Force Development and physical fitness was redefined from "essential for leadership" to "essential for accomplishing the Army's mission." Clearly influenced by the 1970 report of the Physical Fitness Symposium, the 1971 revision contained a new definition of physical fitness ("Special Emphasis Term"): a physically fit soldier has "a healthy body, the capacity for skillful and sustained performance, the ability to recover rapidly from exertion, the desire to complete a designated task, and the confidence to face any eventuality."[74] The concept of rapid recovery from exertion generally reflected the current state of aerobic fitness assessment where step tests were often used to measure cardio-respiratory efficiency as a function of heart rate recovery. AR 600-9 was divided into three major sections: General, Responsibilities, and Training. The training section provided doctrine for basic combat training (BCT), table of organization and equipment (TO&E), and table of distribution and allowances (TDA) units. This section also specified physical fitness testing requirements. "When tests are utilized, the test appropriate to the duty assignment or qualification desired should be administered as outlined in FM 21-20 for men and FM 35-20 for women. DA Form 705, Physical Fitness Testing Record, may be used to record the results."[75] Interestingly the FM 35-20 (1965) failed to specify any fitness tests or testing requirements for women; however later in the Training section 11.b.4, it stated that "The Army minimum physical fitness test—female should be administered to all unit assigned female personnel under 40 years of age."[76] Female personnel were required to achieve the minimum number of repetitions specified for their age group.

On 30 March 1973, as we were nearing the end of the Vietnam Conflict, *Physical Readiness Training* (FM 21-20) was revised and published for the seventh time.[77] The manual was divided into six "parts:" Part 1—Physical Fitness Leadership, Part 2—Physical Readiness Training Programs (program development and design), Part 3—Physical Activities ("conditioning" drills and activities), Part 4—Competitive Conditioning Activities (combatives, team athletics), Part 5—The Army Physical Fitness Evaluation, and Part 6—The Human Body. The major changes in FM 21-20 (1973) came in Part 5 (Chapters 24, 25, 26). Seven separate physical fitness tests comprised the Army Physical Fitness Evaluation (AAPE). There were three basic fitness tests: Advanced Physical Fitness Test; Staff and Specialist Physical Fitness Test; Basic Physical Fitness Test. There were also four special purpose fitness tests: Inclement Weather/Limited Facilities Physical Fitness Test; Minimum Physical Fitness Test; Airborne Trainee Physical Fitness Qualification Test and; Ranger/Special Forces Physical Fitness Qualification Test.[78]

The primary test, the Advanced Physical Fitness Test (APFT), was a derivative of the Physical Combat Proficiency Test that had been used since 1961. The APFT was composed of five events: inverted crawl ("crab walk" for 20 yards); bent leg sit-ups (fingers interlaced behind the head); run, dodge, jump (26 yards); horizontal ladder (20 feet—14 rungs); and the 2-mile run-MR (in fatigues/boots). Male Soldier (17-25) standards for the 2-mile run were 14:41 = 100 pts and 20:33 = 60 pts. To meet the combat readiness requirement a Soldier must score a minimum of 60 points per event and a total of 300 pts. The Staff and Specialist PFT substituted pushups for the inverted crawl and 1MR for the 2MR (1MR scores were: 6:02 = 100 pts and 8:20 = 60 pts). The Airborne Trainee PFQT consisted of chin-ups, sit-ups, push-ups, knee bender, and a 1MR. The Ranger/Special Forces Physical Fitness Qualification Test was a new addition to the 1973 revision. This test consisted of the inverted crawl, sit-ups, push-ups, run/dodge/jump, 2MR, and a combat swim. For Ranger candidates the combat swim requirement was 15m in utilities, boots, pistol belt, first aid pouch, two full canteens, two ammo pouches, harness, and individual weapon. For Special Forces candidate the combat swim was 50m in utilities and boots. A 60-point criterion-referenced standard was established for each event, which was approximately equal to the 75-point level for similar events on other PFTs. For example, on the Ranger/Special Forces PFQT the 60-point standard for the 2-mile run was 16:30 for all Soldiers; there were no age-adjusted scores.[79]

Physical fitness testing requirements remained lower for combat service support Soldiers. "The physical standards to be attained by combat and combat support unit personnel are more demanding than those expected of other personnel due to the nature of the job requirement."[80] The Soldiers in combat and combat support units took the Advanced Physical Fitness Test and were required to score a minimum of 60 points in each of the five events. The standards of fitness for combat service support Soldiers "… are established at a level to insure an adequate degree of fitness."[81] The Soldiers in combat service support units had to complete all five of the events and score a total of 300 points.

Later in 1973 the Army conducted a major reorganization under the aegis of Operation Steadfast. The most significant change resulted in the formation of the Training and Doctrine Command (TRADOC) at Fort Monroe; Combined Arms Center (CAC) at Fort Leavenworth, Logistics Center (LOGC) at Fort Lee, and the Administrative Center (ADMINCEN) at Fort Benjamin Harrison. Army leaders planned for the ADMINCEN "to become the collection point for all matters related to the Army's personnel system and the human dimension of military operations."[82] Although the USAIS (Infantry School) maintained control over PRT doctrine and training, the Army Soldier Support Center at Fort Benjamin Harrison slowly assumed control over various aspects of PRT doctrine. The Family Resource Center took the early lead in PRT doctrine development while ADMINCEN initiated broader organization changes in training and doctrine development to a "schools" model.[83]

Although it had only been two and a half years since the second revision, the *Army Physical Fitness Program* (AR 600-9) was revised and published for the third time on 7 May 1974. Proponency for AR 600-9 was reassigned to the Deputy Chief of Staff for Military Operations. This revision was designed to reflect the recent reorganization of the Army, specifically the formation of the Training and Doctrine Command (TRADOC). Control of physical fitness testing and standards was transferred from the Commanding General (CG) CONARC to the CG-TRADOC. Transferring proponency of PRT doctrine to TRADOC represented the beginning of a significant shift from an infantry-centric to an Army-centric PRT focus, which has plagued Army PRT doctrine ever since. There were no significant changes to training or testing requirements.[84]

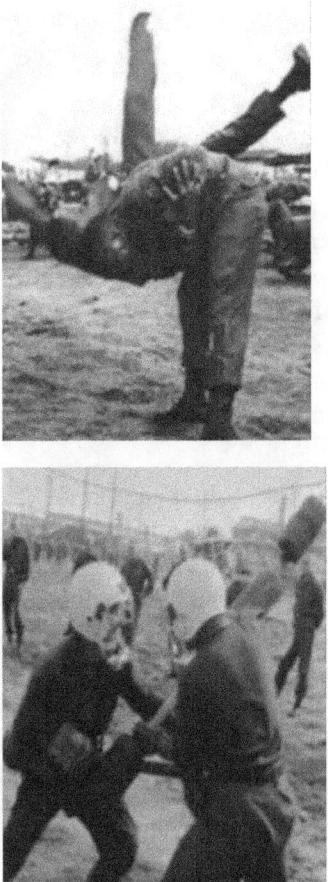
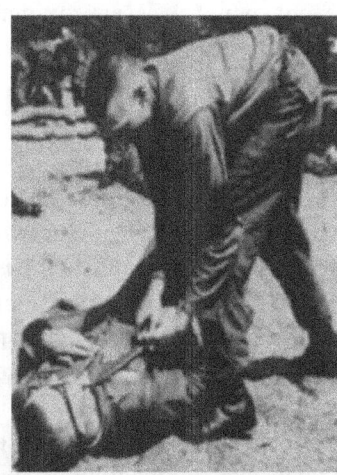
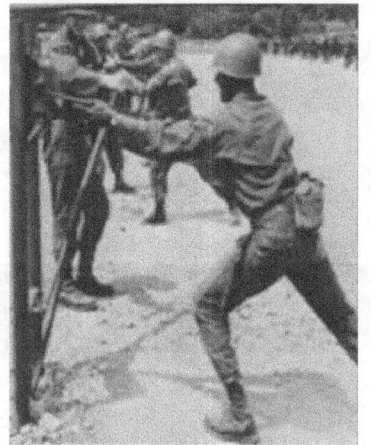

Source: Marshall Gagne Private Collection.

Figure 38. Combatives Training during Basic Training (Fort Knox, 1967).

Two key events for the Army occurred during 1975. First, on 17 February 1975 *Physical Fitness—Women's Army Corps* (FM 35-20) was revised and published for the fourth and final time. As a sign of greater acceptability of women in the Army, the field manual name was changed from *Physical Training—Women's Army Corps* (1965) to *Physical Fitness Training for Women.* Other changes signified a significant transformation in content and perspective. Changes in perspective were most evident by the significant number of photos that depicted women Soldiers engaging in team contact sports and combat-related physical training.[85] A second key event occurred on 7 October 1975 when President Gerald Ford signed Public Law 94-106 opening enrollment in the US Service Academies to women. This single event forever changed Army physical readiness training and assessment policies and practices.

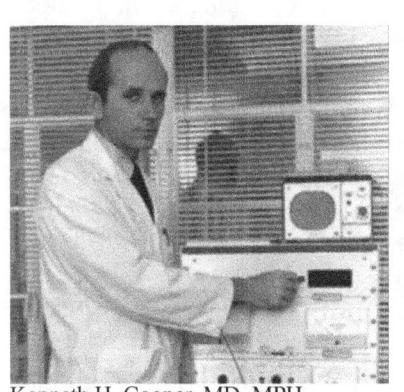
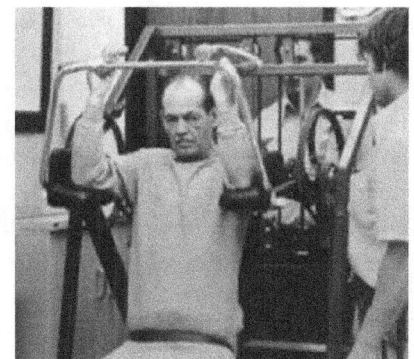

Kenneth H. Cooper, MD, MPH, Founder and Chairman of Cooper Aerobics at Cooper Clinic (c. 1970).

Arthur Jones, Founder of Nautilus, Inc taken during a Colorado Experiment, Fort Collins (1973).

Source: Photo Courtesy of Cooper Aerobics.

Source: Photo Courtesy of www.arthurjonesexercise.com.

Figure 39. Kenneth Cooper and Arthur Jones (c. 1975).

In FM 35-20 (1975) women were introduced to the "stages" of physical training: Beginning, Slow improvement, and Sustaining and the four components of physical fitness: strength, endurance, agility, and coordination. The training programs for women were much more demanding with the introduction of three strength circuits (1) barbells— squat "snatch" to a military press and curls plus body weight exercises; (2) circuit interval training; and (3) an isometric strength circuit. Chapter 6 was entirely devoted to running with specific instructions pertaining to sprinting, formation running, cross-country running, and jogging. The workload concepts of pace and progression were also described.

The most significant change in the 1975 revision came in Chapter 14—"Physical Fitness Testing." Four physical fitness tests were approved for women: (1) Advanced Physical Fitness Test for women (APFT-W)—

80m shuttle run, modified pushups (from the knees); run, dodge, and jump (same test as men); modified sit-ups (crunch), and 1-mile run; (2) Basic Physical Fitness Test for women: same four events as the APFT-W test with a .5-mile run; (3) Staff and Specialist PFT for women: same first four events as the APFT-W with a stationary run; and (4) Airborne Trainee Physical Fitness Qualification test for women: incline chin-up, modified push-up and sit-up, knee bender, and 1-mile run. The incline chin-up device utilized a metal frame with a "foot rest" and a movable chinning bar that could be adjusted according to height. From a seated position the Soldier places her feet on the "foot rest" and grasps the bar with an underhand grip (palms facing the soldier) and arms fully extended and the chinning bar just below shoulder height. Maintaining a straight body (approximately a 450 degree angle) the soldier flexes her arms and pulls up until her chest touches the bar. The score is equal to the maximum number of repetitions. None of the three body-weight tests (incline chin-ups, modified push-ups, or modified sit-ups) were timed. Women were required to score a minimum of 60 points per event for a total of 300 points. Passing scores for the five events in the APRT-W were: incline chin-up = 7; push-ups = 18; run/dodge/jump = 27.5 sec., sit-ups = 20; 80m shuttle run = 26.5 sec.; and 1MR = 9:14. In Change 1, 30 October 1975 a separate scoring form (DA 4415) was created for women.[86] FM 35-20 (1973) previewed many changes that would appear into the next revision of FM 21-20, where Army leaders integrated the men's (FM 21-20) and women's (FM 35-20) physical training doctrine into a single field manual.

Transition of Army PRT to Health-Related Fitness

During the post-Vietnam miasma Army leaders became increasingly concerned with the level of physical fitness and mental toughness of Soldiers as the Army transitioned to an all volunteer force. A critical nuance to this issue was the potentially significant increase in the number of women Soldiers. In July, 1975 the Deputy Chief of Staff—Personnel commissioned the Army Research Institute (ARI) and US Army Forces Command (FORSCOM) to develop the "Women Content in Units Force Development Test," better known as the MAX WAC test.[87] In October 1976 ARI/FORSCOM sampled 40 Army units at 19 posts in the continental US and Hawaii. Although the results indicated that unit content of up to 35% women had no adverse affect on mission performance, Major General Julius Becton, commander of US Army Operational Test and Evaluation Agency (OTEA) disputed those findings. After changing the basic research protocols, OTEA repeated the "women content" study and concluded that a maximum of 20% women per unit was the right percentage to prevent degradation of mission capabilities.[88]

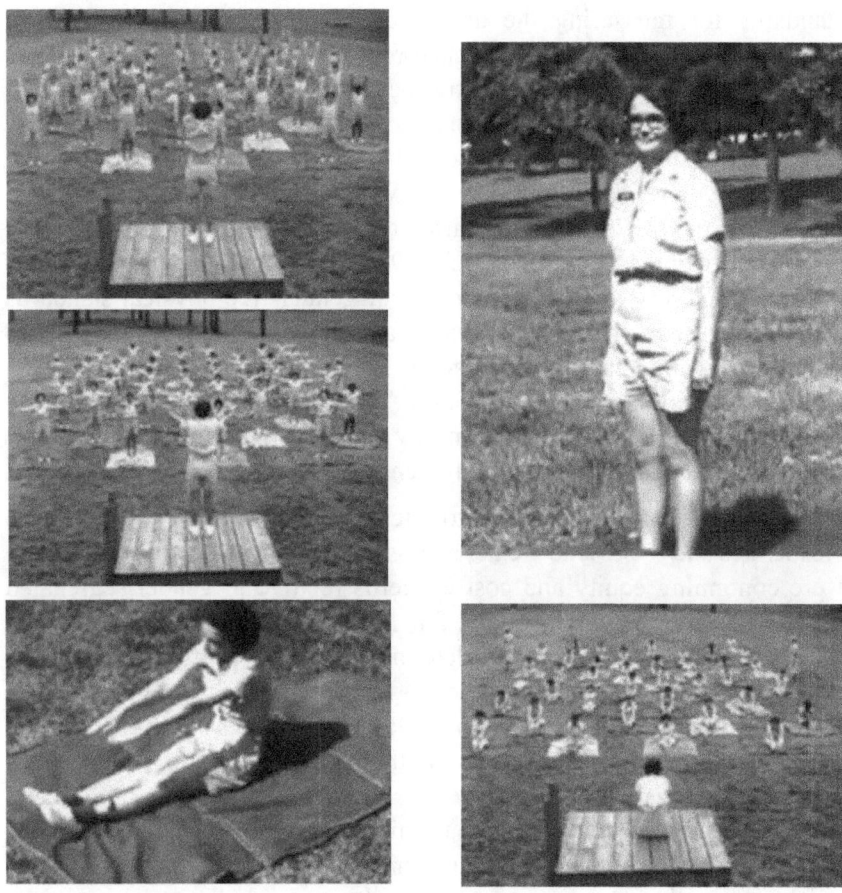

Figure 40. Women's Army Corp PRT (FM 35-20, 1975).

The gender and fitness issue was further exacerbated by the enrollment of women at the US Service Academies in the fall 1976. Increased numbers of women in the Enlisted and Officer Corps resulted in growing pressure for greater opportunities in a wider variety of military occupational specialties (MOS). One of the outstanding issues relative to job performance was the historical perception that women lacked the physical strength and stamina to successfully accomplish warrior tasks and battle drills. "Army commanders had long complained that women were unable to perform many routine physical tasks associated with their assigned specialties."[89] The dichotomy between physical readiness training and assessments required for men in FM 21-20 and PRT required for women in FM 35-20 continued to exacerbate the perception and the reality. In May 1976 the General Accounting Office (GAO) recommended that the Army "develop standards for measuring the ability of personnel to satisfy strength, stamina and operational performance requirements for specialties where such attributes are factors in effective performance."[90] This action resulted from the arbitrary closure of many military occupational specialties (MOS) to women that were presumed to be too physically demanding. With reports like Project 60 (1976), Women in the Army (1977), and Project Athena (1979), the Army tried to determine the range of physical abilities of women Soldiers. In July 1977, the Army Vice-Chief of Staff directed the Army to study the impact of gender-free physical standards that could be used for MOS selection and assignment. With the need to utilize increasing numbers of women in nontraditional MOSs as well as to respond to affirmative action policies, "it became apparent that the Army could qualify and assign new entrants by matching individual qualifications with specific MOS physical requirements regardless of gender."[91]

Based upon the requirement to integrate women into the US Service Academies and to provide greater access to a wider variety of MOSs, there were continuing equity and cost concerns relative to gender-segregated initial entry training (IET). In the fall 1976 the Army conducted a series of Basic Initial Entry Tests to determine the effects of basic physical fitness on integrated physical readiness training. The clinical trials were conducted to determine if women could undergo the same basic training as men regardless of lower levels of strength and cardiorespiratory work capacity. The trials were conducted at Fort Jackson, South Carolina and the results showed that "physical training could be modified for women without changing content or value or lowering male standards. Other results were that the women tested felt more challenged physically, were better prepared for service in units than those who had undergone Women's Army Corps basic training, and could use basic tactical skills and employ weapons necessary for individual and unit survival in a defensive battlefield environment."[92] As a result of these trials TRADOC instituted the Common Entry Level Training (CELT) program. The CELT (mixed-gender unit training) was scheduled to begin at Fort Jackson early in fiscal year 1978. Although men and women were initially segregated by platoons within the same company; Army leaders believed that the more rigorous training in mixed units would provide women better tactical and weapon skills necessary for individual and unit success in a "defensive battlefield environment." The final integration of men and women in initial entry training was completed by the end of fiscal year 1979.[93]

On 30 November 1976 the Army reengaged the growing weight control problem with the fourth revision the *Army Physical Fitness Program* (AR 600-9). The most significant aspects of this revision were the integration of

Weight Control (AR 600-7, 1965) and *Standards for Conduct and Fitness* (AR 632-1, 1972) into AR 600-9 and the introduction of the "Army Weight Control Program" (AWCP).[94] Command authority for implementing AR 600-9 was transferred from the Chief of Staff, Military Operations to the Chief of Staff, Personnel. Chapter 1 was created to establish the regulatory requirements for the Army Weight Control Program (AWCP). The terms "obesity" (excessive accumulation of adipose tissue) and "overweight" (when weight exceeds maximum allowable standards) were defined in section 1-2. Maximal allowable weight tables were removed from *Standards of Medical Fitness* (AR 40-501) and published in the Appendix (p. E3).[95] The physical fitness philosophy was defined in section 1-3a: "It is essential to the readiness and combat-effectiveness of the Army that every soldier be physically fit regardless of age or duty assignment."[96] "Closely related to physical fitness are weight control and military appearance. Corrective measures at all levels of command and staff will be taken, in accordance with this regulation, when officers and soldiers do not maintain acceptable weight and military appearance standards."[97] Indicative of a growing concern over potential harmful effects of exhaustive exercise on older personnel (> 40 years of age), section 1-3.b cautioned commanders to be aware of excessive physical exhaustion; "Pride and competitiveness...may drive individuals beyond their limit of endurance with serious consequences."[98] One example of a sign/symptom of over exhaustion was an exercise pulse rate > 140 beats per minute.[99] The testing section became more generalized (must test at some point during Basic Combat Training and Advanced Individual Training and regular Soldiers must test annually) and less prescriptive (the Army regulation no longer identified specific tests). The Army's weight control program was fully delineated in Chapter 3.[100]

The most significant addition to AR 600-9 (1976) was Chapter 3—"Weight Control." "Excess body fat is a serious detriment to health, longevity, stamina, and military appearance...Members who are overweight or obese must accept the personal responsibility for weight reduction and control..."[101] This chapter further outlined the overweight standard (see Appendix—Weight Tables for Army Personnel), the process of weight loss, the commander's responsibilities, the role of the medical officer, and disposition of chronically overweight personnel. For reference purposes the maximum allowed body weight was: males: 60"—144 lbs, 72"—203 lbs; females: 60"—121 lbs, 72"—175 lbs. Personal complicity to a failure to achieve satisfactory progress could result in discharge from service. The implementation of a "weight control program" would turn out to be prophetic for the Army and for once put them ahead of the physical readiness "curve."

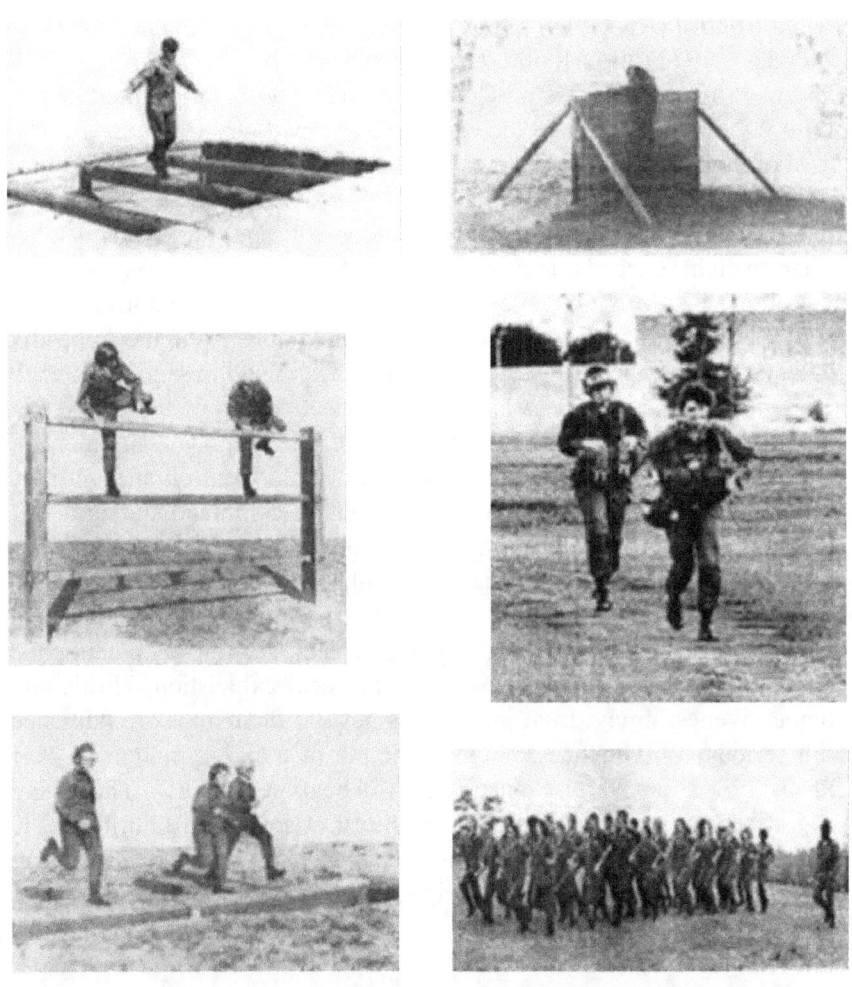

Figure 41. WAC Combat Readiness Training (FM 35-20, 1975).

In 1978 the American College of Sports Medicine (ACSM) established its position stand on exercise frequency, intensity, and duration. In Recommended Quantity and Quality of Exercise for Developing and Maintaining Fitness in Healthy Adults the ACSM outlined the optimal amount of exercise required to achieve and maintain physical fitness in the general population. Using changes in maximum oxygen consumption (VO2max), ACSM differentiate between the amount of exercise needed for general health and the amount needed to improvement your level of fitness. In their position statement, which was updated in 1990 and 1998, ACSM used military readiness as their criterion to established exercise minimums. The ACSM recommended "the frequency (3–5 times/wk), intensity (60–90% of maximum heart rate), duration (20–60 minutes of continuous aerobic activity depending on intensity), and mode (activity using large muscle groups that can be maintained continuously) of the exercise required for development and maintenance of a level of physical fitness similar to that required by all military troops for readiness."[102] In the 1978 version of the position stand, resistance exercise was an additional recommendation—conditioning of the major muscle groups at least 2 d/wk to ensure sufficient strength to perform normal activities of daily living, maintain fat-free mass (FFM), and control body weight.[103]

During the late 1970's Army leaders became more concerned over the rigor of physical readiness training. This issue was exacerbated by concerns over a gendered-integrated initial entry training (IET) program and significant increases in number of women Soldiers and came at the same time Army Chief of Staff General Edward Meyer was expanding initial entry training.[104] On April 28, 1978, the Army formally dissolved the position of Director, Woman's Army Corps and in September 1978 Congress passed a law "that disestablished the WAC as a separate Corps of the Army effective Oct. 20, 1978."[105] Following the work of agencies like the American College of Sports Medicine and the National Strength and Conditioning Association (NSCA) and based upon the Resolutions 8 & 9 of the 1970 Physical Fitness Symposium report, General Donn Starry, Commander-TRADOC, launched a bold initiative to centralize the research and educational components of physical readiness training and thereby standardize PRT doctrine.[106] Four issues drove this effort: (1) a perceived lack of rigor of initial entry training (IET), (2) the complexities of the MOS-related physical fitness tests, (3) the significant increase in the accession of women into the Army, and (4) the lack of currency in the Army physical fitness testing program. "The Army's desire to utilize greater numbers of women in physically demanding, non-traditional occupations has created the need to match individual capacities with occupational demands. Research has been conducted to develop a process by which objectively determined physical demands of MOSs can be converted into gender-free physical fitness standards."[107] The upcoming revision of the Advanced Physical Fitness Test gave Army leaders an opportunity to resolve many of the outstanding issues concerning testing rigor and gender integration by refocusing the Army physical readiness training and assessment.

To jump start this revolutionary change a group of civilian and military physical fitness experts meet at Airlie House, VA in late 1979 to discuss the revision of the Army physical fitness test. In January 1980,

General Starry met with General Meyer to "review the situation." "They agreed that the MOS-related system was too complex and was at the root of the lower standards."[108] In early February General Starry directed the "APRT Study Group" (lead by the USAIS, Fort Benning) to update the Army's PRT doctrine by revising and combining the doctrine currently published in FM 21-20 and FM 35-20 and in doing so developing a new physical readiness test. The new Army Physical Readiness Test had to be gender integrated, easy to administer, and require little or no equipment. The "study group" consisted of representatives from the Army, the Marine Corps, and leading civilian physical educators.[109] Colonel James Anderson (West Point), Colonel Fred Drews (Carlisle Barracks), and Lieutenant Colonel Robert Tetu (from DCSOPS) represented various interests from the Army. The APRT Study Group was tasked to establish a physical fitness test that measured baseline fitness for all Army personnel and could be administered anywhere with no equipment. In late February 1980 the APRT Study Group briefed General Starry on the proposed changes to FM 21-20, the development of a new Army regulation—*The Army Physical Fitness Program* (AR 350-15) and the new Army Physical Readiness Test (APRT).[110]

On 31 October 1980 *Physical Readiness Training* (FM 21-20) was revised and published for the eighth time. This revision represented the philosophical transformation from a Vietnam-era combat readiness focus to a Cold War era nuclear-threat focus. From the Bay of Pigs invasion to the MAD (mutual assured destruction) nuclear deterrence policy, the prevailing attitude among many civil and military leaders was that conventional ground warfare was obsolete. Exacerbated by the problems with an all-volunteer force comprised of an ever-increasing number of women, it seemed prudent to change the Army PRT focus from ground combat readiness to physical fitness and health. This paradigm shift was reinforced by secular advances in fitness development during the 1970 and 1980's with the emergence of Dr. Kenneth Cooper's aerobic movement and Arthur Jones' Nautilus movement. "The most significant impact on Service physical fitness programs in the last 30 years is the body of research dealing with cardio-respiratory endurance or "aerobics." This research, begun by Dr. Kenneth Cooper of the Air Force, has become a primary focus for many unit programs...."[111] This philosophical change was most evident in the transformation of the Army Physical Readiness Test (APRT). The combat-related test items from the 1973 Advanced Physical Fitness Test (inverted crawl, horizontal ladder, and the dodge, run, and jump) were replaced with the push-up. The new three-event APRT purported to measure three areas of soldier fitness: aerobic capacity—

two-mile run, upper body endurance—push-up, and trunk/abdominal endurance—bent knee sit-up.[112] The revised test was gender integrated, required no equipment, was easy to administer, provided normative standards adjusted for physiological differences between men and women, and purported to more accurately measure physical fitness. Soldiers were required to complete the test items in order (push-ups, sit-ups, 2-mile run) in a maximum of two hours, with a min/max rest time of 10/20 minutes provided between each event.[113]

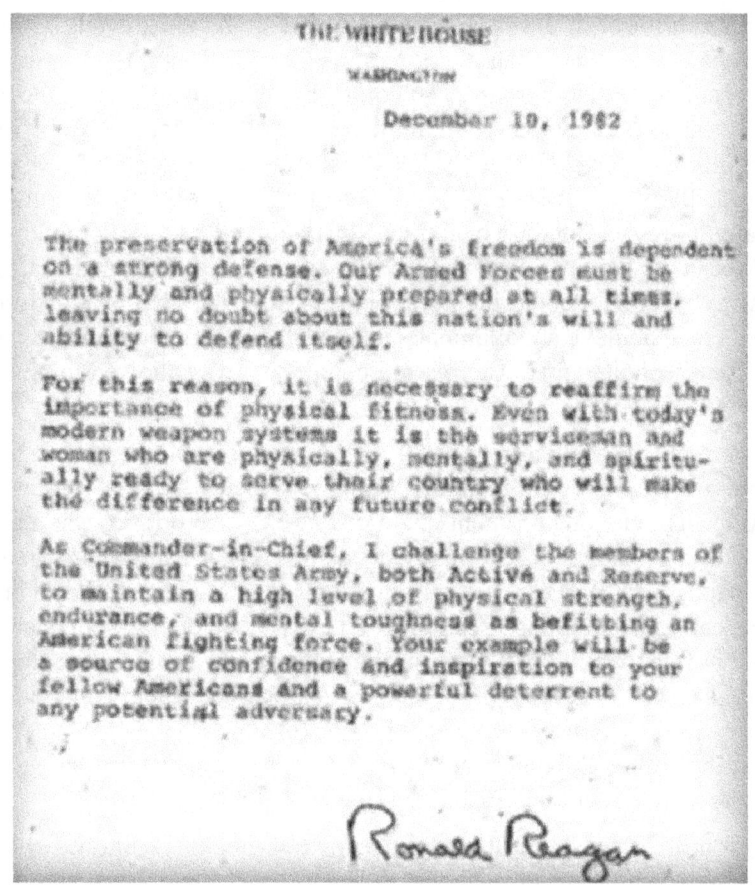

Figure 42. Message from Ronald Reagan—PAM 350-18 (1983).

Once normative data had been collected, the proposed Army Physical Readiness Test (APRT) standards were forwarded to the Cooper Institute for Aerobic Research and Army Research Institute for review. Dr. Cooper applied points to his adjectival ratings for aerobic capacity, e.g., Superior = 100 points, Good = 60 points, and Fair = 50 points. He further stated that 5% of the Army should be able to score 300 points on the APFT ("max" the PT test) and 90% should pass. Lastly he concluded if the Army was presented with healthy recruits, through frequent, progressive and challenging training, the Army could develop Soldiers to meet and surpass the basic minimums.

All soldiers were required to take a record APRT two times a year with a minimum of four months between administrations. The scoring standards were established for men and women in 7-year age groups. The APRT score was determined by converting raw scores to a 100-point scale score for each event. The maximum score on each event a Soldier could earn was 100 points for a total score of 300 points. All Soldiers had to attain at least 60 points (50 points during IET) on each of the three test events to pass the APRT. Minimum scores (60-point score) for 17-25 year old men were PU = 40, SU = 40, 2MR = 17:55; for 17-25 year old women: PU = 16, SU = 27, 2MR = 22:14.[114] This test was administered in fatigue trousers, t-shirt or fatigue shirt and combat boots (commonly referred to as "utes and boots"). Initial assessments indicated that 85% of Army personnel could pass the 3-event APRT and that 5% of soldiers tested could achieve a maximum score, indicating that the standards were sufficiently challenging. The reserve component was allowed to phase in the new APFT over a 2-year period.[115]

In terms of "content" the 1980 field manual symbolized the transient nature of Army physical readiness training in the early 80's. There was a significant reduction in content specificity as FM 21-20 (1973) was reduced from the 31 chapters (350 pages) to eight chapters and approximately 250 pages (1980). There were significant elaborations provided in the "physical considerations" section to address the growing understanding of the physical abilities of women. Women's issues such as bone density, environmental concerns (heat), menstruation, pregnancy and athletic injuries were also discussed (section 1-5). In summary, FM 21-20 (1980) stated that although women are different, "this doesn't mean that women are incapable of achieving satisfactory levels of performance."[116]

From the initial coordination meetings of the APRT Study Group in 1979 and continuing throughout much of 1982, there were significant discussions throughout the Army concerning the training and assessment of soldiers over 40 years of age.[117] General Starry supported the concerns of the TRADOC surgeon concerning the medical safety of Soldiers over 40 taking the 3-event APRT. However, General Meyer (Army Chief of Staff) insisted that all enlisted and officer personnel over the age of 40 would take the 3-event APRT. "The physiological deterioration which accompanies age can be slowed but not halted. There is no reason why persons over 40 should not maintain a degree of fitness commensurate with their age."[118] Four areas were identified that could slow the "deterioration" of aging: heredity, good health habits, exercise, and mental outlook. The level of confusion over this issue was evidenced by the special note in the Preface of FM 21-20, which warned commanders that Soldiers over 40 were not authorized to take the push-up and sit-up events.[119] As counterintuitive as it may seem today from a medical risk perspective, Soldiers over 40 were only authorized to take the 2-mile run test. The ultimate compromise was a phase-in period where medical personnel would review the medical files of personnel over 40 prior to testing. Even with this concern resolved there were no scoring standards for Soldiers 40 years and older in the new FM 21-20 (1980).[120]

The 1980's evolved as arguably the most prolific decade for the development and dissemination of physical readiness doctrine in the history of the US Army. Motivated by Cold War pressures, the recent Soviet invasion of Afghanistan, gender integration issues, manpower issues, and public perceptions of Soldier fitness and physical appearance, President Carter initiated a series of reviews designed to enhance the combat readiness of the Armed Services. With the majority of FM 21-20 (1980) completed by the USAIC study group, on 2 February 1980, President Carter directed the Department to Defense to review all military physical fitness programs.[121] On 17-19 June, 1980 the Secretary of Defense assembled a group of military and civilian "physical fitness experts" at Airlie House to review existing physical fitness policies and practices for the purpose of making short- and long-term recommendations.[122] "Primary attention was given to the medical aspects of fitness, physical fitness programs and testing (especially for personnel over 40 years of age), advisability of establishing an Academy or Institute for Military Physical Fitness, weight control program(s), and nutritional aspects of physical fitness."[123] The two most significant outcomes of the two-day conference were a reaffirmation of physical fitness as a vital component of mission readiness and suggestions for improvements in "screening, research, leadership, and state-of-the-art service-wide programs in fitness as well as positive lifestyles."[124] The second symposium outcome prompted the formation of a Physical Training Study Group chaired by Colonel Travis Dyer. By December, 1980 the Deputy Chief of Staff for Personnel (DCSPER) was already considering new "measures to strengthen and equalize penalties for officers and enlisted personnel who were overweight or out of shape."[125]

One of the significant policy outcomes of the Department of Defense (DoD) *Study of The Military Services Physical Fitness* (which was not published until 1 April 1981) was the issuance of DoD Directive 1308.1, son 29 June 1981.[126] DD 1308.1 directed all services to implement a planned physical fitness program, which included a body weight/composition assessment and management program. "Physical fitness is a vital component of combat readiness and is essential to the general health and well-being of armed forces personnel.[127] The primary objectives of 1308 were:

1. Physical fitness training and activities should be designed to develop skills needed in combat, enhance cohesion in units, promote competitive spirit, develop positive attitudes toward exercise, and promote self-confidence and self-discipline.

2. Physical fitness programs must be carefully planned and supervised, follow the established principals of physical fitness training, and involve the participation of all personnel.

3. Physical fitness programs should improve efficiency in the cardiorespiratory system and/or muscular strength and endurance when conducted with the appropriate amount of regularity, intensity, and duration.

4. Provide a uniform system and standards for weight control and obesity; overweight status to be determined by the percentage of body fatness.

5. The DoD weight control program will enhance the attainment and retention of good health, physical fitness, and a trim military appearance.[128]

After taking office on 20 January 1981 President Ronald Reagan continued ongoing efforts to enhance and modernize the Army's physical readiness training program. On 21 December 1981 Lieutenant General Julius Becton, Deputy Commander for Training—TRADOC, convened a meeting to discuss the way ahead for Army physical readiness training. "Representatives attended from the Deputy Chief of Staff for Operations, The Surgeon General, Fort Benning, the Army War College, West Point, and the Soldier Support Center."[129] After significant discussion among these agencies consensus was achieved concerning the development of a stand-alone organization that would assume responsibility for physical fitness training doctrine. As a result of this meeting the Soldier Support Center at Fort Harrison was given proponency for physical fitness doctrine, the Army War College was tasked to develop a fitness research institute, and the Infantry Center at Fort Benning was tasked to refine the physical fitness test. On 7 January 1982 a coordinating meeting was held at Fort Harrison and the Physical Fitness Task Force was established; the task force would soon evolve into the Soldier Physical Fitness Center.[130]

In an attempt to revitalize the Army's image following the Vietnam Conflict, Secretary of the Army, John O. Marsh, proposed the development of an annual Army "theme" to emphasize some positive aspect of the Army. Secretary Marsh designated 1982 as the Army's Year of Fitness.[131] As part of the Army's transition to a "schools" training model for solving major Army problems and in conjunction with the "Year of Fitness," on 3 May 1982 Secretary Marsh formally created the US Army Soldier Physical Fitness Center (USASPFC) at Fort Benjamin Harrison. The operational element of the USASPFC was the US Army Soldier Physical Fitness School:[132]

> The readiness of the United States Army begins with the physical fitness of the Individual Soldier and the noncommissioned officers and the officers who lead them. We are heirs of high standards that our predecessors established and sustained in peace and war. We will not forget this proud heritage. That is our charge today.[133]

In an attempt to assuage the concerns of the US Army Infantry Center over the transition of proponency for PRT doctrine to Fort Benjamin Harrison, on 8 April 1982 Lieutenant General Julius Becton brokered a memorandum of understanding between Major General Daniel French, Commander—USA Soldier Support Center and the Major General R.L. Wetzel, Commander—United States Army Infantry School. While the USAIS would "assist" with program development, standards, and assessments, the USASPFC would "act as the focal point for the Army Physical Fitness System."[134]

The US Army Soldier Physical Fitness Center (USASPFC) began operations in mid 1982 with three officers, one non-commissioned officer, and two civilians and a budget of $87,000.[135] As a subordinate organization to the Soldier Support Center, the USASPFC was task-organized into three divisions: (1) Training and Doctrine—training analysis, design, and development, (2) Physical Fitness Academy—institutional instruction for physical fitness training, and (3) Sports Division—prepare and implement military competitive activities. These divisions were similar in scope and function to the operational units recommended by the Military Services Physical Fitness study group.[136] For the first time the Army was prepared to properly resource Soldier physical readiness training, research, and education. The "Army Physical Fitness System" was to be composed of five elements: physical conditioning and testing, education, research, nutrition and diet, and weight control.

On 15 July 1982, in a preemptive move to separate the Army's physical fitness doctrine from the weight control doctrine, Headquarters, DA published *The Army Physical Fitness Program* (AR 350-15). AR 350-15 set forth the policies and responsibilities for implementing the Army's physical fitness program and superseded AR 600-9—Chapter 2—"Army Physical Program" (1976), effectively decoupling physical training regulations and body weight/composition regulations.[137] The Deputy Chief of Staff for Operations (DSCOPS) was given responsibility for the Army Physical Fitness Program. The objective of AR 350-15 was to develop and sustain five physical qualities in all soldiers: (1) stamina; (2) quick reactions, flexibility, coordination, and speed; (3) fighting spirit—will to win; (4) self discipline; and (5) a health-enhancing lifestyle. Some interesting components to the program were the requirements to develop (1) an Army-wide database on physical fitness performance, (2) a medical excusal policy for soldiers on profiles (AR 40-501), (3) a heart disease screening for soldiers over 40, and (4) the requirement for the USMA Superintendent to provide technical advice/expertise to DA on physical training.[138] Section II: Implementing the Program outlined training requirements, special fitness programs, and testing requirements and standards. AR 350-15 was relative prescriptive for Initial Entry Training, identifying seven physical skills and describing the program of instruction (POI) as "carefully structured, progressive and challenging."[139]

Active Army members up to the age of 60 were required to take the Army Physical Readiness Test (APRT) twice per year with at least four months between tests. DA Form 705 was the designated "physical fitness scorecard" for the APRT. APRT failures were flagged and entered into a remedial physical training program. Repeated failures "(that is, three consecutive record tests each a minimum of 4 months apart)" were subject to separation from the Service under the provisions of 635-100 (Officers) and 635-200 (Enlisted). Personnel attending military schools were required to pass an APRT in order to attain a certificate of graduation. In an attempt to encourage Soldiers to continually improve their physical fitness, Commanders were encouraged to recognize and reward Soldiers who scored between 275 and 300 on the APFT.[140]

To sustain the momentum initiated by the June 1980 DoD study of Military Services Physical Fitness and the December 1981 TRADOC fitness coordination meeting, the fledgling USASPFC hosted a Physical

Fitness Training Seminar on 19-23 July in Indianapolis, IN. Representatives from throughout the Army (Surgeon General, USA Reserve, Infantry School, USMA, Army War College, etc.) were in attendance. Topics such as running shoes, fitness programs, nutritional drinks, and the Aerobic Institute program were discussed. There was also discussion on the new Army regulation, *The Army Physical Fitness Program* (AR 350-15), which was published on 15 April 1982 and the pending changes to The Army Weight Control Program (AR 600-9).

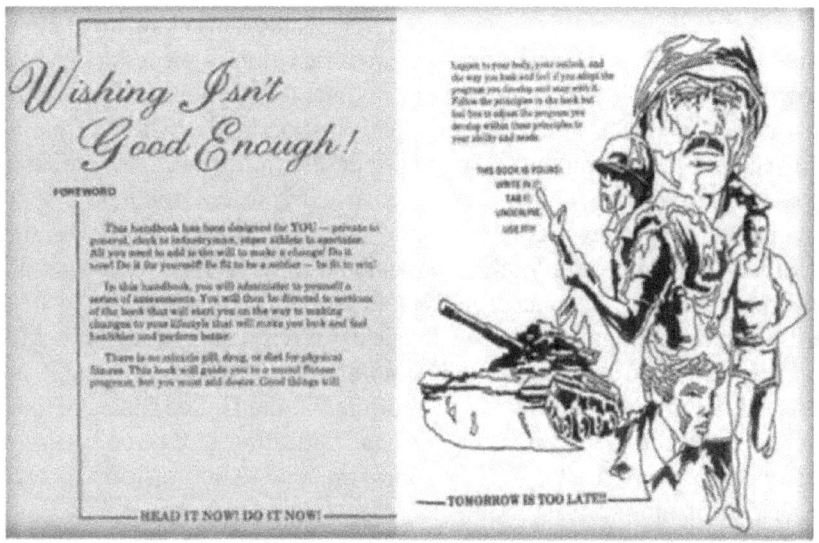

Figure 43. Introduction to DA PAM 350-18 (1983).

As part of the Army Year of Fitness General Glenn K. Otis, Commander, TRADOC took a more active role in fitness development. In September 1982 General Otis sent a communiqué to all commanders outlining his position on Soldier fitness. The message provided guidance on four issues: (1) units will teach Soldiers about physical fitness as well as conduct physical readiness training, (2) all Soldiers enrolled in initial entry training and Army courses greater than 56 days will pass an APRT prior to graduation, (3) running shoes will be permitted for training and testing, and (4) the Soldier Physical Fitness School will prepare a fitness instructional package to be used to educate Soldiers.[141] At the same time a General Officer Steering Committee (GOSC) reported that the Army was losing too many senior leaders to premature medical retirements and sudden cardiac death because "they were physically unprepared for the physical and mental demands of strategic leadership."[142] To resolve these concerns, later in 1982 General Otis established the Army Physical Fitness Research Institute (APFRI) at the Army War College. APFRI's mission was to provide research on and education for senior leaders attending the US Army War College to ensure that strategic leaders would set the conditions for improving force readiness through improved physical fitness.[143]

Following the recommendation of the DoD Military Services Physical Fitness study group (1981), in early 1983 the USASPFC created a program of instruction designed to develop subject matter experts in physical training.[144] The Master Fitness Trainer (MFT) course (with the associated "6P" Army Skill Identifier) was a comprehensive, 4-week resident course taught at Fort Benjamin Harrison by qualified fitness professionals. The program of instruction involved approximately 80 hours of classroom instruction and 80 hours of practical instruction.[145] The curriculum consisted of lessons on the skeletal system, the cardiovascular/respiratory systems, muscle physiology, exercise in extreme environments, sports medicine/injury prevention, strength and cardio-respiratory training, flexibility, and nutrition/body composition. The MFT course was also incorporated into Advanced Individual Training (AIT) for the "03C" military occupational specialty (Physical Activity Specialist). The MFT course was later offered via mobile training teams (MTTs) at CONUS and OCONUS installations and was also offered at the United States Military Academy by the Department of Physical Education in a three course 60 lesson format. From 1985—2002 approximately 10,000 officers received MFT certification at West Point.[146]

On 15 April, 1983 AR 600-9 *The Army Weight Control Program* was revised and published for the fifth time to accomplish two goals: (1) to complete the alignment with AR 350-15, which was published on 15 July, 1982, and (2) to fully comply with DoD Directive 1308.1, which was published two years earlier. Since AR 350-15 assumed regulatory control of the Army physical fitness program, in the 1983 AR 600-9 revision, Chapter 2 was deleted and AR 600-9 became the sole source document for the Army Weight Control Program (AWCP). The Deputy Chief of Staff—Personnel (DCSPER) was given responsibility for the Army Weight Control Program (AWCP).

In an attempt to differentiate between fat and fat-free mass, the new AWCP required that body composition (measured as a percentage of fat mass) be "determined for all personnel-(1) "whose body weight exceeds the screening table weight in appendix A, or (2) when the unit commander or supervisor determines that the individual's appearance suggests that body fat is excessive."[147] There was no mention of how body composition was to be assessed. AR 600-9 stated that "percent body fat measurements will be accomplished by health care personnel (health care personnel are defined in the glossary)."[148] Although the DoD-wide body composition goals were 20% for males and 26% for females, the maximum allowable body fat level ranged from 20-26% for males and from 28-34% for females depending upon age. Extensive guidance was provided to commanders and supervisors relative to proper exercise, nutrition, and weight loss while personnel were enrolled in the AWCP. Failure to make adequate progress was grounds for a bar against reenlistment or discharge from the Army.[149]

On 25 October 1983 the United States launched (Operation Urgent Fury), ostensibly to protect American interests in the Caribbean and rescue American students attending medical school in Grenada. Joint US forces composed of Marines, Army Rangers, and Navy Seals lead the initial assault.[150] Due to the training and combat support by the Cuban Army, resistance was greater than expected. After the initial assault soldiers from the 82nd Airborne participate in "mop-up" exercises. US forces suffered 135 casualties: 19 KIA and 116 wounded.[151] Although the mission was successful with relatively few casualties, there were significant after action discussions relative to the effects of combat loads and heat on physical performance. One of the most glaring problems of the Grenada invasion was the failure by many commanders to maintain load discipline, which lead to ineffective combat Soldiers. "We were like slow-moving turtles. My rucksack weighed 120 pounds. I would get up and rush for 10-15 seconds...and collapse. After a few rushes, I was physically unable to more."[152] Although the Grenada assault force was relatively small and composed primarily of elite troops, the experience served to reinforce the principle of "train as you fight" and the contribution of physical readiness to combat effectiveness.

1982 to 1990 was a period of dynamic growth and productivity for the USASPFC. On 15 October 1982 the Center developed and published the *Commanders Handbook on Physical Fitness* (DA PAM 350-15). Although the pamphlet focused on program design to enhance unit fitness, a comprehensive individual aerobic program chart was presented in Appendix D.[153] During 1983, the Soldier Physical Fitness Center's name morphed into the Soldier Physical Fitness School (SPFS) in order to more accurately reflect its assigned mission of educating the Army in all aspects of physical fitness. On 1 May, 1983 the School developed and published the *Individual's Handbook on Physical Fitness* (DA PAM 350-18). As proscribed in the forward: "this handbook was developed for you...read it now, do it now, tomorrow is too late."[154] In November, 1984 the School developed and published *Family Fitness Handbook* (DA PAM 350-21). PAM 350-21 stressed the importance of the broader Army family and how personal fitness could enhance overall Soldier effectiveness. The USASPFS also developed, revised, and published other Army manuals and materials to support Army PRT and motivate soldiers to maintain their personal fitness: October 1983: *Nautilus Training Principles;* 4 November 1983: *You and the Army Physical Readiness Test* (APRT) (TC 21-450); 28 August 1985: *Physical Fitness Training* (FM 21-20); 30 December 1985: *Army Physical Fitness Program* (AR 350-15); September 1987: *Army Health Promotion Program—Nutrition & Weight Control;* 3 November 1989: *Army Physical Fitness Program* (AR 350-15).

Following long-standing concerns about combat loads (supported by anecdotal reports from Grenada), USASPFS continued their aggressive research program as School personnel (Dr. Michael Bahrke and Lieutenant Colonel John O'Conner, PhD) paired with USARIEM to study "soldier performance and mood states following strenuous road march."[155] The Soldier Physical Fitness School and USARIEM were tasked to provide new load-bearing guidelines in the next revision of Physical Fitness Training (FM 21-20). The SPFS advocated "a minimum of four physical training sessions per week for light infantrymen. These include two sessions of muscular strength/endurance development, a cardio-respiratory workout, and a road march/load-bearing session, which makes increased demands for distance, load, speed, and terrain difficulty."[156]

During the summer of 1983, General William R. Richardson, Commander, TRADOC tasked the SPFS to study/update APFT standards. From October 1983–February 1984, Soldiers were tested at Fort Knox, Fort Jackson, Fort Ben Harrison, and Schofield Barracks. Data for over 4,000 Soldiers were collected and utilized to formulate new testing standards by age and gender. Although the new APRT standards were never implemented other recommendations from this study found their way into PRT policy and doctrine including: 5-year age increments for APFT standards, standards for a fitness badge, and an extended APFT scoring scale.[157] During the standards review in the spring and summer of 1984 the SPFS also reviewed the three items in the current APRT (push-ups, sit-ups, and 2-mile run). After collecting data at Fort Ben Harrison, Fort Sam Houston, and Fort Gordon, the SPFS recommended adding a fourth event to the APFT—pull-ups/flexed arm hang. They further recommended that TRADOC staff this proposal to the MACOMS, OCAR, NGB & DA, send a warning order to the field, and set an implementation data of July 1985, to coincide with the publication of the revised FM 21-20.[158]

By 1985 the SPFS's "table of organization and equipment" included 32 officers, 28 enlisted, and 38 civilian personnel with an annual budget of 5.9 million dollars. SPFS personnel revised and published the ninth revision of *Physical Fitness Training* (FM 21-20) on 28 August 1985. Based upon the proliferation of physical fitness research published between 1980 and 1985, one would have expected significant changes in the 1985 revision of FM 21-20. There were several new chapters – aerobics and running, muscle strength and endurance, and nutrition and fitness, and injuries and information on calculating a target heart rate and the physiological differences between men/women (see Appendix A and B), however there were no significant doctrinal changes in the 1985 revision.[159]

In keeping with the paradigm shift from combat readiness to general physical fitness there were two changes to the Army's fitness test. First, the name "Army Physical Readiness Test" was changed to the "Army Physical Fitness Test" (APFT).[160] Second, Soldiers were approved to "wear attire that is appropriate for physical training (shorts, t-shirts, socks, running shoes)" when training for and taking the APFT.[161] During the revision process, however, the SPFS was unable to convince Army leaders to adopt new minimum performance standards. The only APFT standards presented in the 1985 revision were in Figure 11-1, which depicted a copy of the October 1980 APRT "card" (DA 705).[162] Clearly the absence of new standards had to be resolved quickly, since completing the two-mile run in "running shoes" produced significantly faster times than running in combat boots.

To address another recommendation of the DoD Study of Military Services Physical Fitness, FM 21-20 (1985) provided an extensive discussion of "Soldiers with Profiles." Profiles were classified as temporary or permanent. Soldiers on temporary profiles were scheduled for a 3-event APFT following the termination of their profile; Soldiers were allowed two times the length of the profile not to exceed 90 days to rehabilitate their illness or injury and train for the test. Soldiers with permanent profiles (i.e., were permanently prohibited from performing the 2-mile run) were offered three alternate aerobic events: 800-yard swim, 6.2-mile stationary/conventional (1-speed) bicycle test, or the 3-mile walk. Minimum pass times for each alternate event were published in Figure 11-6 (page 11-10). For an APFT to be considered a valid, record test it had to contain an aerobic event.

On 30 December 1985 *The Army Physical Fitness Program* (AR 350-15) was revised and published for the second time. The Deputy Chief of Staff—Operations (DCSOPS) retained responsibility for the Army Physical Fitness Program and commanders were reminded to "make every effort to design and tailor programs according to what their soldiers may be expected to do in combat."[163] There was a significant increase in specificity as the outcome objectives were increased from five to eight. The term "stamina" was defined as cardiorespiratory endurance, muscular strength and endurance, and anaerobic conditioning. Flexibility, completive spirit, self-discipline, adherence to body compositions standards, and a healthy lifestyle were the other five objectives. Through the SPFS, TRADOC was tasked to develop and field the Army's physical fitness doctrine, training, education programs, and performance standards. Two additional skills were added to the initial entry training POI; forced marching with loads (to include cross-country movement) and strength development (such as rope climbing, pull-ups, and resistance exercises).[164] By 1985 Army leaders were already observing a transition in PRT from a focus on combat readiness to performing well on the 3-event APFT. Commanders were reminded that while physical fitness testing gives Soldiers an incentive to stay in good shape, commanders should use these results only as general indicators of their unit's fitness. "Physical fitness testing will not form the foundation of unit or individual fitness programs…Fitness testing is designed to ensure the maintenance of a base level of physical fitness essential for every soldier in the Army…."[165]

At the same time Commanders were admonished not to allow the APFT to form the core of their PRT programs, the APFT continued to be a graduation requirement for most advanced military schools and a continuation of service. If personnel failed to achieve the minimum APFT standards prior to graduation, the failure was noted in their final academic report and they were designated as non-graduates and returned to their units or to their next assignment.[166] Repetitive APFT failures were subject to a bar from re-enlistment or separation from the Army. "A repetitive failure occurs when a record test is taken and failed, the soldier provided adequate time and assistance to improve his performance, and fails the test again. It should take no longer than 8 weeks of conditioning for a soldier to achieve minimum passing standards on the APRT." Commanders were encouraged to incentivize APFT performance by recognizing Soldiers who score over 270 on the APFT for outstanding performance.

From 1983 to 1984 the SPFS had attempted to answer Army-wide concerns related to APFT scoring standards. There were three major concerns: (1) the scientific authenticity of the criterion-referenced standards that were used to convert raw scores to 100-point scale scores, (2) testing protocols and standards for Soldiers over 40 years of age, and (3) the effects of uniform changes on athletic performance. These concerns were not resolved in time for the 3 August 1985 publication of FM 21-20; therefore Headquarters DA published Change No. 1 to FM 21-20 on 23 June 1986.[167] In Change 1 (1986) age group intervals were reduced from nine to five years, per the recommendation from the SPFS in 1984. By choosing a 5-year age interval, a 37-41 year old interval was established, effectively breaking the sacred 40 year old barrier. Minimum passing scores (60 points) for 17-21 year old men and women change significantly for all three events, especially sit-ups for females and 2MR times for males and females.[168] Minimum 1986 performance scores were (1985 standards): Male: PU = 42 (40), SU = 52 (40), 2MR = 15:54 (17:55); Female: PU = 18 (16), SU = 50 (27), 2MR = 18:54 (22:14).

On 26 September 1986 Headquarters, DA published a consolidated regulatory document entitled *Training in Units* (AR 350-41). As stated in the Summary of Changes, AR 350-41 was designed to provide an overview of Army training goals and philosophy, outline commanders responsibilities, outline training policy and minimum readiness requirements, highlight the training management process, standardize training requirements, and proscribe the "Common Military Training Program." Perhaps since AR 350-15 was already widely used throughout the Army, little attention was given to physical readiness training. Two paragraphs: "physical training" and "training for combat" were presented in Chapter 3: "Forces (Unit) Training"—Section 6: "Physical Fitness." The key element in AR 350-41 for Army PRT was the prescription for "innovative, demanding fitness programs oriented to the physical challenges of combat are essential to any unit physical training strategy."[169] The physical readiness/fitness training issues for the Army were becoming obscured in manuals and regulations. By the end of 1986 to fully understand every aspect of physical readiness training and weight control commanders had to have a working knowledge of DoD Directive 1308.1 (1981), AR 350-1 (1983), AR 350-15 (1985), FM 21-20 (1985), FM 21-20, Change 1 (1986), AR 600-9 (1986), and AR 350-41 (1986).

With the dramatic changes in minimum APFT standards (Change 1, 1986), it was not surprising that Army leaders soon became concerned with Soldier retention. Since the 100-point raw scores also increased significantly, there were also "motivational" concerns relative to a Soldier's ability to earn the Army Physical Fitness Badge (APFB), which was established as an incentive for exceptional performance, or to "max" the APFT (achieve a total score of 300). On several occasions during 1987 Lieutenant General Norman Schwarzkopf (DCSOPS) expressed concerns that Army height/weight and APFT standards were too stringent.[170] "In 1988 the US Army Physical Fitness School (USAPFS) was again tasked to review the current status of physical fitness in active Army personnel (the 1988 Active Army Physical Fitness Survey). Staff members from USAPFS and other Army agencies visited 14 military installations across the United States and administered the Army Physical Fitness Test (APFT) to over 6000 soldiers."[171] The study validated Schwarzkopf's concerns that less than 5% of the Army was achieving a maximum score on the APFT and less than 10% was earning the APFB.[172] Although women were found to perform significantly better than in 1984, data analysis showed higher failure rates among the youngest age groups in both genders. The most frequently failed event for the younger Soldiers was the 2-mile run and older Soldiers were passing at a higher rate. USAPFS recommended new standards that were more age and gender equitable and proposed some recommended changes to the scoring standards. The Office of the Surgeon General non-concurred with the recommendation on the basis that: "morale impact on women, request for "criterion based" standards, increased risk for the 50+ year groups, psychological trauma on those who minimally pass, and a perception that the APFT will be used to downsize."[173] The proposed, more equitable (for some more rigorous) standards were never approved.

The 3-event Army Physical Fitness Test (APFT) quickly became the raison d'être for many Army commanders to the exclusion of battle-focused PRT. Incentives such as the Army Physical Fitness Badge and use of APFT scores on Officer Evaluation Reports (OERs) and Non-commissioned Officer Evaluation Reports (NCOERs) fueled an obsessive focus on the APFT. By the late 1980's Army leaders began to recognize the folly of this pursuit. In 1987 Major Mark Hertling published a thesis at the US Army Command and General Staff College entitled *Physical Training for the Modern Battlefield: Are We Tough Enough.* In Chapter 5 he provided a detailed analysis of US Army fitness levels, in particular addressing the flight from combat-related PRT and assessment to a more "corporate fitness" model.[174] Hertling was particularly critical of the focus of the Master Fitness Trainer curriculum, which he thought spent too much time addressing "unit weaknesses on PT testing and overweight or "special population" Soldiers rather than the development of combat-specific training programs."[175] Hertling concluded his analysis by posing three recommendations: (1) the Army must deemphasize the current three-event PT test as a measure of physical readiness; (2) researchers must provide field commanders PRT programs that will prepare Soldiers for contingency missions; and (3) the Master Fitness Trainer Course should be expanded from four to five weeks to increase the emphasis on physical "readiness" versus physical "fitness."[176]

On 10 June 1987 Headquarters DA published an extensive sixth revision of *The Army Weight Control Program* (AR 600-9). Incorporated into this revision was a detailed explication of the AWCP duties for Master Fitness Trainers (MFT). MFTs were tasked to prescribe proper exercises to assist

Soldiers assigned to AWCP in determining, achieving and maintaining an appropriate personal weight and assist commanders in developing proactive physical fitness programs.[177] There was also a significant change in who assessed body composition; in AR 600-9 (1983) percent body fat was measured by a health care professional (trained physician, nurse, dietician, etc.);in AR 600-9 (1987) percent body fat was measured "by company or similar level commanders (or their designee) in accordance with standard methods prescribed in Appendix B to this regulation.[178] Soldiers will be measured by individuals of the same gender."[179]

Company level commanders were directed to utilize measuring tapes to obtain the circumference measures. Detailed instructions were provided in Appendix B—"Standard Methods for Determining Body Fat Using Body Circumferences, Height and Weight." After obtaining the Soldier's height and weight, the grader would take two circumference measures for men (neck and abdomen) and four circumference measures for women (neck, forearm, wrist, hip). The body fat worksheet (DA Form 5500-R and 5501-R) allowed the grader to convert raw circumference measures into standardized "factor" scores, which could then be used to calculate a Soldier's body composition (percent body fat). Maximum body fat standards were provided by age and gender and remained unchanged from AR 600-9 (1983).[180] A second major addition to AR 600-9 was Appendix C—"Nutrition Guide to the Weight Control Program." This eight page appendix provided a myriad of information such as basic dietary strategies; obesity risks; what are calories, macro- and micronutrients; and portion control. Several 1200-calorie menus were also provided. The assessment of body composition and subsequent compliance with the Army Weight Control Program grew into a significant emotional issue for Soldiers. Failure to meet body fat standards could result in a bar to re-enlistment or extension of enlistment. Soldiers were often flagged "for favorable actions" while on the AWCP. Failure to meet AWCP benchmarks could have negative implications for promotion, professional military or civilian schooling, or assignment to command positions.[181]

On 3 November 1989 Headquarters DA revised and published *The Army Physical Fitness Program* (AR 350-15) for the third time. The DSCOPS retained responsibility for the Army Physical Fitness Program while TRADOC managed the specifics of training doctrine and standards. In the 1989 revision the overarching outcome objective was reversed to read: "enhance combat readiness by developing and sustaining a high level of physical fitness." The number of program objectives was increased from eight (1985) to nine, with the addition of the "ability to cope with psychological stress." HQDA retained the two tests/year APFT requirement and mandated an interval of at least 4 months between testing. In a move to align AR 350-15 with FM 21-20 (1985) alternate aerobic events were specified for Soldiers on permanent medical profiles: 800-yard swim, 6.2-mile bike ride (stationary or 1-speed bike), or the 2.5-mile walk.[182]

The APFT continued to serve as an incentive and a "threat." Although authorized in mid 1986, the Army Physical Fitness Badge was formally introduced in the 1989 revision of AR 350-15. "Soldiers who score 290 or above on the APFT and meet body fat standards will be awarded the Physical Fitness Badge for physical fitness excellence in accordance to AR 672-5-1. Commanders are encouraged to commend soldiers who score over 270 points on the APFT for outstanding performance."[183] Active Army Soldiers without a medical profile were required to remediate an APFT failure within three (3) months; Reserve Component Soldiers were allowed six (6) months. Soldiers who failed to achieve the minimum requirements on the APFT and "displayed no significant, continuing progress" were not allowed to graduate from advanced military schools, were flagged for favorable actions (AR 600-8-2), were barred from re-enlistment, and ultimately were subject to separation from the Service.

From 1985 to 1990 the Army reached the zenith of support for physical readiness programming. The USASPFS was fully resourced by the Army and USARIEM (Institute for Environmental Medicine) and CHPPM (Health Promotion/Preventive Medicine) provided significant research support for program development and assessment. The Master Fitness Trainer program was educating thousands of Soldiers, Officers, and USMA cadets each year, to provide PRT subject matter expertise for unit commanders. Approximately 1000 active and 500 reserve component personnel enrolled in the 4-week resident MFT course at Fort Benjamin Harrison during 1989 and mobile training teams delivered the curriculum to troops in Europe and Korea. TRADOC was even staffing the concept of adding the Master Fitness Trainer program to all Army professional schooling for officers and NCOs in a move to further improve physical readiness training throughout the Army.[184] However, as has been the case throughout Army history, this renaissance in Army PRT would not last.

Notes

1. Paul Cook, "How Did A Lack Of Strategic and Operational Vision Impair the Army's Ability to Conduct Tactical Operations in Korea in the Summer Of 1950?" MA thesis, US Army Command and General Staff College; Fort Leavenworth, 2002, iii; Roy K. Flint, "Task Force Smith and the 24th Division: Delay and Withdrawal, 5-19 July 1950," in *America's First Battles 1776-1965*, ed. Charles E. Heller and William A. Stoff (Lawrence, KS: University Press of Kansas, 1986), 271.

2. William L. Worden, *General Dean's Story as Told by William F. Dean* (New York: The Viking Press, 1954), 12-16; Flint, "Task Force Smith," 269.

3. Gordon R. Sullivan, "A Trained and Ready Army: The Way Ahead," *Military Review* 71: (November 1991): 9.

4. Max Hastings, *The Korean War* (New York: Simon and Schuster, 1987), 78, 81, 87, 94-95.

5. Jonathan House, *Toward Combined Arms Warfare: A Survey of 20th-Century Tactics, Doctrine, and Organization* (Fort Leavenworth, US Army Command and General Staff College, 1984), 149.

6. Although Task Force Smith had some WWII combat veterans only about one man in six had combat experience and most of the men were young, twenty years or less (Roy Appleman, *South to the Naktong, North to the Yalu The US Army in the Korean War* (Washington, DC: Center for Military History, 1992), 61.

7. Theodore Fehrenbach, *This Kind of War: A Study in Unpreparedness* (New York: The MacMillan Company, 1963), 97-106; Clay Blair, *The Forgotten War: America in Korea 1950-1953* (New York: Times Books, 1987), 102.

8. Michael Cannon, "Task Force Smith: A Study in (Un)Preparedness and (Ir)Responsibility," *Military Review* 57 (February 1988): 64; Cook, How Did A Lack Of Strategic, 12, 99; William J. Davies, "Task Force Smith—A Leadership Failure?"(Study Project, Carlisle Barracks, PA: US Army War College, 1992), 7,9; Flint, "Task Force Smith," 266; Michael D. Krause, "History of US Army Soldier Physical Fitness," in *National Conference on Military Physical Fitness-Proceedings Report*, ed. Lois A. Hale (Washington, DC: National Defense University, 1990), 22.

9. Cook, "How Did a Lack of Strategic," 20; Cook was summarizing Cannon, "Task Force Smith," 73.

10. John F. Kennedy, "The Soft American," *Sports Illustrated* 12: (26 December 1960): 15.

11. Cook, "How Did A Lack Of Strategic," 117.

12. Unpublished Graduate Survey conducted by the Department of Physical Education, United States Military Academy, October, 1951.

13. Francis Greene, "Physical Fitness and Physical Training in Korea–Survey of USMA gradates," unpublished; 22 October 1951, 1.

14. Department of the Army, FM 21-20 *Physical Readiness Training* (Washington, DC: US Government Printing Office, 1957), 10.

15. On 26 October 1951 Changes No. 1 (C 1) to FM 21-20 (1950) was published; C1 provided a revision of the confidence obstacle course and the addition of Appendix II – a synopsized version of PRT including a restatement of the purpose, conditioning activities and drills

16. The US perception of technological superiority was crushed on 4 October 1957 when the Soviet Union successfully launched the satellite "Sputnik I" (see history.nasa.gov/sputnik).

17. Hans Kraus would later become the personal physiotherapist to President John F. Kennedy; Ruth Hirshland was the former Ruth "Bonnie" Prudden, who would be an instrumental figure in movement education in the United States throughout the late 20th Century; the primary objective of their research on "hypokinetic disease" was to draw attention to posture and lower back problems in American youth; the connection between Kraus and Hirshland was their love of climbing.

18. Hans Kraus, and Bonnie Prudden, "Muscular Fitness and Health," *Journal of the American Association for Health, Physical Education, Recreation* 24: (December, 1953): 17-19; Hans Kraus, and Ruth P. Hirshland, "Minimum Muscular Fitness Tests in School Children," *Research Quarterly, 25* (1954): 177-178.

19. R. H. Boyle, "The Report that Shocked the President," *Sports Illustrated* (15 August 1955): 31; For all practical purposes the national effort to enhance physical fitness ended with the death of President John Kennedy on 22 November 1963.

20. Julie Sturgeon and Janice Meer. "The First 50 Years 1956-2006–The President's Council on Physical Fitness and Sports Revisits Its Roots and Charts Its Future," (no date), 42 online at: http://www.fitness.gov/50thanniversary/toolkit-firstfiftyyears.htm (accessed 14 September 2011).

21. Department of Defense, *Study of the Military Services Physical Fitness* (Washington DC, 3 April 1981), 3.35; The Army's FY 1954 appropriation budget was cut approximately $5.3 billion (41%).

22. "Move to Close Army School Scored." *The Times-News*, 5 October 1953.

23. John F. Kennedy, "Remarks by Senator John F. Kennedy on Defense Department Appropriations Bill to the Senate on 17 June 1954," JFK Presidential Library and Museum (1954): np; This is a redaction of Kennedy's original speech online at http://www.jfklibrary.org/Research/ Ready-Reference/JFK-Speeches/Remarks-by-Senator-John-F-Kennedy-on-Defense-Department-Appropriation-Bill-to-Senate-on-June-17-1954.aspx (accessed 20 December 2011).

24. "Move to Close Army School Scored." *The Times-News,* 5 October 1953.

25. Department of the Army, FM 35-20 *Physical Training-Women's Army Corps* (Washington, DC: US Government Printing Office, 1956), 5, 103.

26. Department of the Army, FM 21-20 *Physical Readiness Training* (Washington, DC: US Government Printing Office, 1957), 58; Department of the Army, TM 21-200 *Physical Conditioning* (Washington, DC: US Government Publishing Office, 1957), 76.

27. Department of the Army, TM 21-200 *Physical Conditioning*, 5-10.

28. Department of the Army, TM 21-200 *Physical Conditioning*, 466-467; John P. Ladd, "US Army Physical Fitness Testing: Past, Present and Future," Student paper written for the Communicative Arts Program, March 1971, 17-18; The PETB and PAT were taken in utilities and boots.

29. Department of the Army, FM 21-20 *Physical Readiness Training*, 11.

30. There would ultimately be four more fitness "seminars": 1970, 1981, 1990, 2010.

31. *Physical Fitness Seminar Report* (Fort Benning, GA, United States Army Infantry School, April, 1958), i.

32. *Physical Fitness Seminar Report* (1958), 2; The Ranger Department at Fort Benning assumed control of PRT doctrine after the Physical Training School at Fort Bragg was closed in 1953.

33. *Physical Fitness Seminar Report* (1958), 4.

34. *Physical Fitness Seminar Report* (1958), 30.

35. *Physical Fitness Seminar Report* (1958), 31.

36. *Physical Fitness Seminar Report* (1958), 32.

37. *Physical Fitness Seminar Report* (1958), 33.

38. *Physical Fitness Seminar Report* (1958), 34.

39. Kennedy, "The Soft American," 16.

40. Ladd, US Army Physical Fitness Testing, 19; Department of the Army, TM 21-200 *Physical Conditioning*, Change 1 (Washington, DC: US Government Publishing Office, 1959), 1.

41. Soldiers took the Physical Combat Proficiency Test in utilities and boots.

42. Department of the Army, TM 21-200 *Physical Conditioning*, Change 2 (Washington, DC: US Government Publishing Office, 1961), 6-7; Video #65675048110, 1967; Ladd, *US Army Physical Fitness Testing,* 20.

43. Proposed Curriculum Changes." West Point: United States Military Academy, Correspondence from the Master of the Sword to the Commandant of Cadets (Subject: 19 February 1960.

44. Department of the Army, *Your Individual Physical Fitness* (Fort Benning, GA.: US Army Infantry School, no date), document cover; This document was likely published locally in mid 1962; it references two Army publications AR 40-501-C6 (1961) and Army Circular 600-7, Weight Control (1962); AR 40-501-C7 was published in September 1962 and was the precursor to the Army Physical Fitness Program.

45. Department of the Army, *Your Individual Physical Fitness*, 7.

46. Ladd, *US Army Physical Fitness Testing,* 22.

47. Ladd, *US Army Physical Fitness Testing,* 22.

48. *Physical Fitness Seminar Report*, 1958, 32.

49. Department of the Army, *Physical Fitness Training Program for Specialist and Staff Personnel*, DA PAM 21-1, (Washington DC: US Government Publishing Office, 1963), 4.

50. Department of the Army, DA Pamphlet 21-2, *Physical Fitness Program for Women in the Army* (DA Pamphlet 21-2) (Washington DC: Government

Printing Office, 1963), 5; The "5-10 Plan" outlined the exercise program for women that involved five exercises that were to be executed for 10 repetitions.

51. Change 1, AR 40-501, 1961, A3-1; The maximum allowable weight for 18-20 year old women/men at 60"/72 inches in pounds respectively were: 139/163, 191/225.

52. Department of the Army, AR 600-7 *Weight Control* (Washington DC: US Government Publishing Office 1963), 2.

53. "The US Army in Vietnam," in *American Military History*, ed. Vincent H. Demma (Washington, DC: Center of Military History, 1989), 641.

54. Department of the Army, AR 600-9 *Army Physical Fitness Program* (Washington, DC: US Government Printing Office, 1965), 1.

55. Department of the Army, *Physical Fitness Program for Women in the Army* (DA Pamphlet 21-2) (Washington: Government Printing Office, 1965), 5.

56. Department of the Army, AR 600-7 *Weight Control*, (Washington, DC: US Government Publishing Office 1965), 1.

57. Department of the Army, FM 35-20 *Physical Training-Women's Army Corps*, (Washington, DC: US Government Printing Office, 1965), 2.

58. Department of the Army, "The Inclement Weather Physical Fitness Test," Continental Army Command Pamphlet 600-1 (Fort Monroe: US Continental Army Command, 1966), 2.

59. FM 21-20 (1969) represented the first time the term "Physical Readiness Training" was used for the Army's premiere training and doctrine manual.

60. Department of the Army, FM 21-20 *Physical Readiness Training*, (Washington, DC: US Government Printing Office, 1969), 9-11.

61. These five principles were first published in the 1962 USAIS document "Your Individual Physical Fitness."

62. Department of the Army, FM 21-20 *Physical Readiness Training,* (1969), 12.

63. There is a video of the administration of the PCPT online at: http://www.criticalpast.com/video/65675048110_ United-States-cadets_physical-fitness_drill-sergeant_physical-combat-proficiency-test; last accessed 12 March 2012.

64. Department of the Army, FM 21-20 *Physical Readiness Training*, (1969), 213-258.

65. Ken Cooper, *Aerobics* (New York: M. Evans in association with Lippincott, Philadelphia, 1968), 1.

66. On 1 December 1969 the Selective Service conducted two draft lotteries (by birth date and last name) to determine order of call to military service for the Vietnam War.

67. Pamela Cooper, *The American Marathon* (Syracuse, New York: Syracuse University Press, 1999), 157; Merry Lepper's time for the Culver City Marathon was 3:37:07.

68. Charles C. Lovett, *Olympic Marathon: A Centennial History of the Games' Most Storied Race,* (Westport, CT: Praeger, 1997), 125; In 1966 women were not allowed to enter the Boston Marathon; however Gibb snuck onto the

course and completed the 26+ mile race; the women's division was not opened until 1972.

69. Harry C. Beans, "Sex Discrimination in the Military," *Military Law Review* 67; Headquarters–Department of the Army (Pam 27-100-67), Winter 1975): 68.

70. "Physical Fitness Symposium Report" (Fort Benning, GA: United States Infantry School, 1970), 1.

71. "Physical Fitness Symposium Report" (1970), 2.

72. "Physical Fitness Symposium Report" (1970), 5.

73. "Physical Fitness Symposium Report" (1970), 40-42.

74. Department of the Army, AR 600-9 *Army Physical Fitness Program* (Washington, DC: Government Printing Office, 1971), 1.

75. Department of the Army, AR 600-9 *Army Physical Fitness Program*, 2.

76. Department of the Army, AR 600-9 *Army Physical Fitness Program*, 3.

77. Although not specified, the 1973 revision of FM 21-20 was most likely written by personnel at the USAIC, Fort Benning.

78. Department of the Army, FM 21-20 *Physical Readiness Training* (Washington, DC: US Government Printing Office, 1973), 211.

79. Department of the Army, FM 21-20 *Physical Readiness Training* (1973), 211-284.

80. Department of the Army, FM 21-20 *Physical Readiness Training* (1973), 23.

81. Department of the Army, FM 21-20 *Physical Readiness Training* (1973), 25.

82. Richard P. Mustion, "Sustaining Our Army Then and Now," *Professional Bulletin of the United States Army Sustainment PB700-09-06 41:6* (November-December 2009): 1; online at http://www.almc.army.mil/alog/ issues/NovDec09/then_now.html (accessed 20 December 2011).

83. Mustion, "Sustaining Our Army Then and Now," 1.

84. Department of the Army, AR 600-9 *Army Physical Fitness Program* (Washington, DC: US Government Printing Office, 1974), 2.

85. Department of the Army, FM 35-20 *Physical Training-Women's Army Corps* (Washington, DC: US Government Printing Office, 1975), 5; Figure 2 pictures two women running with a combat load during airborne training.

86. Department of the Army, FM 35-20 *Physical Training-Women's Army Corps* (Washington, DC: US Government Printing Office, 1975), 174-202.

87. "Women Content in Units Force Development Test (MAXWAC Test)" (Alexandria, VA: US Army Research Institute for the Behavioral Sciences, 3 October 1977), I-1.

88. Bettie J. Morden, *The Women's Army Corps, 1945-1978* (Washington, DC: Center of Military History, 2000), 371-372.

89. Brian P. Mitchell, *Women in the Military: Flirting With Disaster* (Washington, DC: Regnery Publishing, Inc., 1998), 108.

90. As quoted in James A. Vogel, et al., "A System for Establishing Occupationally-Related Gender-Free Physical Fitness Standards" (Report No.

T 5/80) (Natick, MA: US Army Research Institute of Environmental Medicine, April 1980), 1.

91. Vogel, et al., "A System for Establishing Occupationally-Related", 1.

92. "Department of the Army Historical Summary–Fiscal Year 1977," ed. Karl E. Cocker (Washington, DC: Center of Military History, 1979), 23.

93. "Department of the Army Historical Summary–Fiscal Year 1977," 24; "Department of the Army Historical Summary–Fiscal Year 1979," ed. Edith M. Boldan (Washington, DC: Center of Military History, 1982), 24; At the same time the mixed-gender IET project was underway, the Army also instituted the One Station Unit Training (OSUT) program at Fort Benning, GA (1977). Although initial trails were successful, Congress was not convinced that OSUT was more efficient or effective. From January-May, 1979 extensive trials were conducted at Fort Benning and Fort Knox. As a result OSUT was found to be more cost efficient (resulted in an annual operating savings of $7.3 million) and provided more effective training. OSUT was fully implemented by the end of 1979. (see "Army Historical Summary-1977," 23 and "Army Historical Summary-1979," 25, 26).

94. Karl Friedl, James A. Vogel, Matthew W. Bovee, and Bruce H. Jones, "Assessment of Body Weight Standards in Male and Female Army Recruits" (Natick, MA: US Army Research Institute of Environmental Medicine Technical Report No. T15-90, 1989), 7.

95. When the maximal allowable weight standards were first published in AR 600-9 (1976), the age classifications were removed; weights were listed by gender/height–the max allowable weight for women/men for 60/72" in pounds respectively were: 121/141, 172/203; maximum allowable weights were lowered by approximately 20 pounds per category over the AR 40-501 (1961) standards.

96. Department of the Army, AR 600-9 *Army Physical Fitness and Weight Control Program* (Washington, DC: US Government Printing Office, 1976), 1-1; This statement follows the publication of the recommendations from the two "Physical Fitness Seminars (1958)–Committee 3: Conclusion 11," 32 and "Physical Fitness Seminar (1970)–Conclusion 15," 41.

97. Department of the Army, AR 600-9 *Army Physical Fitness and Weight Control Program* (1976), Section 1-3.a.2., 1-1.

98. Department of the Army, AR 600-9 *Army Physical Fitness and Weight Control Program* (1976), 1-1.

99. From a current perspective relative to the work capacity of an 18-21 year old, an exercise heart rate of 140 beats per minute would only be considered a moderately strenuous work.

100. Department of the Army, AR 600-9 *Army Physical Fitness and Weight Control Program* (1976), 3.

101. Department of the Army, AR 600-9 *Army Physical Fitness and Weight Control Program* (1976), 3-1.

102. "Physical Fitness Policies and Programs," in *Assessing Readiness in Military Women: The Relationship of Body Composition, Nutrition, and Health* (Washington, DC: National Academic Press; 1998), 63.

103. "Physical Fitness Policies and Programs," 63; Michael L. Pollock, et al., "Position Stand: The Recommended Quantity and Quality of Exercise for Developing and Maintaining Cardiorespiratory and Muscular Fitness, and Flexibility in Healthy Adults," Medicine & Science in *Sports and Exercise* 30: (June 1998): 501.

104. Online at http://www.army.mil/women/newera.html; (accessed 13 March 2012); By 1978 there were approximately 18,000 WACs serving in the Army Reserve and 25,000 in the Army National Guard. "In August 1982, the Secretary of Defense ordered the increase in Army enlisted women's strength from 65,000 to 70,000 and officers from 9,000 to 13,000, including medical personnel."

105. Online at http://www.army.mil/women/newera.html (accessed 13 March 2012).

106. "Physical Fitness Symposium Report" (1970), 42.

107. Vogel, et al., "A System for Establishing," vi; After women were admitted to the United States Military Academy initiated several physical training studies: "Project 60–A Comparison of Two Types of Physical Training Programs on the Performance of 16-Year-Old Women" (1976) and "Project Athena–A Longitudinal Study of the Integration of Women into the Corps of Cadets" (1976).

108. "Department of the Army Historical Summary–Fiscal Year 1980," Edited by Lenwood Y. Brown (Washington, DC: Center of Military History, 1983), 45.

109. Stephen McGugan, "The Cadet Physical Fitness Test: Overachieving Or Overdemanding?" Paper completed for LD720, American Military History, West Point, NY, 1997.

110. Department of the Army, AR 350-15 *The Army Physical Fitness Program* (Washington, DC: US Government Publishing Office, 1982), 1; "Soldier Physical Fitness Center: An Historical Review" (USAPFS Archived Historical Documents, undated) 42.

111. Department of Defense, "Study of the Military Services Physical Fitness" (Washington, DC 1981), 3-36.

112. Department of the Army, FM 21-20 *Physical Readiness Training* (Washington, DC: US Government Printing Office, 1980), E-3; "Superintendents Annual Historical Review," (1981), 56; Hardyman, 1988, 48; McGugan, The Cadet Physical Fitness Test, 5.

113. Department of the Army, FM 21-20 *Physical Readiness Training* (1980), E-12, E-15.

114. Department of the Army, FM 21-20 *Physical Readiness Training* (1980), E-3; The 2-mile run was run in boots, therefore the 60-point time standards were significantly higher than would be expected in running shoes

115. Hardyman, 1988, 48.

116. Department of the Army, FM 21-20 *Physical Readiness Training* (1980), 1-6.

117. Most civilian and military personnel who were involved with the Soldier Fitness School and the development of the 1980 and 1985 FM 21-20 *Physical Readiness Training* attribute this attitude to concerns expressed by senior military leaders (i.e. general officers) relative to their ability to meet minimum Army fitness standards.

118. Department of the Army, FM 21-20 *Physical Readiness Training* (1973), 28.

119. Department of the Army, FM 21-20 *Physical Readiness Training* (1980), i.

120. See AR 40-501, C35 *Standards of Medical Fitness*, 1987, 10-25 for additional information on the "Army Physical Fitness Program for Active Members Age 40 and Over."

121. Department of Defense, "Study of the Military Services Physical Fitness," 1-1; Krause, "History of US Army Soldier Physical Fitness," 23.

122. Department of the Army Historical Summary – Fiscal Year 1980, 46.

123. Department of Defense, Study of the Military Services Physical Fitness, 1-1.

124. *National Conference on Military Physical Fitness–Proceedings Report*, ed. Lois Hale (Washington, DC: National Defense University, 1990), 2.

125. "Department of the Army Historical Summary–Fiscal Year 1980," 46.

126. "Department of Defense, Study of the Military Services Physical Fitness," 3-13; Department of Defense, "Directive on Physical Fitness and Weight Control Programs (Directive No. 1308.1)" (Washington DC, 1981), 1.

127. Department of Defense, Directive 1380.1 (1981), 1; Hodgdon, 1992, p. 57-58; James Hodgdon, *A History of the US Navy Physical Readiness Program from 1976 to 1999* (Arlington, VA: Office of Naval Research, 1999), 6.

128. Department of Defense, Directive 1380.1 (1981), 1, Encl. 1, 1 Encl. 2, 1; James Hodgdon, "Body Composition in the Military Services: Standards and Methods," in *Body Composition and Physical Performance–Applications for the Military Services,* ed. Bernadette M. Marriott and Judith Grumstrup-Scott (Washington: DC: National Academy Press, 1992), 57-58; Hodgdon, *A History of the US Navy Physical Readiness Program*, 6.

129. "Soldier Physical Fitness Center: An Historical Review" USAPFS Archived Historical Documents, undated, 42; From additional materials to include a "Director Survey" form, this document appears to have been written/compiled by Dr. Mel Parks of the US Army Physical Fitness School.

130. Soldier Physical Fitness Center (1982), USAPFS Archived Historical Documents, undated, 1.

131. TRADOC Information Pamphlet: "An Imminent and Menacing Threat to National Security," (Fort Monroe, VA: TRADOC Public Affairs Office, 2008), 8.

132. Throughout the 10-year tenure of the Soldier Physical Fitness School at Fort Ben Harrison the "name" and acronym attributed to the center/school varied based upon the speaker; the "nom du jour" was most often the Physical Fitness School.

133. The Honorable John O. Marsh, Jr, Secretary of the Army, 8 February, 1982, speaking before the Committee on Armed Services, House of Representatives, Second Session, 97th Congress.

134. Department of the Army, "Memorandum of Understanding between the US Army Soldier Support Center and the US Army Infantry School, Subject: Army Physical Fitness System," 8 April 1982, Lieutenant General Julius Becton, Deputy Commander for Training.

135. TRADOC Information Pamphlet, 2, 8.; By 1983 the USAPFCS staffing had increased to 9 officers, 6 NCOs, and 20 civilians.

136. TRADOC Information Pamphlet, 1.

137. On 15 February 1983 AR 600-9 was reissued as "The Army Weight Control Program."

138. Department of the Army, FM 350-15 *Army Physical Fitness Program* (Washington, DC: US Government Printing Office, 1982), 2-3.

139. Department of the Army, FM 350-15 *Army Physical Fitness Program* (1982), 4.

140. Department of the Army, FM 350-15 *Army Physical Fitness Program* (1982), 6.

141. USAPFS Archived Historical Documents: "Soldier Physical Fitness School: An Historical Review," undated, 46; The SPFS developed a package called the "Training Support Package–Physical Fitness Training: Total Fitness," which was the principal supporting document in the mandatory 2-4 hour course on total fitness which was to be included in all TRADOC schools.

142. Online at https://apfri.carlisle.army.mil (accessed 1 December 2011).

143. Online at https://apfri.carlisle.army.mil/web/aboutUs.cfm (accessed 1 December 2011).

144. Department of Defense, "Study of the Military Services Physical Fitness," 3-20.

145. Personal communication with Colonel Gregory L. Daniels, Master of the Sword, 2 February, 2012; Colonel Daniels attend the 4-week residence course at Fort Benjamin Harrison in March, 1985 as Second Lieutenant Daniels representing the 2/320th Field Artillery, 101st Airborne Division.

146. Historical Records, West Point, NY: Department of Physical Education, United States Military Academy (unpublished records).

147. Department of the Army, AR 600-9 *Army Weight Control Program* (Washington, DC: US Government Printing Office, 1983), 3.

148. Department of the Army, AR 600-9 *Army Weight Control Program* (1983), 3.

149. In AR 600-9 the body weight table in the Appendix was no longer a criterion-referenced measure of "weight control" problems (i.e., they were no longer "maximum allowable weights); the body weight table published in AR

600-9 was used as "screening" tool to identify those Soldier who required a body composition assessment; maximum allowable body weights for accession into the Army were still published in AR 40-501; these criterion values differed by approximately 20 pounds by age/height/ gender; screening weights for 17-20 year old women/men for 60/72" respectively were: 111/132, 190/160.

150. Reynold A. Burrowes, *Revolution and Rescue in Grenada: an Account of the US Caribbean Invasion* (New York: Greenwood Press; 1988), 79.

151. Dorothea Cypher, "Urgent Fury: The US Army in Grenada," in *American Intervention in Grenada: The Implications of Operation "Urgent Fury,"* ed. Peter M. Dunn and Bruce W. Watson (Boulder, CO: Westview Press; 1985), 106.

152. James M. Dubik., and T.D. Fullerton, "Soldier Overloading in Grenada," *Military Review* 66 (January, 1987): 39; Stephen J. Townsend, "The Factors of Soldier's Load," Master's thesis, Command and General Staff College, Fort Leavenworth, 1994, 1.

153. *The Commander's Handbook on Physical Fitness* (Washington DC: Government Printing Office, 1982), 25.

154. *The Individual's Handbook on Physical Fitness* (Washington DC: Government Printing Office, 1983), ii.

155. Joseph J. Knapik, et al., "Soldier Performance and Mood States Following a Strenuous Road March" (Natick, MA: US Army Research Institute of Environmental Medicine, 1990), 1.

156. "Department of the Army Historical Summary–Fiscal Year 1988," ed. Cherly Morai-Young (Washington: Center of Military History, 1993), 41.

157. "History of the Present APFT," (USAPFS Archived Historical Documents, undated), 4.

158. "History of the Present APFT," (USAPFS Archived Historical Documents, undated), 5.

159. Department of the Army, FM 21-20 *Physical Readiness Training* (1985), A-1, B-1.

160. Department of the Army, FM 21-20 *Physical Readiness Training* (1985), 11-1; The sample score card (DA705) presented in Figure 11-1, 11-2 and 11-3 still uses the term Army Physical Readiness Test.

161. Department of the Army, FM 21-20 *Physical Readiness Training* (1985), 11-2.

162. Department of the Army, FM 21-20 *Physical Readiness Training* (1985), 11-3.

163. Department of the Army, FM 350-15 *Army Physical Fitness Program* (1985), 4.

164. Department of the Army, FM 350-15 *Army Physical Fitness Program* (1985), 4.

165. Department of the Army, FM 350-15 *Army Physical Fitness Program* (1985), 5.

166. Department of the Army, FM 350-15 *Army Physical Fitness Program* (1985), 6.

167. DA Form 705–the Army PFT card was subsequently reissued in June 1986.

168. The 2-mile run times decreased significantly to reflect the advantage of running in running shoes instead of combat boots.

169. Department of the Army, FM 350-41 *Army Forces Training* (Washington, DC: US Government Printing Office, 1986), 9.

170. H. Norman Schwarzkopf, *It Doesn't Take a Hero* (New York: Bantam Books, 1992), 271.

171. Joseph J. Knapik, et al., "Army Physical Fitness Test (APFT): Normative Data on 6022 Soldiers (Technical Report No. T94-7)" (Natick, MA: US Army Research Institute of Environmental Medicine, 1994), 2; John S. O'Connor, Michael S. Bahrke, and Robert G. Tetu, "1988 Active Army Physical Fitness Survey," *Military Medicine* 155: (1990): 579.

172. Knapik, et al., "Army Physical Fitness Test (APFT)," 13; Extrapolating from the raw data on pages 14 and 22 for 17-21 year-old Soldiers, the following percentages would tab/max by event in 1988: Men– PU–7.5%/2%, SU–4%/<1%, 2MR–10%/1%; Women: PU–7.5%/2%, SU–5%/<1%, 2MR–7%/4%.

173. Louis F. Tomasi, P. Rey Regualos, Gene Fober, and Matthew Christenson, *Age and Gender Performance on the US Army Physical Fitness Test* (Fort Benning, GA: Army Physical Fitness School, 1995), 1.

174. Mark Hertling, *Physical Training and the Modern Battlefield: Are We Tough Enough?* Fort Leavenworth, School of Advanced Military Studies Monograph, US Army Command and General Staff College, 1987, 35.

175. Hertling, *Physical Training and the Modern Battlefield: Are We Tough Enough?*, 35.

176. Hertling, *Physical Training and the Modern Battlefield: Are We Tough Enough?*, i.

177. Department of the Army, AR 600-9 *Army Weight Control Program* (1987), 3.

178. Department of the Army, AR 600-9 *Army Weight Control Program* (1987), 3; Body weight screening values for 17-20 year old women/men for 60/72" respectively were: 116/132, 190/167, which represented a slight increase in screening weights for women published in AR 600-9 *Army Weight Control Program* (1983).

179. Department of the Army, AR 600-9 *Army Weight Control Program* (1987), 4.

180. Maximum allowable percent body fat standards for 17-20 year old Soldiers were: men = 20%, women = 28%.

181. Department of the Army, AR 600-9 *Army Weight Control Program* (1987), 11.

182. Department of the Army, FM 350-15 *Army Physical Fitness Program* (1989), 5.

183. Department of the Army, FM 350-15 *Army Physical Fitness Program* (1989), 6.

184. "Department of the Army Historical Summary–Fiscal Year 1989," ed. Vincent H. Demma (Washington, DC: Center of Military History, United States Army, 1998), 253.

Chapter 7
Return to Combat—Focused Physical Readiness Training.

Due to declining federal revenues in 1988 and 1989, which were exacerbated by the financial costs of the first Gulf War (1990-91), the Army was forced to take under consideration several cost-saving initiatives. During the initial Base Closure and Realignment Commission (BRAC) hearings of 1989, it seemed likely that Fort Benjamin Harrison would be closed. In April 1990 Headquarters-Department of the Army (HQDA) initiated Project Vanguard and in May 1990 the Vanguard Task Force, headed by Major General John R. Greenway, began assessing ways to improve effectiveness and lower operating and sustainment costs. With Fort Ben Harrison's closure imminent the Vanguard TF recommended closing the USASPFS and reassigning its duties to the Academy of Health Sciences at Fort Sam Houston. After much discussion with HQ TRADOC, the decision was made to reduce USASPFS's manpower and mission and place it under the command of the US Army Infantry Center (USAIC) at Fort Benning.[1] Along with significant reductions in personnel, the resident Master Fitness Trainer course and associated "6P" Army skill identifier were also eliminated.[2] Under the direction of the USAIC and now relocated at Fort Benning, PRT focus began a slow but inexorable shift away from health-related fitness to combat-focused fitness. The name of the United States Army Soldier Physical Fitness School changed slightly during this transition to the US Army Physical Fitness School.

On 30 September 1992 *Physical Fitness Training* (FM 21-20) was revised and published for the tenth time. The 1985 chapter on "fitness leadership and instructor training" was deleted and the information was moved to Chapters 1 and 10 (Introduction and Developing the Unit Program). The 1992 edition added two new chapters on Body Composition (Chapter 5) and Physical Training During Initial Entry Training (Chapter 11). Chapter 6—Nutrition and Fitness was significantly expended from 1985 and included a section on nutrition for optimal performance.[3] The materials from the "Additional Activities" chapter (1985) were relocated into Chapters 7-9; Circuit Training and Exercise Drills, Obstacles Courses and Additional Drills, and Competitive Fitness Activities. FM 21-20 (1992) grew from 11 to 14 chapters.

The 3-event APFT was continued in the 1992 revision. The total performance score was determined by converting raw scores to a 100-point scale-scoring table for each event. The point scale was adjusted based on age and gender. The maximum score a Soldier could earn on each event was 100 points for a total score of 300 points. All soldiers were required to score at least 60 points on each of the three test events in order to pass the APFT. Soldiers who fail a record APFT were required to retest within 3-months. Soldiers failing to remediate an APFT failure on a "90-day" retest were subject to a bar from reenlistment or separation from the Army. The minimum scores (60 point score) for 17-21 year old men and women remained unchanged from the 1986 scoring revision: Male: PU = 42, SU = 52, 2MR = 15:54; Female: PU = 18, SU = 50, 2MR = 18:54.

On 19 March 1993 *Training in Units* (AR 350-41) was revised for the second time. AR 350-41 (1993) marked the termination of the stand-alone Army Physical Fitness Program regulatory document, which had been in existence since the early 1960's. In this consolidation effort, the contents from AR 350-15 were published in their entirety as AR 350-41, Chapter 9—"Physical Fitness." Physical fitness, which provides the foundation for combat readiness and unit readiness, "begins with the physical fitness of Soldiers and the Noncommissioned Officers and Officers who lead them."[4] AR 350-41 (1993) reiterated that commanders and supervisors must conduct exercise periods with sufficient intensity, frequency, and duration to attain the overarching objective of enhancing combat readiness. This objective was to be measured by nine criteria: cardio-respiratory endurance, muscular strength and endurance, anaerobic conditioning, flexibility, body composition, competitive spirit to win, self discipline, ability to cope with psychological stress, and a healthy lifestyle. All personnel in the active Army, the Army National Guard and US Army Reserve were required to participate in year round collective or individual physical fitness training programs. Active Army personnel, full-time Guardsmen, and full-time Reservists were required to participate in vigorous physical fitness training 3 to 5 times per week during the unit's normal duty-day.[5] The initial entry training "skills list" presented in Section 8 (AR 350-15, 1989) was incorporated into Section 9-6-a of AR 350-41 as the military skills list critical to support the unit's mission essential task list (METL). Active duty, Guard, and Reserve Soldiers were required to take an APFT at least twice each year with a minimum of four months separating record tests. Profiled Soldiers were encouraged to rehabilitate their illness or injury and take a record 3-event test. Alternative aerobic events were specified for Soldiers on permanent medical profiles. AR 350-41 reiterated the ancillary role of the APFT as an assessment tool to be used by Commanders to establish a baseline level of fitness for all Soldiers. This baseline level, according to Colonel Stephen D. Cellucci, Commandant, USAPFS "is the minimum physical capacity required to wear the green uniform."[6] Cellucci further stated that Army leaders at every level need to understand the role of the APFT as one baseline field fitness test. Unit programs must be designed to help Soldiers gain and maintain optimal levels of performance required in combat.

In late 1991, as part of the TRADOC's "Women in the Army" initiative, General Frederick Franks, Commander, TRADOC directed the Physical Fitness School to again study and review the APFT standards. The purpose of this study was: (1) to ensure the APFT measured baseline Army physical fitness; (2) to provide scientific review of the APFT; and (3) to assess gender equity in the scoring standards. The USAPFS established an APFT Update Study Committee to conduct the review. Participating agencies included: the United States Army Research Institute of Environmental Medicine (USARIEM), Army Research Institute (ARI), and the Office of the Surgeon General. The Army Physical Fitness School repeated the 1988 "Active Army Physical Fitness Survey" using a random sample of 2,588 active-duty soldiers stratified by age, gender, and MOS. The researchers measured APFT performance between September 1994 and March 1995 at various test sites throughout the Army. USAPFS personnel also measured heights and weights and calculated body mass indexes for the soldiers.

Average performance by all Soldiers had increased significantly since 1984. Only 12.5% of the sample failed the APFT, with a relatively equal failure rate for men and women. A disproportionate percentage of Soldiers less than 27 years of age failed (29.7%), while only 8.5% of career Soldiers greater than 27 years of age failed. Tomasi, et al. reported that men "maxed" the push-up event at greater rate than women and that the women's sit-up and 2-mile run standards were too low. Women "maxed" the 2-mile run (i.e., scored 100 points) at twice the rate of men. Tomasi and colleagues made eight recommendations; the more salient were: (1) adjust the "effort scales" to ensure "equal effort" by both genders, (2) move towards one performance standard for both genders, (3) relax the APFT Badge standards from 290 to 270 – 90-points in each event, and (4) establish scoring standards for Soldiers 52-56, 57-61, and over 61 years of age.[7] In response to the results of this survey, a recommendation was submitted to the Army Chief of Staff to modify the requirements for passing the Army PFT. The proposal included a slight increase in the minimum push-up standard for men and women, equalizing the minimum sit-ups standard for men and women, and decreasing the minimum 2-mile run standard for men and women. Approved changes were to be published in the 1998 revision of FM 21-20.[8] The authors concluded that the Army needed to recognize the physical capabilities of women and establish standards that reflect an "equal level of effort."[9]

On 1 October 1998 *Physical Fitness Training* (FM 21-20) was revised and published for the eleventh time as Change 1-1992. The 3-event

APFT remained unchanged and there were no changes in PRT content or doctrine. In accordance with AR 350-41 (1993), all Soldiers were required to take a record APFT two times a year. A record APFT must at a minimum include an aerobic event. FM 21-20 (1998) prescribed three alternate aerobic events (800-yard swim, 6.2-mile bike, 2.5-mile walk) for those Soldiers who are unable to run due to a permanent or long-term medical condition. The proscribed uniform for the APFT was the Army physical fitness uniform (APFU) and running shoes. The recommended changes to the APFT scoring standards made by the 1995 USAPFS study group were generally ignored. The only change in APFT standards (1998) was for 17-21 year old women Soldiers when the 60-point push-up standard increased from 18 to 19 repetitions.

Developing PRT Doctrine for the 21st Century

The most comprehensive revision of Army physical training doctrine occurred with the publication of *Physical Fitness Training* (FM 21-20) in 1985. Although FM 21-20 was re-issued in 1992 and again 1998, the changes were primarily cosmetic. Throughout the 1990's there was constant turmoil relative to the mission, authority, and responsibilities of the US Army Physical Fitness School and support for the physical readiness mission by the Army. Similar to the reductions in force that occurred following WWI and WWII, during the Clinton administration there were again significant reductions in Army manpower. "Since Bill Clinton assumed office, Department of Defense (DoD) employment has fallen 152,500 or 17 percent. DoD employment has fallen from 32 percent of total federal employment in 1989 to 27% today...Of every 100 federal jobs eliminated over the past four years, 94 were military personnel."[10] These reductions took a significant toll on the USAPFS in both civilian and military personnel.

As early as 1975 the Headquarters—Department of the Army (HQDA) published AR 350-1, *Army Training*. This regulation provided the conceptual framework for Army training and was divided into chapters regarding the Army Training System, Army Training Management, Common Military Tasks, the Army Standardized Program, etc. To fill the gaps in Army doctrine, from 1975 to 2000 various "commands" produced command-specific versions of 350-1. In October 1998 and again in October 2002 FORSCOM published FORSCOM Regulation 350-1 *Training—Active Duty Training for FORSCOM Units*. In Chapter 3-6 FORSCOM provided broad guidance relative to physical training. Physical Fitness Training (PFT) programs were to be based upon "wartime mission needs as defined by the battle focus process and unit and individual METL tasks."[11] Program criteria were aligned with the nine objectives published in AR

350-41, *Training in Units* (1993) with one additional objective of smoking cessation. Forces Command directed that all Soldiers and leaders were to participate in their unit PRT programs "except for medical or remedial considerations that require an individually tailored program."[12] Even though the Master Fitness Trainer (MFT) program was in the process of being terminated, leaders were encourage to make maximum use of MFTs to design "well-rounded, innovative, and imaginative unit PFT programs."

Similar to FORSCOM, the US Army in Europe (USAREUR) published its version of AR 350-1, *Training—Training in the Army in Europe* in November 2000 (July 2002 and October 2005). *Training in the Army in Europe* was considerably more sophisticated and Chapter 4-4(d) outlined physical fitness training expectations for USAREUR units. Physical fitness programs (PFPs) were designed to promote combat readiness and enhance overall fitness. All personnel were required to take a record APFT biannually and commanders were required to ensure the safety of PFPs by employing MFTs under the supervision of an officer or senior NCO. The reference documents for UASREUR PFPs were FM 21-20, AR 350-1, AR 600-9, and Command Policy Letter 8.[13]

In a second move to streamline Army regulations by merging regulatory documents, on 9 April 2003 Headquarters-DA revised AR 350-1, *Army Training and Education*. Materials from *The Army Physical Fitness Program* (AR 350-15, 1989), *Training in Units* (AR 350-41, 1993), and *Army Training* (AR 350-1, 1983) were merged and AR 350-41 was terminated.[14] Policies governing the Army Physical Fitness Program were presented in Chapter 1-21, individual fitness standards were presented in Chapter 3-9, and policies governing unit PRT were presented in Chapter 4-9. AR 350-1 (2003) maintained the nine overarching objectives of the Army Physical Fitness Program (APFP) published in AR 350-41 (1993) and added a 10th objective: motor efficiency—coordination, agility, balance, posture, speed, power, and kinesthetic awareness.[15] There were no changes in the nine military skills required for unit physical training (4-9, p. 72). The APFP was administered by Deputy Chief of Staff-G3 with support from the Deputy Chief of Staff-G1 (weight control), Office of the Surgeon General, TRADOC, Army War College, and others.

The USAPFS had begun work on a new PRT doctrine soon after the revised FM 21-20 (1998) was published. Their intent was to publish a significantly revised PRT doctrine in a new field manual—FM 3-25.20. Around 2000, the USAPFS suffered additional personnel cuts, which further exacerbated attempts to meet its doctrinal and training mission. By the end of FY 2001 they could no longer resource the 6P (Master Fitness Trainer) Army Skill Identifier (ASI) and all resident instruction and the mobile training teams were terminated. The MFT course, which taught the basic science of exercise as well as the application of PRT doctrine, was the hallmark of Army fitness doctrine and training since its inception in 1983 at Fort Benjamin Harrison. With a significant portion of the new PRT field manual (FM 3-25.20) completed, two events delayed the publication of FM 3-25.20 for nearly eight years. The first event was the attacks of 11 September 2001 and the subsequent deployment of US combat troops as part of Operation Enduring Freedom (OEF). The second event was a somewhat innocuous request from Lieutenant General Van Alstyne, Deputy Commanding General for Initial Entry Training, TRADOC to propose a new physical readiness test to accompany FM 3-25.20.[16] In early 2003 the USAPFS proposed a 6-item physical readiness test as a potential replacement for the 3-event APFT. The six test items proposed in an "in progress review" to the TRADOC Commander were: standing long jump (2 trials), power squats (max repetitions in 1-min), heel hook (max repetitions in 1-min), agility run (12x25 yards), push-up (max repetitions in 1-min—no rest), and a 1-mile run. Test items were to be administered sequentially with a minimum of five minutes and a maximum of 10 minutes rest between each event. The test required four soldiers in a "testing cohort" (1-scorer, 1-timer, 2-spotters) and had to be completed in a maximum of two hours.

After the briefing the proposed test found its way onto the internet and went "viral" throughout the Army. Although the USAPFS had not intended to staff a new physical readiness test in FM 3-25.20, feedback from Army was so negative and vociferous that the publication of FM 3-25.20 was temporarily suspended. During this hiatus the historical struggle between TRADOC and the US Army Infantry School over who "owned" physical readiness doctrine resurfaced. In late 2005 General Wallace, Commander, TRADOC concluded that housing the USAPFS at Fort Benning exacerbated the confusion over who controlled PRT doctrine. To eliminate further confusion over PRT doctrine proponency the decision was made to move the USAPFS to Fort Jackson sometime in 2007. In addition to delineating proponency, the move to Fort Jackson would also incorporate the USAPFS into the emerging nexus of the Victory University and the Directorate of Basic Combat Training under the Physical Fitness Division.

On 13 February 2006 Headquarters-DA revised and published *Army Training and Leader Development* (AR 350-1), which superseded AR 350-1 (9 April 2003). Most notable in this revision was the inclusion of regulatory policy related to the Army combatives training program (Section 1-23). Combatives was defined as "instruction of hand–to–hand and rifle–bayonet fighting and is key in ensuring Soldiers are mentally prepared to engage and kill the enemies of the United States in close combat."[17] AR 350-1 (2006) established FM 3–25.150 (2002) as the Army's instructional guide for combatives training. Physical training regulations were presented in Section 1-24.[18] The major change from the 2003 revision was the reduction in APFT testing requirement for US Army Reserve forces from twice to once per year. Additional guidance was provided concerning APFT testing for Soldiers 55 years and older and physical training programs for deploying units.

On 27 November 2006 Headquarters-DA issued a change to *The Army Weight Control Program* (AR 600-9), which had just been published in September 2006 as a revision to AR 600-9 (1987). Basic policies and procedures did not change. The two primary objectives were designed to insure Soldiers: (1) were able to meet the physical demands of their combat mission, and (2) presented a trim military appearance. The Deputy Chief of Staff, G1 retained proponency of the AWCP with support from the Surgeon General, while commanders and supervisors implemented the AWCP. The assessment of body composition was accomplished through multiple circumference measures with a measuring tape. Although commanders could "tape" a Soldier based upon a visual inspection, body weight measures in excess of "screening weights" were generally the impetus to "tape" a Soldier. Criterion-referenced body weights were presented in Table 3-1.[19] There was one significant change from AR 600-9 (1987) in the circumference measures used to compute body composition for women. In AR 600-9 (1987) circumference measures for women were: neck, forearm, waist, and hips; in the 2006 revision the three approved circumference measures were: neck—just below the larynx, waist—anatomical waist at the narrowest point below the ribs, and hips—over the greatest protrusion of the gluteal muscle (buttocks). Maximum allowable body fat percentages by age/gender (M/F) were: 17–20 years: 20%/30%, 21–27 years: 22%/32%, 28–39 years: 24%/34%, and 40 years & older: 26%/36%.[20] Failure to make progress in the AWCP had significant implications for Enlisted and Office personnel relative to re-enlistment, promotion, civil schooling, and selection for command.

In early 2005 with the publication of FM 3.25-20 delayed and the Soldier Fitness School preparing to depart Fort Benning, the 75th Ranger Regiment established a center to development a new physical readiness training program for the Ranger Regiment. Considering the lessons learned during Operation Enduring Freedom (OEF) and Operation Iraqi Freedom (OIF) the Ranger leadership recognized the need to revise their physical training model and chose as their archetype the "combat tactical athlete". In response to the perceived need for higher levels of combat readiness demonstrated by engagements such as the Battle of Takur Ghar (Roberts Ridge), 75th Ranger Regiment leaders initiated the "Ranger–Athlete–Warrior" (RAW) program.[21] The initial objectives were to control PRT injuries, improve physical performance, and consolidate PRT efforts into a single program of instruction. In 2006 a planning team produced a RAW training manual (RAW v.1.0) with initial objectives and lessons learned. In 2007 the planning team produced RAW v.2.0, which addressed feasibility, acceptability, and suitability. In 2008 the regimental commander assembled a training staff that included physical and occupational therapists, a dietician, and an exercise physiologist to facilitate the development and implementation the "Ranger Athlete Warrior" (RAW) program. The training staff proposed a "master fitness training" model to "train representatives from each battalion (one per company) to become PRT subject matter experts (SMEs). These SMEs, along with the BN physical therapists, would serve as the primary resources within the BN for RAW training, scheduling, and assessments.[22] The end-state objectives of the RAW program were designed to ensure all rangers: (1) achieve a level of physical fitness commensurate with the physical requirements of ranger missions (functional fitness); (2) understand and choose sound nutritional practices (performance nutrition), (3) employ mental toughness skills to enhance personal and professional development (mental toughness); and (4) receive screening/education for injury prevention and prompt, effective, and thorough treatment/rehabilitation of injuries when they do occur (sports medicine). The training staff established a conceptual PRT framework, which was presented in the Infantry Task/Physical Component Matrix.[23]

In January of 2008, senior Ranger leaders approved a battery of RAW athletic and tactical assessment "tasks." These assessments were implemented across the Regiment to provide data that would guide future changes in the program.[24] The 10 assessment "tasks" were designed to measure strength, endurance, and mobility:[25]

1. Illinois Agility test—quickness and agility.
2. 4kg medicine ball toss—total body power.
3. Metronome Push-up – muscular endurance of upper body/core.
4. Pull-up—strength and endurance of grip and upper body (overhand grip).
5. 300 Shuttle Run—anaerobic endurance.
6. BEEP test—aerobic endurance.

7. Heel Clap—strength and endurance of grip/pulling/core.[26]
8. 185-pound bench press—upper body push strength.
9. 254-pound Dead Lift—total body lift strength.
10. Ranger Physical Assessment Test (RPAT)—all components of tactical fitness; 3 mile run + combat focused obstacle course (including a 185 SKEDCO pull), to be completed in one hour.

Infantry Task/Physical Component Matrix

Task	Strength	Muscular Endurance	Aerobic Endurance	Anaerobic Endurance	Flexibility	Motor Efficiency
Footmarch	X	XXX	XXX	X	X	X
Climbing	XXX	XX	X	XXX	XX	XXX
Sprints to Cover	XX	X	X	XX	XX	XXX
Crawl	XX	XXX	X	XXX	XX	XXX
Carrying	XXX	XX	X	XX	X	XX
Run	X	XX	XXX	X	X	X
Total	12	13	10	12	9	13

X = Low Demand
XX = Moderate Demand
XXX = High Demand

Figure 44. Ranger-Athlete-Warrior-Task Matrix.

As a result of the surge in Army manpower needs associated with Operations Enduring Freedom and Iraqi Freedom from 2001-2005, there was a significant increase in the number of marginally fit Soldiers accessed into the Army.[27] These marginally fit Soldiers were significantly more likely to become injured during initial and advanced military training. By 2005 there were a plethora of research studies and working groups focused on resolving the PRT "injury" problem. In 2006 the Department of Defense Injury Prevention and Performance Optimization Research Initiative allocated $5.3 million to funded research to determine injury reduction protocols for the Air Assault course at Fort Campbell, KY. The typical injury rate at the two-week Air Assault course was about 53%. In an attempt to reduce training injuries, the 101st Airborne Division entered into a partnership with the Neuromuscular Research Laboratory (NMRL) at the University of Pittsburg. After collecting data on strength, flexibility, aerobic capacity, and balance the NMRL, through the efforts of lead researcher Dr. Scott Lephart, came to the conclusion that there were fundamental flaws in the 101st Airborne Division's physical training program. By early 2009, Lephart had developed the Eagle Tactical Athlete Program (ETAP), which resulted in significant improvements in overall functional fitness. "Division-wide implementation of ETAP began in May 2009 utilizing the "Train the Trainer" strategy...utilizes an Instructor Certification School (ICS), which is a 4-day school designed to teach Non-Commissioned Officers (NCOs) how to implement ETAP with their respective units."[28]

In the fall of 2007 the USAPFS moved its headquarters to Fort Jackson, S.C. There were further reductions in personnel and the director's billet was changed from an Active Component Army officer to a civilian GS13 (formerly an AC-O6 billet, which had been down-graded to an AC-O5 billet in 1999). During 2007 the Physical Fitness School continued to work on the revised field manual and produced a final draft of FM 3-25.20 dated December 2007; however the draft was never approved for publication. During the summer of 2009 TRADOC established a revised command group for Initial Military Training (IMT). Lieutenant General Mark Hertling was selected as the deputy commanding general (DCG) in charge of Initial Military Training (IMT), which gave him command responsibility for the USAPFS. Based upon his lifetime interest in physical readiness training to include a master's degree in exercise science from Indiana University, a 3-year tour of duty in the Department of Physical Education at the United States Military Academy, and a PRT master's thesis at the Army War College, Hertling's initial guidance to the USAPFS Director, Mr. Frank Palkoska, was to complete and publish the PRT manual. After several attempts to identify a proper product type and series, Lieutenant General Hertling finally approved the publication of a new PRT manual as a training circular—TC 3-22.20 *Army Physical Readiness Training*. The "training circular" product was historically linked to the "training manual" designator used in the 1957 revision of FM 21-20, which resulted in the publication of the extensive training manual, *Physical Conditioning* (TM 21-200).

On 18 December 2009 *Army Training and Leader Development* (AR 350-1) was revised and superseded AR 350-1 (2006); this regulation is currently in force. There were several minor administrative changes that pertained to fitness assessments for various reactivated or recalled Soldiers. Recalled retirees on a temporary assignment are required to take an APFT and Soldiers over 55 are permitted to take an alternate cardio event without a medical excusal. Section 1-25, "Modern Army Combatives Training" was significantly enhanced. The US Army Combative School (a tenant of the US Army Infantry School—FT Benning) has proponency for Army combatives training. "Combatives training is a fundamental building block for preparing Soldiers for current and future operations and must be an integral part of every Soldier's life."[29] Four levels of instructor certification were established to ensure the development of a professional combatives instructor cadre that is essential to sustaining the combatives program.

During 2010, the 75th Ranger Regiment revised their PRT manual and published RAW PT v.4.0 (which is now in force).[30] There were no fundamental changes in scope or philosophy; however there were some significant changes to the fitness assessment "tasks." Two items were deleted (bench press, and "BEEP" test) and two new tasks were substituted: the 5-10-5 Pro Agility test was substituted for the Illinois Agility Run test and the standing broad jump was substituted for the 4kg medicine ball toss. Lastly the dead lift weight was lowered from 254 to 225 pounds, which completed the eight (8) item assessment "task" battery the Rangers use to measure strength, endurance, and mobility.[31]

1. 5-10-5 Pro Agility test—quickness and agility.
2. Standing Broad Jump—total body power.
3. 225-pound Dead Lift – total body lift strength.
4. Pull-up—strength and endurance of grip and upper body (overhand grip).
5. Metronome Push-up—muscular endurance of upper body/core.
6. Heel Clap—strength and endurance of grip/pulling/core.
7. 300 Shuttle Run—anaerobic endurance.
8. Ranger Physical Assessment Test (RPAT)—all components of tactical fitness; 3 mile run + combat focused obstacle course (including a 185 lb. SKEDCO pull), to be completed in one hour.

RAW v.4.0 provided numerous exercises designed to improve the six components of the Physical Tasks matrix. Following the base-build-peak periodized training model developed by Tudor Bompa and popularized by Joe Friel, v.4.0 presented detailed multi-week training programs for the "transition" phase (3 weeks), foundation phase (4-12 weeks), and various endurance and strength build phases. The basic workout model consists of three components: "preparation," exercise, and "recovery," which follows the exercise model presented in FM 3-22.20.[32] Perhaps the most significant addition to RAW v.4.0 was the section on performance nutrition. Dietary meal plans based upon a total energy intake of 3,000 and 4,000 kcal were presented based upon a macronutrient ratio of: 65% carbohydrate, 20% protein, and 15% fat.[33] RAW v.4.0 emphasized the benefits of rest and recovery and despite the elimination of the majority of the commonly held principles of exercise from TC 3-22.20 retained a robust list of eight principles of exercise: regularity, progression, overload, variety, recovery, balance, specificity, and precision.

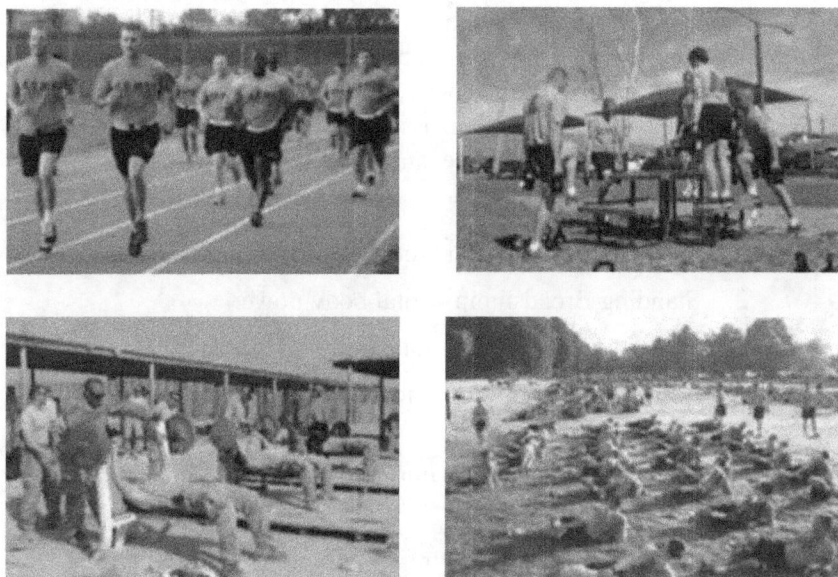

Figure 45. OEF/OIF Physical Readiness Training.

On 1 March 2010, Training Circular 3-22.20 was published by Headquarter, Department of the Army under the signature of General George W. Casey and superseded FM 21-20 (1992) and Change 1 (dated 1 October 1998). This manual is the approved physical readiness training doctrine for the active Army, Army National Guard, and US Army Reserve. TC 3-22.20 represents a comprehensive revision of Army PRT with a focus on preparing Soldiers, leaders, and units for the physical challenges of fighting in the full spectrum of operations. "Combat readiness is the Army's primary focus as it transitions to a more agile, versatile, lethal and survivable force."[34] TC 3-22.20 supports the ARFORGEN (Army Forces

Generation) model that utilizes the "reset," "train/ready," "available" phases to frame readiness training. Soldiers are trained to standards in mobility, strength, and endurance in the initial conditioning phase (future soldier), toughening phase, and the sustaining phase. The three overarching principles of PRT training are precision (adherence to optimal execution standards), progression (systematic increase in intensity, duration, and volume), and integration (using multiple training activities to achieve balance and appropriate recovery).

Training Circular 3-22.20 provides detailed guidance on conducting physical training. Leaders are to prepare Soldiers for physical training using the Preparation Drills. These 10 exercises are designed to warm and stretch muscles and prepare the body for vigorous exercise.[35] Chapter 9 presents various strength and mobility activities and Chapter 10 presents activities for endurance and mobility. Upon completing a vigorous exercise session, Soldiers use the five Recovery Drills for passive stretching and to bring the body back to a steady-state condition. Supplemental conditioning programs are provided for special circumstances and populations such as weight control, prolonged deployments, APFT improvement, reconditioning, etc. At the time of publication the 3-event Army physical fitness test was still the approved fitness test as described in Appendix A-1.

Shortly after the publication of TC 3-22.20, Lieutenant General Hertling provided additional guidance relative to the revision of the Army Physical Fitness Test (APFT). During a visit to the United States Military Academy, where Hertling served on a panel to review the final "senior" project for the Class of 2010 Kinesiology majors, he discussed his plans for a new Army physical readiness test. By June 2010 the USAPFS established a process for the revision of the APFT. On 26-27 October, 2010 the Physical Fitness School hosted an APFT Working Group for the purpose of revising the APFT. The agenda included an overview of Army PRT, a discussion of physical readiness attributes, defining physical readiness measures, defining test constructs, lastly developing potential courses of action for a new PR test. Nineteen professionals, representing the Armed Services, the US Service Academies, civilian universities, USARIEM, US Army Public Health, and the Army War College, attended the working group conference. The product of the conference was an initial draft of two new Army fitness tests—the Army Physical Readiness Test (APRT) and the Army Combat Readiness Tests (ACRT) and a timeline/process to finalize test construction and standards development.

The review and development process was tentatively scheduled for most of 2011; however, when Lieutenant General Hertling was selected as the new Commander, US Army in Europe and Seventh Army, the suspense for the development of the new APRT/ACRT was moved forward. With USAPFS as the lead, a five-item physical readiness test emerged in December, 2010 when Lieutenant General Hertling briefed General Martin Dempsey, Commander, TRADOC. The five test items were: standing long jump (2 trials)—explosive power, rower (1-min with no rest)—abdominal endurance, shuttle run (60 yards)—explosive power and agility, push-ups (1-min with no rest)—upper body muscular endurance, and the 1.5-mile run—cardiorespiratory endurance. Beginning in the summer 2011, the USAPFS initiated a feasibility pilot study for the 5-event APRT. Major General Richard Longo, Deputy Commanding General, Initial Entry Training, TRADOC replaced Hertling in late March, 2011 and initiated a formal review of the pilot study results in order to formulate a recommendation for the new APRT.

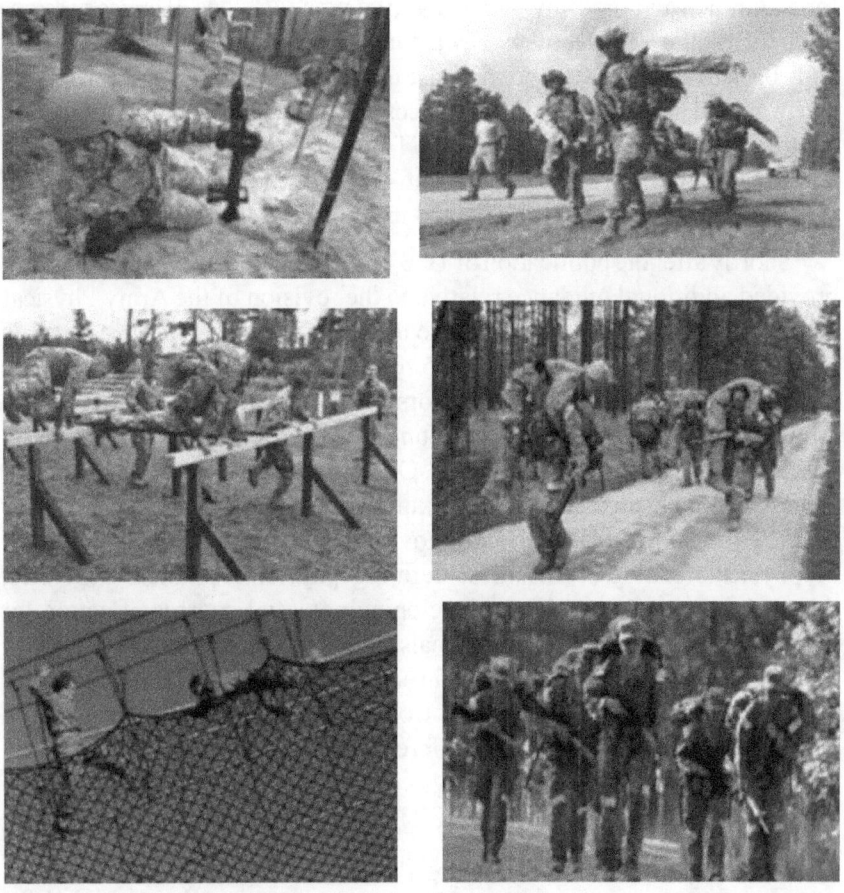

Figure 46. OER/OIF Combat Readiness Training.

In late 2011 as the results of the pilot study significant concerns emerged relative to the efficacy of the 5-event APRT and the feasibility of a functional ACRT test, to include concerns by the Command Sergeant Major of the Army. Shortly after assuming the duties as DCG-IMT on 2 March 2012 Major General Bradley May requested a pause in the APRT implementation in order to facilitate further review. May requested a supplementary external review by USARIEUM, the Department of Physical Education-West Point, and an independent university consultant. Each review expressed concerns about the developmental process and the potential testing events. These concerns were sufficient to convince TRADOC to terminate the current efforts to field a new APRT/ACRT and to initiate a comprehensive empirical study of baseline Soldier physical readiness requirements. Guidance from Army leaders was to link the performance assessment events to the physical requirements of Warrior Tasks and Battle Drills (WTBD) and Common Soldier Tasks (CST). Mr. Michael Haith from Human Dimension Integration (TRADOC) and Dr. Whitfield East from the Department of Physical Education (West Point) were selected as the co-leads for the baseline study. In October 2012 a working group with representatives from Army Public Health, Army Institute of Environmental Medicine, United States Military Academy and Uniform Services University meet at Fort Eustis for a 2-day working session to outline the study timeline. In December, 2012 General Cone (Commander, TRADOC) approved a 3-part Soldier Physical Readiness Requirements Study.

Part One involves a systematic review of current scientific research on physical training, to include injury prevention, physical standards development, physical training and assessment doctrine, and practices within the Army, sister services, and other militaries and vocations. Special attention will be given to these topics as they relate to age and gender. The findings of the systematic review will be used to influence how we assess baseline physical readiness, inform current Army physical training practices and doctrine, suggest ways to mitigate performance injuries, and shape the Master Fitness Training certification curriculum and instruction.[36] Part Two of the baseline study will involve identifying the physical requirements of WTBDs and CSTs and potential general and functional fitness assessments that can be used to measure these tasks. In Part Three the task measures will be validated through rigorous empirical assessments, which will yield a final battery of fitness assessment events. Once the final fitness events have been approved, the study team will undertake a performance analysis to establish criterion-referenced standards that will be applied to all Soldiers. The entire baseline Soldier physical readiness requirements study is expected to take 24-27 months

Notes

1. Richard P. Mustion, "Sustaining Our Army Then and Now," *Professional Bulletin of the United States Army Sustainment PB700-09-06 41:* (November-December 2009): online at http://www.almc.army.mil/alog/ issues/NovDec09/then_now.html (accessed 20 December 2011), 1; *Department of the Army Historical Summary, Fiscal Years 1990 and 1991,* ed. Scott W. Janes (Washington: US Army, Center for Military History, 1997), 31.

2. *Department of the Army Historical Summary, Fiscal Years 1990 and 1991,* 65, 124.

3. Department of the Army, FM 21-20 *Physical Fitness Training* (Washington, DC: US Government Printing Office. 1992), 99.

4. Department of the Army, FM 350-41 *Training in Units* (Washington, DC: US Government Printing Office, 1993), 16.

5. Department of the Army, FM 350-41 *Training in Units* (1993), 16.

6. Louis F. Tomasi, et al., *Age and Gender Performance on the US Army Physical Fitness Test* (Fort Benning, GA: Army Physical Fitness School, 1995), 2.

7. Tomasi, et al., *Age and Gender Performance*, 8-9.

8. Tomasi, et al., *Age and Gender Performance*, 1-2, 8-9; "Physical Fitness Policies and Programs," in *Assessing Readiness in Military Women: The Relationship of Body Composition, Nutrition, and Health* (Washington, DC: National Academic Press; 1998), 65.

9. Tomasi, et al., *Age and Gender Performance*, 1.

10. Stephen Moore, and James Carter, *The Strongest Economy in a Generation—If You're a Government Worker,* 15 November 1996, on http://www.cato.org/pub_display.php?pub_id=6254 (accessed 15 March 2011).

11. Department of the Army, Regulation 350-1, *Training: Active Duty Training for FORSCOM Units-FORSCOM* (Fort McPherson, Georgia: United States Army Forces Command, 2002), 19.

12. Department of the Army, Regulation 350-1, *Training: Active Duty Training for FORSCOM Units*, 19.

13. Department of the Army, Regulation 350-1, *Training: Training in USAREUR–USAREUR*, (Heidelberg, Germany: United States Army Europe Command, 2002), 31.

14. AR 350-15 *Army Physical Fitness Program* had already been superseded by AR 350-41 (1993).

15. Department of the Army, AR 350-1, *Army Training and Education* (Washington, DC: Government Printing Office, 2003), Section V: 1-21, 11.

16. Personal correspondence from Mr. Frank Palkoska, Director, USAPFS, 18 September 2011.

17. Department of the Army, AR 350-1, *Army Training and Leader Development* (Washington, D. C.: Government Printing Office, 13 January 2006), 11.

18. Department of the Army, AR 350-1, *Army Training and Leader Development*, 13.

19. Department of the Army, AR 600-9 *Army Weight Control Program* (Washington, DC: US Government Printing Office, 2006), 4. Body composition screening weights for 17-20 year old women/men for 60/72" respectively were: 128/132, 184/190, which represented significant increases in the maximum screening body weights for women from AR 600-9 (1987).

20. Department of the Army, AR 600-9 *Army Weight Control Program* (2006), 4-5.

21. During the Battle of Takur Ghar, a Ranger Quick Reaction Force (QRF) was deployed to rescue troops under attack at a forward observation post that had been overrun by insurgents; the second element of the Ranger QRF was off-loaded on Takur Ghar about 800 meters east and 2000 meters below the summit; fighting over rough terrain with several feet of snow, through a barrage of mortar and small arms fire, the Ranger QRF fought their way to the summit to rescue US troops.

22. RAW PT, v.3.0, (Fort Benning, GA: 75th Ranger Regiment, 2008), 1; "Further, Faster, Harder" (RAW Historical Briefing Slides) (Fort Benning, GA: 75 Ranger Regiment, 2011), Slides 2, 16.

23. "Further, Faster, Harder," Slide 4; Danny McMillian, "Ranger Athlete Warrior Program: A Systemic Approach to Conditioning," Infantry 96:3 (May-June 2007): 7.

24. Online at https://www.benning.army.mil/tenant/75thRanger/physical.htm (accessed 1 September, 2011); RAW PT v.3.0, 13 May, 2008, 72.

25. RAW PT, v.3.0, 72-79.

26. This test event was developed by the US Army Physical Fitness School in 2003 and was called the "heel hook" and is similar to the "ankles to the bar," a test event used at the United States Military Academy; online at: http://www.youtube.com/watch?v=-0Lywt1YDfk (accessed 3 January 2012).

27. During the summer surges of 2003 and 2004 approximately 10% of all Soldiers reporting to Fort Jackson failed the 1-1-1 (1-min push-ups, 1-min sit-ups, 1 mile run) initial physical fitness test; this could amount to as many as 150 Soldiers per week.

28. Online at http://www.pitt.edu/~neurolab/research/dod/dod.htm (accessed 10 January 2012); Allison M. Heinrichs, "University of Pittsburgh Strengthens Army Training," *Tribune-Review*, 23 August 2009; Jack Kelly, "Training to Prevent Injuries Gains Strength at an Army Base," *Pittsburgh Post-Gazette,* 02 September 2009; By the fall of 2011 over 1300 NCOs had enrolled and been certified through the 101st Airborne Instructor Certification School.

29. Department of the Army, AR 350-1, *Army Training and Leader Development* (Washington, DC: Government Printing Office, 2009), 13.

30. RAW PT, v.4.0, (Fort Benning, GA: 75 Ranger Regiment, 2010), 1.

31. RAW PT, v.4.0, 69-72.

32. A camera-ready copy of FM 3-22.20 was circulated in December,2007, however it was never authorized for dissemination

33. RAW PT, v.4.0, 102-3.

34. Department of the Army, TC 3-22.20 *Army Physical Readiness Training* (Washington, DC: Government Printing Office, 2010), xvii.

35. Some form of "warm-up" drill has been used by the Army since 1885 when Herman Koehler introduced "setting up" exercises at the United States Military Academy and Water Camp introduced his "daily dozen setup" during World War I.

36. Physical Fitness Training Information Paper, prepared for General Raymond T. Odierno, 4 January 2013.

Chapter 8
Summary, Analysis, and Discussion

To have good soldiers, a nation must always be at war.
—Napoleon Bonaparte

Summary and Analysis

"Safe behind its ocean barriers and supported by the intellectual ideals of its enlightenment-trained founders, America resisted the creation of a large standing military force as both unnecessary and dangerous to its liberty."[1] The founding fathers set the conditions for the Continental Army over 200 years ago with the decision to maintain a relatively small "standing" Army and plans to meet military threats through an intensive mobilization of civilian personnel. Constrained by this condition, the Army has endeavored with little success to establish a comprehensive and sustainable physical readiness training doctrine that enables all soldiers to develop and maintain the level of physical fitness required for combat readiness. "Every war in which the US has been involved since 1860 has revealed the physical deficiencies of our soldiers during the initial mobilization…casualties in initial engagements were attributed to the inability of our soldiers to physically withstand the rigors of combat…"[2] Due to the absence of a systemic and pervasive PRT doctrine with consolidated and enduring support from Army leaders, the Army's emphasis on physical readiness training has followed a sinusoidal pattern of surge and consolidation through multiple force mobilizations and times of peace. During the periods of rapid force mobilization military and civilian leaders bemoan the poor health and fitness of the civilian population and the extraordinary task of conditioning conscripts and volunteers for combat. During the periods of force consolidation political and economic influencers have caused national leaders to casually abandon the physical lessons learned from the Battle of the Somme to Task Force Smith, from the Ia Drang Valley to the Korengal Valley. Throughout its 200+ year history the United States Army has consistently failed to provide PRT programs and resources to adequately prepare soldiers for combat. Army leaders have essentially relegated physical readiness to the "and other duties as assigned" category of training.

> *The success and general efficiency of every military establishment is, in a very large degree, dependent upon the physical fitness, endurance, and condition of the individual units of which it is composed.*
>
> —William Lee Nash, Major General, USA

During the Army's first 100+ years the physical readiness training banner was born through force of will by charismatic military and civilian leaders. Early on, the nexus of Army physical readiness training was the United States Military Academy at West Point. With early influencers like Alden Partridge, John Kelton, Edward Farrow, and Herman Koehler, USMA "trained the trainers" who would ultimately bear the responsibility for physically training our Soldiers. Through their influence a young Second Lieutenant Franklin Bell (1878 USMA graduate) began a career-long advocacy of physical readiness training, which resulted in the first Army-wide General Order (No. 44) requiring Commanders to systematically develop and implement physical training programs for their soldiers. Although throughout the 1800's the Prussian and US Armies continually demonstrated the link between success in combat and individual soldier fitness, it was not until the post WWI years that the US Army truly embraced the contributions of physical conditioning as a force multiplier in combat.

At the onset of WWI the United States faced its first large-scale mobilization against a foreign enemy, which marked a significant turning point for Army PRT. Through the guidance of President Woodrow Wilson, Raymond Fosdick (Chairman, Commission on Training Camp Activities) engaged Dr. Joseph Raycroft (noted medical doctor and director of health and physical education at Princeton University) to lead the Army's efforts to train millions of volunteer and conscript Soldiers. Through the lessons learned from our European allies prior to 1918, Army PRT sharpened its focus on combat readiness, which culminated with the publication of *Mass Physical Training* (1920). Shortly after the Treaty of Versailles in 1919 and with his failed attempt to have the United States join the League of Nations, Wilson's influence waned as did the influence of Joseph Raycroft. Three lasting contributions from the WWI "training camps" program were: (1) the 3-month basic combat training model, (2) the "mass athletics" model promulgated by Raycroft, and (3) the founding of the Physical Training and Bayonet School at Camp Benning. This school served as the precursor to the Physical Fitness Schools that reemerged in 1946 at Fort Bragg and the Soldier Physical Fitness School that reemerged again in 1982 at Fort Benjamin Harrison. The implementation of the "physical training school" model began a long-term struggle between the US Army Infantry School and the Army over control of physical readiness training.

Due to forced consolidations during the Interwar Years, the Physical Training and Bayonet School was terminated and much of the impetus to enhance PRT was lost. During this interregnum the Army instinctively turned back to West Point for PRT guidance and Koehler's last publication, West Point Manual for Disciplinary Physical Training (1919), became the foundation for the next three Army PRT manuals—Training Regulation 115-5 (1928); *Basic Field Manual* (1936); and FM 21-20 (1941). All three manuals were published under the guidance of the Superintendent—United States Military Academy. Although the Army's physical readiness training program was successful in sustaining the professional Army, in virtually every after action review following WWI, WWII, and the Korean War military and civilian leaders expressed chagrin and angst over how poorly our citizen-Soldiers were prepared for the physical rigors of combat. "Of the first two million men examined under Selective Service, fully half were found unfit for military combat service."[3]

At the onset of WWII research in the science of exercise, conducted by civilian educators like Dudley Sargent, Charles McCloy, A.A. Esslinger, and Thomas Cureton, enhanced Army physical readiness training programs through more progressive program designs, improved conditioning drills, and the introduction of organized sports and combatives. The nexus of Army PRT again focused on developing combat readiness. The prime movers for Army PRT during WWII were Colonel Leonard Rowntree and Colonel Theodore Bank. These officers were critical to the formation of the Victory Corps and the insinuation of the science of exercise into Army PRT. With over 400,000 wartime casualties, WWII provided a surfeit of data to assess military preparation, training, and strategy. The analysis of these data clearly demonstrated the limitation of current Army PRT doctrine as published in FM 21-20 (1941) and resulted in the rapid action publication *Physical Training, Training Circular 87* (November, 1942).

One of the best examples of the transient nature of the Army's physical readiness training doctrine came from the leadership of the 2d Army during the ramp-up to WWII (1941-1942). In a 1941 training memorandum 2d Army Commander, Lieutenant General Benjamin Lear directed commanders to provide minimal emphasis on physical training and cautioned that excessive fatigue and exhaustion were to be avoided. Less than a year later Lieutenant General Lear directed that "physical hardening was to be brought to such a state that infantry units…are physically and emotionally prepared for the realities of the war."[4] His successor Lieutenant General Fredendall continued to emphasize physical conditioning when he directed that "All troops should undergo a course of training paralleling that of our Ranger Battalion...it would involve maximum physical hardening...."[5] The universal conclusion by Army leaders following WWII was you had to be fit to fight, and you had to train hard to be fit.

> *If all soldiers were physically hardened to the extent of being 'tough guys'... military operations would be a success.*
> —Lieutenant General Lloyd Fredendall, 1 June 1943

> *"Success in battle goes to the troops 'who can take one more step and fire one more shot' than the enemy."*
> —Colonel Lewis A. Walsh, Commanding Officer 517 Parachute Regimental Combat Team, 1944

With the print still fresh on the after action reviews following WWII and Korea proclaiming the benefits of physical readiness training to combat effectiveness, as a result of resource consolidation and indifference, Army-wide "interest" in PRT doctrine and training waned. By the end of 1953 the Physical Fitness School (FT Bragg) was terminated to save $225,000. As was the case in the early 1920's, the US Army Infantry School (USAIS) at Fort Benning stepped in and assumed responsibility for Army PRT doctrine and training. "The Ranger Department is charged with this Army-wide responsibility...the responsibility to monitor physical training Army-wide," make recommendations for policy and doctrine, prepare training literature and aids, conduct PRT research, and provide instruction to Officers and NCOs.[6] Over the next 30 years the USAIS worked to better understand and apply the science of exercise to physical readiness training. They conducted periodic seminars (1958, 1970, 1980), where military leaders and civilian exercise scientists worked to improve the quality of physical training programs and instruction. However, much of the Army's leadership still viewed physical conditioning as a wartime requirement and thus failed to ensure that Soldiers were properly prepared for the physical challenges of combat during the long intervals of peace.

Even with the significant rise in national consciousness regarding secular physical fitness that began in the late 1950's through the efforts of Presidents Eisenhower and Kennedy and the Council on Physical Fitness and Sport, significant reforms in Army PRT doctrine were not forthcoming. It was clear that military leaders "appreciated" the role of physical conditioning to success in combat; however as is so often the case, the universal acceptance of the need for well conditioned soldiers failed to translate into direct actions to ensure mission accomplishment. Based upon the continuous ebbs and flows in the US Army's commitment to physical readiness training, it is clear the Army has never truly institutionalized the importance of sustained combat readiness.

Beginning in the early 1970's two major paradigm changes significantly influenced Army PRT doctrine and assessment that would coalesce in the surge of the early 1980's. The first change resulted from the naissance of secular physical fitness. Americans were jogging for exercise and fun while reading Ken Cooper's new book *Aerobics* and Arthur Jones' Nautilus machines were popularized by the 1977 docudrama *Pumping Iron,* staring a young Arnold Schwarzenegger. The entire country became fixated with marathon mania and Frank Shorter and Bill Rodgers became national heroes. Through the birth of the fitness industry, as regulated by the American College of Sports Medicine, millions of Americans embarked upon their personal fitness journey. The second major paradigm change resulted from congressional legislation that allowed women to enroll at the nation's service academies. The United States was again at peace and some of the Vietnam War scars were on the mend when President Gerald Ford signed legislation opening enrollment in the US Service Academies to women on 7 October 1975. Sans the Army Nurse Corps, prior to 1976 women were mostly relegated to a limited number of administrative and clerical military occupational specialties.[7] Once women were enrolled at West Point, the Army faced two growing problems: (1) how to provide greater leadership opportunities that would qualify women Officers for advancement to higher rank and (2) how to develop a "separate but equal" physical readiness assessment process that would make women Officers competitive for positions of higher leadership.[8] Although women's physical readiness training and assessment had made significant progress since 1943, women still suffered from the perception as the "weaker sex" that the Army was preparing for non-combat roles.

As a result of these two paradigm changes, from 1979 to 1981 Army leaders formulated a plan to change the focus of PRT and assessment from "combat readiness" to health-related fitness and weight control.[9] The guidance from Army leaders prior to the publication of the 1980 revision of FM 21-20—*Physical Readiness Training* was to develop and implement a gender integrated physical readiness program and assessment. Prior to 1980 most men took the Advanced Physical Fitness Test, which purported to measure combat readiness by testing the inverted crawl, run-dodge-jump, horizontal ladder, bent leg sit-ups, and the two-mile run (in boots). Most women took the Advanced Physical Fitness Test, which was composed of the 80 meter shuttle run, run-dodge-jump, modified push-ups (from the knees), modified sit-ups, and one-mile run.[10] Due to a myriad of factors including the low intensity level of women's PRT and the parochial expectations and beliefs about the strength and endurance capabilities of women, Army leaders concluded that the men's Advanced Physical Fitness Test was too challenging for women, especially the horizontal ladder.[11] The perception that women were incapable of achieving any degree of functional fitness, even on a relative scale with men, caused the post-Vietnam ensemble of all-male Army leaders to make an unfortunate mistake.

Rather than doing due diligence to develop a common function fitness test and perhaps expecting more of women Soldiers in the physical domain, Army leaders scrapped the functional fitness assessments proscribed by FM 21-20 (1973) and FM 35-20 (1975) in lieu of a genderless physical fitness test. Based upon the parochial views of women at the time, this was simple solution to a complex social and physiological problem. Several concrete examples demonstrate just how misinformed Army leaders were about the physical capabilities of women Soldiers. We now know that the variation in aerobic capacity between men and women is about 10-12% for any distance—100meters to 100 miles. However, in FM 21-20 (1980) the delta between the 100-point performance time for men (13:05) and women (17:10) for the 2-mile run (17 year old) was 31.21%. To assuage concerns over massive numbers of women failing the 2-mile run (in boots), Army leaders set the 60-point (failure) time for women at 22:10. This baseline "run" time is just slightly faster than a brisk walking pace. The gender bias and associated lack of knowledge about women's anatomy and human performance was even more evident in the 60-point performance score for women's sit-ups = 27 repetitions. The 60-point sit-up performance score (1980) was so egregiously inaccurate that in FM 21-20 (1985) the 60-point performance score for sit-ups for 17 year old women was raised to 52 repetitions—a 93% increase.

The combination of a transition to a health-related fitness, concerns about women's strength and endurance, and the expanding role of women in the Army engendered the development of the 3-event Army Physical Readiness Test (APRT). The transition to a health-related fitness focus was reinforced by the resurrection of the US Army Soldier Fitness Center at Fort Benjamin Harrison by order of the Secretary of the Army, John O. Marsh, on 26 April 1982. The transition was completed when FM 21-20 (1985) was published and the title was changed from *Physical Readiness Training* (1980) to *Physical Fitness Training* (1985) and the APRT became the APFT. These name changes were more than symbolic; they represented a fundamental shift from combat-focused PRT to health-related PRT and assessment.

Although Army doctrine clearly identified the 3-event APFT as a tool for Commanders to determine a Soldier/unit's general fitness, it rapidly became the raison d'être for unit fitness. In an attempt to increase the emphasis on physical fitness, Army leaders inadvertently exacerbated the preoccupation with the 3-event test when they insinuated APFT performance into rank advancement and job selection through its inclusion in officer evaluation reports (OER) and non-commissioned officer evaluation reports (NCOER). Through selective attention, Soldiers and Commanders became more and more focused on APFT performance and less and less focused on combat-related and mission essential fitness. Throughout the 1980s and 90s it was relatively common for unit APFT reports to be the first item of business at quarterly training briefs.

Due to difficult economic times from 1988-89, the Army initiated cost-savings efforts based upon recommendations by the Vanguard Task Force. One of the BRAC casualties in 1990 was Fort Benjamin Harrison. As Fort Ben Harrison prepared to close, there were significant discussions concerning the disposition of the USAPFS. Initial plans were made to decentralize PRT doctrine and distribute authority to instillation commanders across the country. After significant discussions between the US Army Infantry Center (USAIC), Army Medical Department (AMEDD), and Training and Doctrine Command (TRADOC), the decision was made to move the US Army Physical School to Fort Benning and place it under the command of the USAIC.[12] The move from Fort Ben Harrison to Fort Benning marked the beginning of an inexorably slow 20-year transition from an emphasis on physical fitness back to an emphasis on combat readiness.

Army PRT doctrine drifted throughout the 1990s, as Army leaders were primarily preoccupied with concerns over age and gender equity in APFT standards and rising body fat concerns. The four USAPFS Commandants that served during the 1990s had no background in exercise science, and military and civilian resources dwindled. With the loss of personnel such as Tomasi, O'Connor, Bahrke, and Thomas most of the ongoing research was contracted out to CHPPM, USARIEM, and West Point. Although FM 21-20 was revised in 1992 and again in 1998, there were no substantial content changes and the 3-event APFT remained the Army's physical fitness test. The confounding factor for Army PRT during this 20-year period was the precipitous decline in youth fitness and concomitant increase in childhood obesity throughout the United States. During the late 1990s the US Army Recruiting Command found it increasing difficult to meet their recruiting mission as a result of a thriving economy and a decreasing number of qualified recruits due to poor fitness levels and excessive body fat.13 Unfit and overweight recruits also caused significant PRT issues in Basic Combat Training (BCT) as injury and attrition rates increased sharply and graduation rates declined.[14] With no resolution to these fitness and obesity issues by 2000, the Army initiated a decade of research and discussion on pre-accession physical fitness assessment, injury reduction, and attrition mitigation.[15]

When Muslim extremists attached the World Trade Center and Pentagon on 11 September 2001, the United States and the Army were once again at war. As has been the case throughout the history of the Army, we were unprepared to respond from a physical readiness perspective. The strength, power, endurance, and agility components of post WWII PRT were drowned out by the need to do more pushups and sit-ups. Through a lack of focus on warrior tasks and battle drills, the US Army was again playing catch-up. Fortunately as with the First Gulf War large scale combat operations were brief; in less than 30 days (19 March 2003 to 14 April 2003) joint US Forces defeated a poorly trained and disjointed Iraqi Army.[16]

Unfortunately sustained combat operations in Iraq and Afghanistan required to "win the peace" proved more onerous. Through repetitive deployment cycles of ever increasing lengths, acute and chronic orthopedic injuries, and the dwindling pool of qualified recruits, many active and reserve component units prepared to deploy significantly under strength. "An example representing this high degree of operational change is the tremendous number of soldiers and pieces of equipment that were cross-leveled into undermanned and underequipped RC [Reserve Component] units and then quickly trained and validated for deployment to Operation ENDURING FREEDOM (OEF) and OIF."[17] These manning issues had significant implications for many Army units. The testimony of personnel, in the Article 15-6 hearing s that followed the Abu Ghraib Prison incident, demonstrated the deep impact of waning forces generation:

> Because both of the USAR [US Army Reserve] units were significantly under strength before being deployed to Iraq, they received many soldiers from other USAR units country-wide to fill up their ranks. This process is known as "cross-leveling." Although it has the benefit of filling the ranks, it has the disadvantage of inserting soldiers into units shortly before deployment who had never trained with those units. The soldiers did not know the unit. The unit and the unit leadership did not know the

soldiers. The Army has always stressed 'you train as you fight.'[18]

Poor physical readiness also had a direct impact on combat operations during OEF/OIF. Grueling operations in inhospitable climates and unforgiving terrains against battle-hardened insurgents forced the Army to refocus physical readiness training. Company-grade Officers returning from command in Iraq and Afghanistan generally relate similar conclusions about physical readiness training and Captain Nick Billotta's reflections serve as a good exemplar of the physical needs in full spectrum combat operations.[19] From July, 2008 to July, 2009 Captain Bilotta served as the Alpha Company commander in RC East, Afghanistan. Alpha Company's area of operational (AO) was in Kunar Province; its company observation post (OP) was at 7,000 feet elevation, with an elevation range from 4,000 to 12,000 feet. The terrain was uncompromising and the enemy unforgiving. During the "fighting season" Alpha Company's Soldiers were in direct contact with the enemy on almost a daily basis. Due to significant loss of life, Alpha Company's AO was designated "the most violent place on earth." Captain Bilotta identified four elements that "mattered most" during his deployment: (1) communications, (2) medical support, (3) use of enablers, and (4) physical fitness. In discussing the physical needs of his soldiers, he concluded that many military operations failed because individual soldiers couldn't carry their combat loads in the rugged terrain. His summed up the need to be physically fit by stating: "it may not be the most important thing we do in a day, but it's the most important thing we do everyday." When asked, what was the single most important physical attribute required of soldiers during his command, Captain Bilotta replied, "stamina."

Discussion

> *In all history the relation between intellectual, political, and physical superiority has been a constant.20*
> —James E. Pilcher, The Building of the Soldier, 1892

Army Training and Leader Development (AR 350-1) states: "Commanders will conduct physical fitness programs that enhance Soldiers' abilities to complete Soldier or leader tasks that support the unit's FSO METL."[21] The primary mission of the US Army is to "fight and win the nation's wars"; all other concerns must subordinate to this end. Since its inception on 14 June 1775 the US Army has struggled to develop and implement a coherent physical readiness training program designed to prepare Soldiers for combat. Due to the myriad of organizational complexities the Army's PRT mission is complex and multidimensional. However, the solutions to these complexities, acknowledged time and again by Army and civilian fitness professionals, are clear and unequivocal. To successfully accomplish this mission the Army needs to address four outstanding issues:

Physiological needs of the modern combat Soldier:

The US Army cannot clearly define and operationalize the physiological needs of the modern combat Soldier. This physiological tableau must be scientifically based and sufficiently broad to prepare Soldiers for full spectrum combat operations in varying terrains and climates. Once the Army establishes the requisite physiological needs for combat, it can then develop applicable training programs and criterion-referenced assessments and standards to measure physical readiness and ensure success of our combat mission.[22] These performance assessments and concomitant standards can then serve as the sole determinant of combat readiness. By establishing a physiological basis of combat, the Army may bring some resolution the gender issues that have plagued Army PRT since the late 1970s.[23]

To sharpen our focus on how we think about physical readiness training and assessment in the Army, we can address five embedded issues. Using a macro/micro approach we must first define the physiological needs of the modern combat soldier. Although the US Army Physical Fitness School, the 75th Ranger Regiment (Ranger Athlete Warrior) and to a lesser degree the 101st Airborne Division (Iron Eagle Tactical Warrior) have made some progress in PRT development over the past six years, the Army has yet to empirically define the physiological needs of the modern combat Soldier. We have a myriad of first-person anecdotal reports from Soldiers, commanders, and fitness professionals that describe the physical nature of combat, but we have no empirical evidence. The closest we came was in 1942-43 when Drs. Esslinger and McCoy worked with Colonel Ted Bank developed a "combat focused" PRT program and then tested their program against known measures of endurance, stamina, and coordination and against existing Army PRT programs. These results provided the foundation for TC 87—*Physical Training* (1942) and DA Pam 21-9—*Physical Conditioning* (1944). To demonstrate the lack of empirical data, we have but to consider three rudimentary PRT questions. For the modern combat Soldier: (1) what is the proper balance between muscular strength and cardiorespiratory endurance; (2) which is more crucial to combat operations aerobic work capacity or anaerobic work capacity; and (3) what degree of mobility is required/expected based upon current combat loads?

Without empirically-based answers to these rudimentary questions, Army physical readiness training and assessment is just a "guess." Until we know the physiological needs of combat, we will continue to "rearrange the deck chairs on the Titanic" by refining, revising, and refocusing PRT programs and assessments based upon current fitness trends, attempts to reduce injuries and attrition, or the predilections of Army commanders and leaders.

Once we define the physiological needs of the modern combat soldier, we can then establish a cogent and coherent conceptual framework for physical readiness training. The intuitive context, the raison d'être, is combat performance. To function optimally in combat a Soldier must first develop a baseline of physical fitness that can be applied to mission essential or functional tasks. The marriage of physical and function fitness in PRT development will establish the contextual framework of functional combat fitness. The PRT framework or "form" can then support the PRT context or function (i.e., "train like you fight").

At the third level, need and context give way to an operational framework. This framework should be built around the concept of physical work capacity (PWC); i.e., the ability to perform physical work in a functional environment. The standard metric of physical work capacity is work volume, which is defined as the product of work intensity and work duration. Work intensity is a function of resistance (speed) x repetitions (distance) + rest. In producing combat-ready troops, Soldiers must be trained throughout the intensity physiologic spectrum with accommodations for proper rest/recovery. This PRT framework is perhaps easier to visualize graphically:

A proper operational framework takes us to the fourth level, which will allow the USAPFS to development periodized training plans that address the functional needs of combat by addressing the three physiologic systems. To perform optimal physical work Soldiers must develop and integrate all three physiologic systems: (1) neural—the brain sending efferent impulses to the muscles to incite muscle action, (2) portal—the heart and lungs sending oxygen and macronutrients to the muscles to provide fuel for metabolism, and (3) mechanical—the muscles, connective tissue, and bones providing structure for movement. The integration of these systems will allow us to develop a periodized training plan (i.e., a long range roadmap for physical readiness training) that incorporates the seven basic principles of exercise (regularity, progression, overload, recovery, balance, variety, and specificity) to optimize physical development and reduce organic injury.

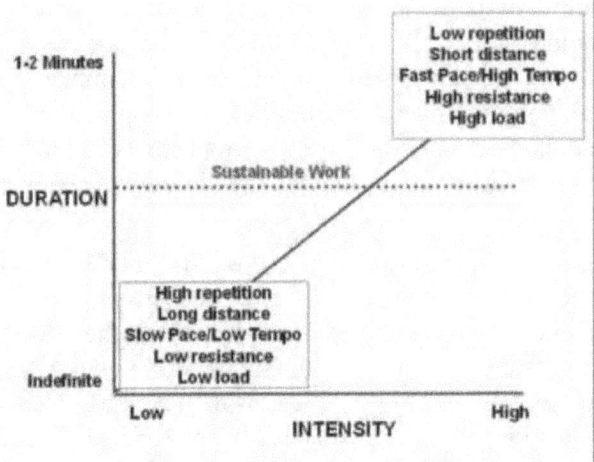

Figure 47. Physical Work Capacity Continuum.

The fifth developmental level addresses training frequency (how often we train) and training volume (how long/hard—duration x intensity). These components must be strictly coordinated with training recovery (i.e., the time required for a Soldier to rest between work bouts). Training recovery is in turn regulated by two factors: the physiologic characteristics of the individual Soldier and their current physiologic status. Failure to understand the rate at which a Soldier recovers and his/her current physiologic status and to incorporate that knowledge into the development and execution a periodized training plan will ultimately lead to organic failures.

There are many manifestations of a dysfunctional periodized training plan. In some cases Soldiers fail to develop adequate baseline levels of physical fitness. In other cases the lack of specificity results in a failure to acquire appropriate levels of functional fitness. However, one the most revealing symptoms of a dysfunctional PRT plan is a high number of organic failures (injuries), which seems to be the case in the Army.[24] For CY2004 Ruscio et al. estimated that Service members (DoD-wide) had over 2 million injury visits for acute and chronic (overuse) injuries affecting approximately 900,000 Service members at a cost of hundreds of millions of dollars and resulting in over 25,000,000 days of limited duty.[25] In 2006 the Department of Defense recorded an estimated 743,547 musculoskeletal injuries at a cost of over $2.2 billion.[26] To better understand how relatively minor changes in a physical readiness training plan can mitigate injuries (and therefore attrition), saving millions of dollars in lost productivity; it is instructive to compare combat basic training for the Marines and the

Army. The annual injury rate for Marine Corps Depot, Paris Island is approximately 11.7% per year. The historic BCT injury rate for the Army is approximately 17% per year. There are two primary differences in Army and Marine PRT programs that result in lower injury rates at the Paris Island Depot. First, Marine Corps basic training is 12 weeks versus 10 weeks for the Army. The additional two weeks allow the Marine Corps to increase training volume at a slower rate (i.e., moderating increases in overload and increasing recovery time). Second, the Marine Corps utilizes a DEP (delayed entry program) fitness development program that requires recruits to participate in organized physical training prior to shipping to the MEPS (prehabilitation). While in DEP, "Marine Corps Recruiters will help them prepare physically, and will provide information to help them adjust to their future in the Marine Corps."[27] While extending the length of combat basic training or deploying a pre-enlistment PRT program would not be trivial endeavors for the Army, minimizing training injuries, reducing recruiting costs, decreasing BCT attrition rates, and reducing rehabilitation costs make the benefits of a holistic, research-based PRT program worth the cost.

Resourcing PRT: facilities, equipment, and time

For over 100 years military and civilian fitness professionals have counseled the Army on the need for proper facilities, equipment, and time to conduct PRT. Each year the Army loses hundreds of millions of dollars in productivity due to organic injuries in basic or advanced combat training and Soldier attrition due to a lack of resources.[28] These losses can be significantly minimized with access to proper facilities and equipment and adequate training time:

> Soldiers are combat systems, and the gym and the PT field is the motor pool and maintenance facility for that combat system. Fitness is an integral part of readiness and survivability on the battlefield.[29]

The contributions of physical readiness to combat performance are not in disputable. High levels of physical conditioning provide Soldiers with three significant performance advantages: (1) an increased high and low intensity work capacity, resulting in increased functional fitness, (2) an increased mental toughness and perseverance (will to win), and (3) a decreased risk of injury, resulting in increased survivability due to all-cause morbidity and combat-related injuries. The salient question is, when so many military and civilian leaders proclaim the importance of physical readiness, why has the Army continually failed to properly resource physical readiness training? Terms, like "pentathelete" and "Soldier athlete," are common place in Army parlance and Army training manuals laud the benefits of high levels of physical conditioning. In addition we clearly know "what right looks like" relative to performance training. Why then does the Army continually under resource PRT facilities, equipment, and time. Although counterintuitive, the simple answer is physical readiness training is not important to the Army; however, answers to complex organizational issues are rarely simple. The Army is a large, diverse organization with finite resources.[30] In a resource constrained environment, the sheer size of the force makes it difficult to provide proper facilities, equipment, and time.[31]

During the ramp-up to WWI from 1916-1918, the Army was tasked to in-process, house, clothe, feed, and train large numbers of volunteer and conscript soldiers. At that time and in that place the Army's only training model was the Turnverein (playground) model, where large numbers of students/athletes gathered outdoors and participated in group calisthenics, exercises, and drills. Even with Colonel Herman Koehler's lifelong efforts to encourage the Army to build suitable gymnasia and weight rooms on each Army instillation, there were few facilities available for physical training at the start of WWI; certainly relative to the large number of Soldiers that required training. Almost 100 years later the Army still utilizes the playground/Turnverein model to mitigate the "limited facilities"—"large numbers" issue. By arranging Soldiers in large unit formations on outdoor fields the Army has eliminated the need for gymnasia and weight rooms and also minimized personnel needs by optimizing the leader-to-lead ratio. Historic "facility" constraints also forced the Army to adopt a "unit physical training" (unit PT) model to implement its physical readiness training program. Although there are arguably some team-building benefits from "unit PT," a platoon- or company-sized extended rectangular formation is not a productive exercise environment.

In 1913 Captain Merch B. Stewart, who would ultimately serve as the 33rd Superintendent of the United States Military Academy, proposed the solution to the "unit PT" problem. In the introduction to his book *Physical Development of the Infantry Soldier* he stated:

> In the training of the soldier, the greatest benefit is not derived by indiscriminate and impartial use of these exercises. Each individual soldier presents a special problem in physical training; each should be studied and diagnosed as to his particular requirements and each should be given the training his condition requires.[33]

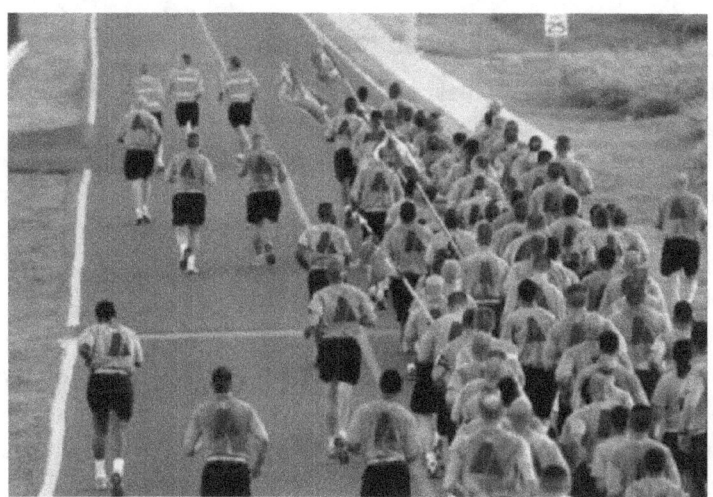

Figure 48. Unit Formation Run. [32]

When is the last time an athletic team exercised as a unit? The answer is—never. You may see teammates lifting or running together and you will certainly see players executing "skill drills" (mission essential tasks) as a unit; however modern athletes never exercise/train as a "unit." Virtually all athletes train in alone (with a strength or running coach) or dyads or in very small groups of three, four or five. The "dyad/small group" model allows athletes to optimize their exercise bout to ensure proper warm-up and maximize overload and progression through appropriate use of duration and intensity. Individualized exercise prescriptions allow athletes (and potentially Soldiers) to achieve physical performance outcome goals in the most effective and efficient manner.

Regardless of adherence to precision and progression as specified countless Army PRT manuals (including the current TC 3-22.20), the Army's "unit PT" model makes it virtually impossible to address the intensity and duration needs of the individual Soldier and therefore hinders progression. Also, due to the limitations on facilities and instructors, large unit PT sessions tend only to focus on two fitness domains: muscular endurance and cardio-respiratory endurance. Soldiers are constrained by the "unit PT" model to sub-maximal, repetitive, body weight exercises. In a 2003 survey of 2,000 active duty Officers and NCOs, a significant number of respondents stated that "unit PT" interfered with their personal exercise prescription to the point it diminished their overall physical readiness.[34] Clearly some units (Army Rangers, Special Forces, Delta Force, etc.) have resolved these issues by limiting physical readiness training to very small groups (often just a battle buddy or a squad-size element) and by developing ancillary PRT programs and assessments that address the METL needs of the individual combat soldier (the Ranger-Athlete-Warrior program and the Iron Eagle Challenge—101st Airborne Division are just two examples). We see more and more "rogue" PT programs throughout the Army as various "units" build their own "CrossFit" facilities, purchase their own "Bowflex" equipment, and implement the exercise program de jure like P90X in an attempt enhance combat readiness. The focus of all of these PRT programs is the individual Soldier.

The "numbers" issue also creates problems scheduling PRT. The Army's solution has been to execute PT outside the duty day (at 0630), on a patch of dirt proximal to the Company area, with limited/no equipment. Although convenient for the Army, the 0630 PT schedule is problematic on many levels. Since the "duty day" generally starts at 0900, starting PRT at 0630 conveys to active component Soldiers the notion that PRT is an ancillary duty, not to be confused with their "real job," which happens during the duty day. 0630 is also likely the worst time of the day to conduct physical training; the body is less hydrated and muscles are cold, stiff, and generally out of fuel. Many of the early Army PRT leaders recommended 1000 (or 1-2 hours after breakfast) as the optimal time to conduct physical training.[35]

The "numbers" issue also exacerbates facility and equipment availability for training and assessment. Pull-up/dip bars are often the only "equipment" available to units. During the 1980 APRT revision, one of the primary considerations for event selection was "no equipment," therefore the Army jettisoned the run-dodge-jump and horizontal ladder. During the 2010 revision of the APFT command guidance again specified a minimal need for equipment, even casting doubt on the feasibility of including pull-ups in the APRT. Large unit formations make it impractical to provide proper equipment to facilitate the development of strength and power.

In a resource constrained environment, the daunting problem is how can the Army optimize PRT to improve the physical readiness of combat troops? Perhaps leaders my find one solution by answering this question: which Soldiers actually need to be "combat ready"? Does the Army really need every Soldier to have the same level of physical work capacity and functional fitness? Does a 68G—Patient Administrative Specialist or a 91B—Wheeled Vehicle Mechanic need to have the same level of combat readiness as an 11B—Infantryman? In seeking an answer to this question, it may be beneficial to analyze force structure relative to PRT training and expectations in the US Navy. The current strength of the active duty Navy is approximately 460,000; somewhat comparable to the Army. The Marine

Corps makes up approximately 40% of all active duty Navy personnel (around 200,000 troops). Based upon their combat mission the Marine Corps has designed and implemented a significantly more aggressive physical readiness training and assessment program than the Navy at large. If we consider the Marine Corps to be the combat arms element of the US Navy, perhaps Army leaders might extrapolate that split-operations (split-ops) model to Army PRT. If key leaders can identify those Soldiers with a direct combat or tactical mission, it may be more judicious to design, resource, and implement a unique combat-focused PRT program for this smaller population.

In the 2008 revision of FM 3-0—*Operations*, the Army reorganized warfighting functions into six combined arms elements: mission command, movement and maneuver, intelligence, fires, protection, and sustainment. Although each element of combat power is crucial to overall mission success, the likelihood of mission command, intelligence, and sustainment personnel directly engaging the enemy in combat is relatively small. The Army may benefit by formally recognizing this needs dichotomy as it pertains to PRT. In the past the Army has used terminology such as "combat" and "combat support/support services." It might be useful to differentiate personnel assigned to strategic and upper echelon operational levels as "combat operations support" and personnel assigned to lower echelon operational and tactical levels as "combat operations" with regard to PRT. The Army could then develop a differentiated PRT model similar to the Navy to more judiciously utilize resources and better meet the distinctive needs of these two populations.

This would not be the first time the Army utilized multiple PRT training and assessment models. During the 1960s the Army had at least three physical readiness training and assessment models: (1) the male combat Soldier (FM 21-20), (2) the male Staff and Specialist Personnel (DA Pam 21-1), and (3) the female Soldier (FM 35-20 & PAM 21-2). Semantics aside, perhaps the terms "tactical" and "operational" more appropriately classify the multi-echeloned PRT needs of the Army. This prioritization of effort would allow the Army to design and execute at least three levels of physical readiness training: (1) Basic PRT for initial military training (BCT, AIT, OSUT), (2) Operational PRT for Soldiers in combat support operations, and (3) Tactical PRT for Soldiers with a direct combat mission. Recent efforts by the Australian Defense Force (ADF) have resulted in a similar "tiering" of physical readiness. Under the auspices of establishing "physical employment standards" (PES) the ADF established three levels of military performance: basic fitness assessment (similar to Initial

Entry Training), "all Corps" assessment, combat arms assessment, and commanding officer fitness assessment [36]

Basic PRT could be designed to develop baseline fitness levels in Soldiers during initial military training (IMT) and would follow the highly prescriptive program set forth in TC 3-22.20.[37] Considering the generally poor initial physical status of many recruits, the use of body-resistance exercises with minimal equipment like pull-up/dip bars and kettle bells would likely suffice to prepare Soldiers for Operational and Tactical physical readiness training. Due to the need for significantly greater command and control during IMT, the Army could use the Drill Sergeant School to properly train NCOs on the exercise principles of precession, progression, and integration. It would likely be appropriate and useful to develop a Basic PRT assessment for all IMT Soldiers as an indicator of their readiness to move on to Operational/Tactical PRT. The results of Basic PRT would greatly enhanced by extending the length of basic combat training to 12 weeks, similar to the Marine Corps (13 weeks), the Australian Defense Force (80 days), and the British Army (14 weeks) and by initiating a PRT program while a recruit is in the delayed entry program (DEP).[38]

Operational PRT (O-PRT) could be designed to sustain/enhance the fitness foundation obtained during initial military training for Soldiers assigned to non-combat roles. O-PRT would utilize a highly individualized approach with a greater emphasis on physical fitness and weight control. As a general rule there would be no unit physical training. Unit PT sessions would be used to enhance unit cohesion, while the preponderance of O-PRT would be conducted by the individual Soldier on their personal time. "A personal [fitness] program significantly improves a soldier's performance in a selected component of fitness, and the benefits may compensate for any shortfall not obtained in group sessions."[39] Personal time, before, during, or after the duty day, could be used for physical training. Soldiers assigned to the O-PRT program would participate in periodic fitness assessments using traditional physical fitness tests such as push-ups, dips, pull-ups, crunches, and low intensity endurance runs. Operationally-specific norm-referenced scales, based upon a criterion-referenced pass/fail standard, would be used to determine compliance with PRT requirements and expectations. Regularly scheduled Army weight control body composition assessments would also be conducted. Soldiers should be allowed/encouraged to access Moral-Welfare-Recreation (MWR) or private training facilities and personal trainers to ensure regularity and progression in their PRT plan. Due to the distributed nature of O-PRT, the Commander may require Soldiers to submit a quarterly training plan and/or an accountability log to ensure compliance with stated fitness goals. Fitness assessments for O-PRT Soldiers should be conducted on a quarterly basis.

> *It appears very probable that the conditions of a future war will force us to outfight the enemy rather than out produce him.*
>
> —Lieutenant Colonel Frank Kobes, USMA, 1958

Tactical PRT (T-PRT) could assume a decidedly more combat-readiness focus, concentrating on the development of speed, power, agility, strength and stamina to enhance the successful execution of warrior tasks and battle drills. Due to the reduced requirements and manpower savings from O-PRT and reduced loss of productivity associated with B-PRT, the Army could re-allocate these resource savings to tactical PRT. Appropriate resistance, combative, and non-impact cardio training facilities could be developed at the division or battalion level. Individual exercise prescriptions would be established for every tactical soldier and most T-PRT would be conducted in small homogeneous teams (buddy teams or squads). Developmental guidelines and model programs would be provided by the US Army Physical Fitness School. With a focus on physical fitness and functional fitness, T-PRT would be assessed with two distinct tests. The USAPFS is currently working on the Army Physical Readiness Test (APRT) and Army Combat Readiness Test (ACRT), which may adequately assess tactical PRT. The proposed APRT contains 5 test items designed to measure speed, power, endurance, and agility. The proposed ACRT is a high intensity, short duration functional fitness assessment designed on obstacle course format.[40] If physical readiness assessments can be segregated by mission needs, we could increase the specificity of T-PRT assessments, thereby increasing content validity by allowing the assessment to focus only on combat readiness. Based upon the current USAPFS model, Soldiers preparing for combat operations would take the APRT and ACRT once each year, approximately six months apart and must take a pre-deployment ACRT within 30 days of deploying.

Education and training for PRT instructors.

In 1983 the Army established an instructor training program (Master Fitness Trainer), with an associated Army skill identifier (03C); however the MFT program was terminated in 1989 due to lack of support from key leaders.[41] The prevalence of "rogue" PRT programs, sanctioned by unit commanders, creates the potential for serious performance and injury problems for the Army. Resolution #8 of the 1970 USAIS Physical Fitness Symposium (FT Benning) recommended "that an Army Physical Fitness

Institute to train selected officers and enlisted men would contribute immeasurably to the Army Physical Fitness Program."[42] Many modern armies utilize certified physical fitness instructors to develop, implement, and monitor basic and tactical PRT.

The Australian Defense Force (ADF) is an excellent exemplar. The ADF established a Physical Training School (ADFPTS) at CERBERUS (Westernport, VIC) in 1989. The school conducts a myriad of physical training courses to include the initial and advanced Physical Training Instructor (PTI) and Military Fitness Leader (MFL) courses. "PTIs are qualified to design, conduct, evaluate and review the unit's physical training programs to develop physically conditioned personnel to support commanders in executing their operational tasks."[43] The PTI instructor course is 18 weeks where participants are taught the theoretical and practical aspects of physical training including topics such as advanced anatomy and physiology, exercise physiology, morphology and testing, group exercise leadership, nutrition, first aid/athletic training, sport leadership, and sport psychology. Duties of a PTI are as follows:

1. Plan and conduct physical training instructional sessions.
2. Provide individual and group physical training programs.
3. Provide initial management of sports injuries.
4. Conduct physical training assessments.
5. Conduct obstacle course training.
6. Implement and monitor occupational health/safety in the physical training environment.
7. Apply, supervise and manage injury prevention strategies.
8. Promote health and fitness awareness.
9. Officiate, coach and coordinate sporting competitions.
10. Provide advice to the Commanding Officer on physical training, injury prevention, rehabilitation and Military Self Defense.
11. Instruct and supervise Military Self Defense.
12. Instruct on Combat Fitness Leaders Courses.
13. Rehabilitation of soldiers; and education on health and fitness.[44]

The PTIs rank structure is equivalent to US Army ranks of E2-E6 and WO1-WO2 and is considered a military occupational specialty. The ADF also certifies Combat Fitness leaders (CFL) who are Soldiers embedded in their units that are uniquely trained and qualified to lead combat-focuses physical training. CFLs are alwsays under the supervision of a PTI. Although PTIs would be beneficial to any tactical unit, they would be especially useful at the basic and advance training schools, which would significantly reduce the workload for Army Drill Instructors.[45]

By way of analogy, understanding the modern Division I (D1) football team might help us understand the benefits of a certified physical training instructor to the US Army. The physical training program for a D1 football team is directed by a certified strength and conditioning coach. This coach designs a periodized training program based upon the needs of each position (linemen, cornerbacks, running backs, etc.). The strength and conditioning coach then explains the training program to the athletes and position coaches, and then provides any technical assistance pertaining to execution. Under the direction of the position coach, the athlete executes the periodized training program while participating in periodic evaluation to assess progress.

How is this model applicable to the Army? A large D1 football team generally has around 120 athletes, approximately the same size as an Army Company. The certified Company "physical training instructor" (C-PTI) would be analogous to the certified strength and conditioning coach. The C-PTI would in turn follow Captain Merch Stewart's recommendation that each Soldier be "studied and diagnosed as to his particular [training] requirements and each should be given the training his condition requires."[46] Once each Soldier has his/her periodized training plan, a platoon sergeant or team leader would manage implementation and adherence. By maintaining small, homogeneous training cells Soldiers could optimize the duration and intensity of every workout, therefore ensuring optimal overload, progression, and recovery. These smaller training cells would also maximize the use of facilities and equipment by scheduling off-cycle training that doesn't conflict with other cells in the Company:

> …it was apparent from [my] experiences of the World War that a course of training should be planned…to qualify [Officers] as physical directors and instructors of their future commands. They must learn, not only how to perform themselves, but how to teach others. They must understand the means by which then can most speedily and efficiently bring their men to the necessary physical condition.[47]

Another important facet of the physical training instructor issue is Officer PRT education. Traditional officer candidates can acquire these skills, abilities, and knowledge during their undergraduate education. ROTC cadets could complete a course of study (or perhaps a minor) in exercise fitness/leadership that address the topics included in the ADF PTI course. West Point cadets currently enroll in a 1.5 credit hour Fundamentals of Personal Fitness and a 1.5 credit hour Army Fitness Development course (unit fitness), which address most of the topics in the ADF PTI curriculum. A master fitness trainer-like curriculum, either resident or through distance learning, could to be developed and implemented in the Officer Candidate School program of instruction to ensure all Officers have a fundamental understanding of the science of exercise training, prescription, and assessment. These certified Second Lieutenants would design and supervise the Platoon/Company-level physical readiness plan, while providing support and mentoring to the "physical training instructor" NCO.

PRT Research and Development for the Army

Research and development are the seed corn of any organization. The evolutionary nature of the physical requirements for combat makes it imperative that the Army commit to a comprehensive PRT research and development program by resourcing a centralized and unified effort.[48] On numerous occasions military and civilian leaders have articulated the need for a comprehensive research program to support the development of physical readiness training doctrine. Resolution #2 of the 1970 USAIC Physical Fitness Symposium recommended "that a national research and documentation center is needed to serve as a national focal point for research on physical fitness."[49] In the 1980 *Department of Defense Study of the Military Services Physical Fitness,* the assembled working group recommended that the Department of Defense establish an Armed Forces Physical Fitness Academy (PFA). The mission of the PFA was to: develop physical training programs and assessments, train a cadre of physical training instructors; conduct and direct interservice physical fitness research, maintain contact with foreign Army PT organizations, and establish a career field (MOS) for physical training instructors.[50] The "physical fitness academy" concept was implemented with the founding of the Soldier Physical Fitness Center in 1982. In the coordinating memorandum signed by Lieutenant General Julius W. Becton, Deputy Chief for Training (TRADOC) the role of the Soldier Physical Fitness Center was to provide physical fitness programs and testing for combat units by providing information, research, and consultation. From 1983-1990 the School was sufficiently resourced to manage PRT doctrine, develop and implement the Master Fitness Trainer certification program, and maintain a broad-based research initiative. With the pending reduction in resources and scope mandated by the Vanguard Task Force in 1991, the Physical Fitness School began a two decade decline relative to the research mission even though the 1991 coordinating memorandum stated that "the mission of the USAPFS will include: fitness doctrine preparation and writing; research of the fitness needs of the Army; standardization of fitness requirements within the Army; fitness policy development; and training assistance to the Army."[51]

Until recently there were at least seven (7) organizations (civilian and military) conducting PRT research and development for the Army: the Institute for Environmental Medicine (USARIEM), the Center for Health Promotion and Preventative Medicine (CHPPM), the Army Research Lab (ARL), the Army Research Institute (ARI), University of Pittsburg—Neuromuscular Research Lab, the Army Physical Fitness Institute (APFRI), and the Department of Physical Education at the United States Military Academy. With meager resources the 75th Ranger Regiment has attempted to fill the void in applied PRT research for the last six years. However, these efforts have been indiscriminate and fragmented, regularly engaging "pop-up targets" (IET attrition, IET injury rates, Air Assault injury rates, etc.) rather than pursuing a systematic, long-range research agenda. These disjointed efforts by disparate organizations often produce redundant and overlapping research in an attempt to resolve dissonant PRT problem. The Eagle Tactical Athlete Program, developed by the University of Pittsburg and implemented in the 101st Airborne Division, is the best exemplar of this fragmented process.

For the Army to regain the momentum in PRT there is a need to resource a modern, comprehensive combat-focused fitness research program that will drive physical readiness training and assessment. We have but to compare the secular advances in the science of exercise and human performance over the past 30 years with current Army PRT doctrine to understand the gross disparity. Here are four basic research questions that demonstrate the depth of our lack of understanding: (1) what are the baseline physical attributes that constitute combat readiness; (2) what are the frequency, duration, and intensity of training required to illicit these physical attributes, (3) what fitness measures best assess these physical attributes; and (4) what resources (trainers, facilities, and equipment) are required to facilitate acquisition of these physical attributes in a timely manner while mitigating organic failures. We currently cannot answer even these basic questions to any degree of scientific acceptability. Only PRT doctrine grounded in the science of exercise and human performance can prepare Soldiers, leaders, and units to fight in the full spectrum of operations.

The most precious and irreplaceable resource in the US Army is the individual Soldier. We must do all we can to develop and preserve this resource. Throughout the history of the Army physical readiness training has been universally recognized as a force multiplier that enhances combat effectiveness, resilience, and survivability on the battlefield. We spend billions of dollars each year developing and producing tactical weapons and funding the associated training necessary to deploy them. Although we have the most technologically advanced Army in the world, our commitment to physical readiness training is derisory by comparison. As the Army moves to a smaller, lighter, more mobile force in the fight against the global war on terrorism, a long-term, comprehensive commitment to the highest quality physical readiness training is mandatory to ensure our future success.

> *Nations have passed away and left no trace, and history gives the naked cause of it--one single, simple reason in all cases; they fell because their people were not fit.*
>
> —Rudyard Kipling

Notes

1. Richard W. Stewart, *American Military History Volume I: The United States Army and the Forging of a Nation, 1775-1917*, ed., (Washington, DC: Center for Military History, United States Army, 2005), Epilogue, 387.

2. Department of the Army, FM 21-20 *Physical Readiness Training* (Washington, DC: US Government Printing Office, 1980), 1-2.

3. Lyle M. Spencer, and Robert K. Burns, *Youth Goes to War* (Chicago: Science Research Associates, 1943), 165.

4. Bell L. Wiley, and William P. Govan, *History of the Second Army* (Study No. 16) (Washington, DC: Historical Section, Army Ground Forces, 1946), 108, 111.

5. Wiley and Govan, *History of the Second Army*, 122.

6. *Physical Fitness Seminar Report*, (Fort Benning: United States Army Infantry School; April 1958), 2.

7. Brian P. Mitchell, *Women in the Military: Flirting with Disaster* (Washington, DC: Regnery Publishing, Inc., 1998), 11; "In 1965, 70 percent of enlisted females were in administrative and clerical work...."

8. Mitchell, *Women in the Military*, 11; "Until 1976 the highest pay grade or rank a woman could hold in any of the services was O-6."

9. Most professionals associated with Army PRT over the past 30 years acknowledge that the shift in PRT from combat readiness (i.e., functional fitness) to personal health and fitness was the most detrimental change to Army PRT. With the stereotypical perception of women's physical capabilities vice upper body/core strength and functional fitness in 1980, it is beyond speculation to conclude that the health-related PRT focus and 3-event APFT were designed in part to make the PRT "fair" for women. This perception and the resultant actions have likely done more to harm women and to the Army than any other single event other than overt discrimination. A relatively significant number of military personnel are satisfied to meet the minimum physical requirements for service. As such, if you set the "bar" too low, as has been done for the pass/fail standards for women relative to physical performance, you establish a caste of second-class Soldiers. By way of presenting a single data point that supports this assertion, during the fall term 2011 women USMA cadets averaged 96 points and 92 points respectively on the push-up and 2MR test; men averaged 93 and 88. The average 3-event total for women = 284 (n=909) and men = 271 (n=4882). The delta between the average women's 2MR time = 15:38 and men = 13:39 equals approximately 2 minutes, which is a 14.52% delta. By normative comparisons of men and women on runs of this length, the delta should be about 10.5%; these disparities can be attributed to improper standards, which are insufficient to extrinsically motivate women to achieve optimal performance.

10. Department of the Army, FM 35-20 *Physical Training-Women's Army Corps* (Washington, DC: US Government Printing Office, 1975), 174.

11. A similar change occurred at the United States Military Academy when the parallel bar "traverse" (one of the 11 obstacles in the Indoor Obstacle Course

Test) was eliminated (cadets assumed an extended-arm support position on a set of Olympic parallel bars and "hand walked" the length of the bars) and was replaced by the balance beam "traverse."

12. The USAPFS was to be placed on the TDA for the USAIC and the USAPFS Commandant was to be rated by the Commander, USAIC and senior rated by TRADOC Deputy Commanding General for Combined Arms.

13. US Army Recruiting Command failed to meet their recruiting mission in 1998, 1999, and 2005; data online at http://www.usarec.army.mil/hq/apa/goals.htm (accessed 6 December 2011).

14. Joseph J. Knapik, et al., "Seasonal Variations in Injury Rates during US Army Basic Combat Training," *Annals of Occupational Hygiene* 46: (2002): 18; Time loss injury rates for Army BCT were 18.9% for a fall sample and 37% for a summer sample.

15. "Physical Fitness and Musculoskeletal Injury," in *Assessing Fitness for Military Enlistment: Physical, Medical, and Mental Health Standards,* ed. Paul R. Sackett and Anne S. Mavor (Washington, DC: The National Academies Press, 2006) 106-108. In October 2003 the Center for Accessions Research, US Army Accessions Command hosted it's third Initial Entry Training Accession Working Group Meeting at Fort Sam Houston. One of the primary objectives of the Attrition Working Group was to assist in developing an effective IET attrition reduction strategy.

16. Online at http://warchronicle.com/iraq/news/timeline_iraq_war.htm (accessed 22 July 2011); original source www.cnn.com. During the First Gulf War the 'Rand Study" reported that units were deploying at 63% strength against the required Duty MOS Qualification rate (Bruce R. Orvis, et al., *Ensuring Personnel Readiness in the Army Reserve Components* (Santa Monica, CA: The Rand Corporation, 1996), 7); These issues grew in the mid 2000's during OEF and OIF as the Army instituted "stop loss" actions to assist under-strength units that were deploying.

17. Joseph E. Whitlock, *How to Make Army Force Generation Work for the Army's Reserve Components* (Paper, Army War College Fellowship, The University of Texas at Austin, August, 2006), 11.

18. Anthony R. Jones, AR 15-6 *Investigation of the Abu Ghraib Prison and 205th Military Intelligence Brigade* (Department of the Army, 23 August 2004), 32.

19. Captain Nick Bilotta serves on the faculty of the Department of Military Instruction (USMA) and briefed the Department of Physical Education regarding his Company command in Afghanistan on 15 February 2011.

20. James E. Pilcher, "The Building of the Soldier," *The United Service* 7: (April 1892): 322.

21. Department of the Army, AR 350-1 *Army Training and Leader Development* (Washington, DC: Government Printing Office, 18 December 2009), 152.

22. A relevant example of how similar organizations accomplish this goal is the Houston, TX Fire Department. The Houston Fire Department uses a job-

related physical ability test designed to determine if an applicant has the requisite strength and endurance needed to perform the job duties of a firefighter. These job duties require balance, coordination, strength, endurance, and cardio-vascular fitness. Applicants are tested over seven (7) timed, pass/fail events while wearing gloves and an air pack because firefighters are required to wear Self-Contained Breathing Apparatus (SCBA) and other heavy protective clothing while functioning at emergency incidents. The events include:

- Balance Beam Walk-within 30 seconds, one must walk the entire length of the beam.
- Ladder Extension-within 1 minute, an applicant must fully extend and lower the fly section of a 24' aluminum extension ladder by using the hand-over-hand method.
- Stair Climb-within 3 minutes 30 seconds, an applicant must pick up, shoulder hold, and carry two (2) 50' sections of hose, tied in a "Brown Fold," then climb and descend six (6) flights of stairs.
- Equipment Hoist-within 1 minute, an applicant standing on the 3rd floor of the drill tower, using the hand-over-hand method, must hoist one section of 2 ½" hose (44 lb.) from the ground up to the 3rd floor window, and then lower the hose back to the ground.
- Portable Equipment Carry-within 1 minute, an applicant must pick up an equipment/accessory box (Hurst, or Amkus, extrication tools) (70 lb.) from a 2' stand and carry it 50' in one direction, turn around to carry it back 50' and then place the box on a 3' stand.
- Rescue Attempt-within 30 seconds, an applicant must carry or drag a 150 lb. human dummy, 30 feet.
- 1.5 Mile Run-within 13 minutes 7 seconds, an applicant must run 1.5 miles.

23. The Marine Corps has a combat obstacle course test (CFT), requirement for all members and has initiated steps to eliminate the flexed-arm hang for women from the PFT; see "Female Marines may face pull-ups for PFT," *Marine Corps Times*, 10 July 2011, D. Lamothe; *Marine Corps PT: not equal, not fair*; W. Easter, 2009.

24. Based upon the April 2009 *Armed Forces Medical Surveillance Monthly Report,* there were 7.8 million ambulatory visits for illness and injury during 2008; the largest percentage (> 24%) of visits were caused by musculoskeletal and connective tissue injuries—generally construed to be "overuse" injuries (approximately 1.9 million visits); Larkin, 2010, 41-42.

25. Bruce Ruscio, et al., "DOD Military Injury Prevention Priorities Working Group: Leading Injuries, Causes and Mitigation Recommendations" (Washington, DC: Office of the Assistant Secretary of Defense for Health Affairs, February 2006), 1, 4, 7; "Preventing Injuries in the US Military: The Process, Priorities, and Epidemiologic Evidence" (Aberdeen Proving Ground, MD: Army Center for Health Promotion and Preventive Medicine, December 2008), Section 1-1, A(2), 1-2.

26. Christopher P. Larkin, "Combat Fitness a Concept Vital to National Security," MS paper, Department of Defense: Joint Forces Staff College, 18 June

2010, 100; Major Larkin extrapolated these data, which were derived from the folSlowing source: Armed Forces Health Surveillance Center. "Ambulatory Visits among Members of Active Components, US Armed Forces, 2008," *Medical Surveillance Monthly Report* 16: (April, 2009): 10.

27. Online at http://www.marines.com/main/index/making_marines/recruit_training/delayed_entry_program (accessed 15 September, 2011); Army injury rates will be systemically higher than the Marine Corps because significantly more women attend Army BCT and women are injured at a higher rate than men.

28. Ruscio, et al., *DOD Military Injury Prevention*, 1.

29. Thomas C. Lowman, "Does Current Army Physical Training Doctrine Adequately Prepare Soldiers For War?," MA thesis, Command and General Staff College, KS, 2010), 113; Lowman was quoting Colonel Henry Arnold III, 4 IBCT, 1ID through direct correspondence.

30. The force size of the active duty Army is approximately 550,000 Officers and enlisted Soldiers.

31. By comparison the GAO estimated the Army spent approximately $11.5 billion dollars between FY 2001 and FY 2010 to design, develop, store, and distribute the Army Combat Uniform (ACU); between FY 2005-2010 the Army will have spent over $1.24 billion dollars in production and procurement of ACUs, "Warfighter Support: Observations on DOD's Ground Combat Uniforms," *Government Accounting Office Report: GAO-10-669R Warfighter Support*, 2010, 48).

32. "Unit training runs" a common site on many Army Posts, are normally conducted at a 9:00-10:00 pace; yet even at this slow pace (which would be categorized as a "junk mile" pace for most Soldiers) there are Soldiers "falling out" on either side of the formation making formation runs inappropriate for virtually all Soldiers involved from an "overload" perspective.

33. M.B. Stewart, *The Physical Development of the Infantry Soldier*, (Menasha, WI: George Banta Press, 1913), 5.

34. Maureen K. LeBoeuf, and Whitfield B. East, "Case No. 2: Physical Readiness and Assessment," in *The Future of the Army Profession*, ed. Lloyd J. Matthews (Boston: McGraw Hill Primis Custom Publishing, 2006), 486.

35. Herman J. Koehler, *Manual for Physical Training for use in the United States Army* (New York: Military Publishing Company, War Department, 1914) 10; Joseph Raycroft, *Mass Physical Training for use in the Army and Reserve Officer Training Corps*, (Washington, DC: US Infantry Association, 1920), 2.

36. "Physical and Employment Standards." Australian Defense Force: Major Ryan Holmes, March 2011, slides 6-7; The combat arms assessment consisted of four tests: 10k forced march (110 min.), box lift and place (30kg), jerry can carry (225 m), and the fire and move simulation (16x 6m).

37. Basic PRT is for soldiers in BCT, AIT, OSUT.

38. Belinda R. Beck, "Stress Fractures," ACSM Current Comment (Indianapolis, IN: *American College of Sports Medicine*, 2007), 1, online at: http://www.acsm.org (accessed 3 May 2011); Note: based upon the *American College of Sports Medicine* "Current Comment" on stress fractures, it takes about

six weeks of adaptive exercise before bone density and connective tissue improve enough to help prevent stress-reaction injuries; "Bones are most susceptible to stress fracture when weakened by remodeling-related porosity, a primary stage in the adaptive response of bone to changes in patterns of loading," 2.

39. Combat Fitness Handbook, *Australian Army, Land Warfare Procedures–General–LWP-G 7-7-4*, Commonwealth of Australia (Australian Army), 2009, 19.

40. The RPAT (Ranger Physical Activity Test) can provide initial guidelines for the components of a functional combat readiness test (RAW PT, v4.0, 72).

41. Researchers from the University of Pittsburgh, Neuromuscular Research Lab (NMRL) concluded that the only viable way to implement their Eagle Tactical Athlete Program (ETAP) was to develop a certified cadre of fitness instructors; "The objective of Phase II is to enroll Division NCOs into the ICS [instructor certification school] and phase-implement the ETAP into Division PT. In Phase IIA, the NCOs will learn the theory and implementation of the updated PT program (ETAP) and at the completion of the course be certified as Eagle Tactical Athlete Training Leaders," "Neuromuscular Research Laboratory Newsletter," (Department of Sports Medicine and Nutrition, University of Pittsburg, 2009), 2.

42. "Physical Fitness Symposium Report," (Fort Benning: United States Infantry School, October 1970), 42.

43. Combat Fitness Handbook, Australian Army, *Land Warfare Procedures*, 21.

44. Combat Fitness Handbook, Australian Army, *Land Warfare Procedures*, 22.

45. This text was extracted from an Australian Defense Force job announcement for a Physical Training Instructor (NCO), 23 March 2011: A Physical Training Instructor (PTI) is a Royal Australian Army Medical Corps (RAAMC) soldier who is responsible for the provision of physical conditioning and rehabilitation to the Australian soldier and the ADF in a variety of settings. The PTI is employed in the prevention of injuries, delivery of Military Self Defense and the Combat Fitness Leader Courses (CFLC). Also, the PTI delivers the Defense Injury Prevention Program (DIPP), conducts fitness assessments and physical training of Australian Defense Force members and coordinates sporting events and other specialist activities; online at: defencejobs.gov.au/army/jobs/PhysicalTrainingInstructor/JobDetails (accessed 11 June 2011).

46. Stewart, *The Physical Development of the Infantry Soldier*, 5.

47. Douglas MacArthur, *Reminiscences* (New York, NY: McGraw Hill Book Company, 1964), 81.

48. See the Recommendations Sections for the 1958, 1970, and 1981 "Physical Fitness symposia."

49. "Physical Fitness Symposium Report (1970)," 41.

50. Department of Defense, "Study of the Military Services Physical Fitness" (Washington DC; 1981), 3-34.

51. Memorandum for Record: Subject: "Relocation of the Physical Fitness School," 9 July 1991.

Appendix A
Chronological Summary of Significant Activities for the US Army Soldier Physical Fitness Center

1980 2 February, President Carter requested the Secretary of Defense to assess the physical fitness programs for all Armed Services.

1981 3 April, findings of the DoD Study of Military Services Physical Fitness were published.

21 December, Lieutenant General Julius Becton, TRADOC Deputy Commander for Training, convenient a meeting at Fort Monroe on to discuss plans for a physical fitness center.

1982 7 January, Secretary of the Army John O. Marsh created a Physical Fitness Task Force at the Soldier Support Center, Fort Benjamin Harrison, IN and signed a resolution forming the US Army Soldier Physical Fitness Center; the operational component of the Soldier Physical Fitness Center was the Physical Fitness School (PFS); there were two branches of the PFS: (1) Academy–dealing with research and pedagogical aspects of the mission (i.e., the master fitness trainer program), and (2) Doctrine–dealing with regulatory aspects of the mission (i.e. FM 21-20).

3 May, the USASPFC was activated; Lieutenant Colonel Joe DiEduardo was appointed as the first Commandant; Director of the Academy–Lieutenant Colonel Larry Hicks was responsible for developing the Master Fitness Trainer course (MFT); Director of Doctrine-Lieutenant Colonel Mark Saunders was responsible for doctrine development; Major William Schutsky was the Director of Instruction.

1983 January - July, Colonel Clyde D. Lynn, was appointed Commandant of the USASPFC; personnel attended the DoD Committee for Physical Fitness Conference in San Diego (24-15 Feb); Director of the Academy–unknown; Director of Doctrine-Lieutenant Colonel Robert (Bobbie) Hoffman; the Center's name was changed to the Soldier Physical Fitness School (SPFS) to more accurately reflect its assigned mission of education the Army in all aspects of physical fitness.

1983 2d Quarter, MFT pilot course was administered.

May, USASPFS began offering the 4-week resident MFT course to senior NCOs and Company grade officers from throughout the Army; there were 30 faculty in the Physical Fitness Academy;

October, USASPFS hosted the semi-annual meeting of the DoD Committee for Physical Fitness; USASPFS Academy provided

Advanced Individual Instruction (AIT) for all 03C–Physical Activities Specialist (approximately 50% of the 03C AIT training involved enrollment in the MFT course).

1983   July, Colonel Walter Wilms, (AR) was appointed Commandant of the USASPFS; 14 September–SPFS personnel attended the US Military Symposium on Fitness Planning Conference, Carlisle Barracks; Director of the Academy–unknown; Director of Doctrine-Lieutenant Colonel Robert (Bobbie) Hoffman.

1987   Colonel Robert Tetu was appointed Commandant of the USASPFS; Director of the Academy-Lieutenant Colonel Oliver Johnson, Director of Doctrine-Lieutenant Colonel Jack O'Conner; the 03C MOS category was terminated.

1990   25-26 January, Lieutenant Colonel John S. O'Connor, Ph.D. (Director of Training) reported on the status of the USAPFS at the National Conference on Military Fitness, Washington, DC.

1991   Colonel Bruce J. Wicks (SF) was appointed Commandant of the USAPFS; Director of the Academy–Lieutenant Colonel John O'Conner; Director of Doctrine–Mr. Edward Tarantino; after the decision was made to mover the Center to Fort Benning, Lieutenant Colonel Sam Pride was appointed as the Interim Director of the Center for Colonel Wicks during the move to Fort Benning.

The Army Chief of Staff approved the Vanguard Taskforce recommendations, which included elimination of USAPFS in FY92; during subsequent negotiations between TRADOC and HQDA a solution was found to save the School by transferring it to the US Army Infantry Center (USAIC–Fort Benning; the transfer occurred between July 1991 and June 1992. When the "Center" moved to Fort Benning they dropped the Center designation and became the US Army Physical Fitness School. The "Academy" mission of the USASPFS was also terminated as part of the move to Fort Benning.

1992   Colonel David White (IN) was appointed Commandant of the USAPFS. Director of Doctrine–Major Marcus Alexander; Director of Training–Mr. Frank Palkoska; with the demise of the "Academy" the 4-week resident MFT course was discontinued; however Mobile Training Teams and the Department of Physical Education, USMA continued to train Soldiers and Officers and award the 6P MFT ASI until 2002; USAPFS was assigned to "update APFT standards" to ensure standards require "equal effort" by both genders. Dr. Louis Tomasi (Research Physiologist USAPFS), Dr. Gene Fober (Army Research Institute) in cooperation with USA.R.I.E.M. personnel led the effort; the

USAPFS supervised the publication of FM 21-20 (1992).

1993   Colonel David White (IN) was assigned to update the physical fitness uniform; Dr. L. Tomasi was the lead investigator; the project was designated "Improved Physical Fitness Uniform."

1994   Colonel Jeanne M. Picariello (ANC) was appointed Commandant of the USAPFS.

1997   Colonel Stephen D. Cellucci (AR) was appointed Commandant of the USAPFS; the new PT standards and APFU (PT uniform) were approved by Army Chief-of-Staff (General Reimer).

1998   USAPFS supervised the revised publication of FM 21-20.

1999   Lieutenant Colonel William Rieger (IN) was appointed Commandant of the USAPFS.

2001   All mobile training teams for MFT course were terminated; 6P Army Skill Identifier was removed from the Army Training Requirements and Resourcing System (ATRRS).

2002   the USAPFS developed a revised FM 21-20, to be published as FM 3-22.20.

2003   As part of the FM 21-20 revision Lieutenant General Van Alstyne requested a draft proposal for a new Army physical fitness test; due to excessive injuries during Initial Military Training, Lieutenant General Dennis Cavin (USAAC) provided guidance to USAPFS to fix Initial Military Training PRT program of instruction; "futures" track (FM 3-22.20) was put on hold to work exclusively on "current" issues, which, along with significant negative reactions to the newly proposed APFT, effectively terminated the revision/publication of the FM 3-22.20.

2006   Mr. Frank Palkoska was appointed Director of the USAPFS.

2007   USAPFS moved to Fort Jackson, S.C. as part of the Directorate of Basic Combat Training.

2010   USAPFS published Training Circular (TC) 3-22.20 as the replacement training doctrine for FM 21-20.

Appendix B
Chronological Summary of Publications for US Army Physical Fitness Training and Assessment

1825 – *Elementary Course in Gymnastic Exercises*–Captain P. H. Clias, Royal Military Academy, Woolwich, England.

1840 – *Infantry Tactics or Rules for the Exercise and Maneuvre of the United States Infantry*, Winfield Scott.

1861 – *Rifle and Light Infantry Tactics (for the exercise and maneuvers of troops when acting as light infantry or riflemen)*; prepared under the direction of the War Department–Brevet Lieutenant Colonel W. Joseph Hardee, US Army Vol. 1; Philadelphia: J.B. Lippincott & Co., 1861.

1862 – *Infantry Tactics for the Instruction, Exercise, and Maneuvers of the Soldier, A Company, Line of Skirmishes, Battalion, Brigade, or Corps*; Brigadier General Silas Casey, Vol. II; New York: D. Van Nostrand, 1862.

1864 – *Handbook of Calisthenics and Gymnastics*-James M. Watson.

1867–*Manual of Physical Exercises*–William Wood; Harper: New York.

1868 – *A Military System of Gymnastic Exercises and a System of Fencing for Use by Instructors*; Archibald MacLaren, London: Her Majesty's Stationary Office.

1869 – *A System of Physical Education–Theoretical and Practical*; Archibald MacLaren, Oxford: Clarendon Press Series.

1879 – *Manual of Drill and Calisthenics*–J. Laughlin Hughes (Toronto).

1881 – *A Military System of Gymnastic Exercises and a System of Swimming*, Edward S. Farrow; Instructor–Department of Tactics and Master of the Sword (1882-1884), New York: Metropolitan Publishing Co.

1882 – *Manual of Calisthenics*– James M. Watson; New York: E. Steiger & Co.

1887 – A *System of Callisthenic Exercises for use in School of the Soldier*, Herman J. Koehler; West Point: US Academy Press.

1891 – *A B C of the Swedish System of Educational Gymnastics*, Hartvig Nissen, Philadelphia: F.A. Davis, Publisher.

1892 – *Manual of Callisthenic Exercises*–Herman J. Koehler, War Department; US Army: Government Press.

1897 – *Physical Drill for Foot Troops*–Captain Constantine Chase, 4th Artillery, US Army. Washington: Government Printing Office. (close order drills with weapons, bayonet, and Indian clubs).

1898 – *Manual of Physical Drill*–Major Edmund J. Butts, US Army, New York: D. Appleton and Company.

1904 – *US Army Exercises: Rearranged for General Use*–Private Frank Idone, US Army.

1904 – *Manual of Gymnastic Exercises: Prepared for Use in Service Gymnasiums*–First Lieutenant Herman J. Koehler, Washington: Government Printing Office.

1904 – *Physical Training Manual for Use in Public Schools, Normal Schools, and Gymnasia*–Carl Zeigler, M.D. Superintendent of Physical Training and Hygiene for Cincinnati Public Schools.

1909 – *A Manual of Physical Exercises*, General John P. Hawkins, US Army.

1909 – *Manual of Physical Exercise; a Health Hand-book*; Arte R.T. Winjum, Battle Creek, MI.

1913 – *Physical Development of the Infantry Soldier*, Merch Bradt Steward, Menasha, WI: Banta Press.

1914 – *Manual of Military Training*, J. A. Moss, Menasha, WI: Banta Press.

1914 – *Manual of Physical Training for use in the United States Army*, War Department Document No. 436, Office of the Chief of Staff (written by Lieutenant Colonel Sladen, Major Koehler, Captain Matthews (US Army) and sanctioned by Major General Leonard Wood, Chief of Staff, War Department.

1917 – *Field Physical Training of the Soldier–Special Regulations, No. 23*, Captain Herman Koehler, United States Military Academy, West Point.

1917 – *Manual of Military Training*, Major James A. Moss, 2d Edition, Menasha, WI: Banta Press.

1917 – *The Plattsburg Manual–A Handbook for Military Training*, Captain O. O. Ellis and Captain E.B. Garey, New York: The Century Co.

1917 – *Military Instructors Manual* (Chapter 3: Physical Training), Captain James Cole and Major Oliver Schoomaker, New York: Edwin N. Appleton.

1918 – *Extracts from the Manual of Physical Training for use in the United States Army*, War Department, Lieutenant Colonel Herman Koehler–West Point.

1919 – *Army Physical Training*, Colonel William Henry Waldron, US Army, New York: Henry Hold & CO.

1919 – *West Point Manual of Disciplinary Physical Training*, Lieutenant Colonel Herman Koehler–West Point, Instructor at United States Training Camps and Cantonments, 1917-18; Instructor at Business Men's and Militia Camps,1915-16; sanctioned by SECWAR Baker; E.P. Dudley & CO: New York.

1920 – *Mass Physical Training*–for use in the Army and the Reserve Officers' Training Corps; United States Infantry Association: Washington, DC (forward by Major General William G. Haan– Chief, War Plans Division).

1923 – *Manual of Military Training*, Moss, J.A. and Lang, J.W., 4th Edition, Menasha, WI: Banta Press.

1924 –*Standards for Physical Qualifications for Entrance into the National Guard–NGR-28* (31 Dec 1924).

1927 – *Physical Examinations–NGR 27* (1 April 1927).

1928 – *Physical Training (Training Regulation 115-5) Part I–general training without equipment. Part II–with special equipment.* Published under the supervision of Brigadier General Merch Brandt Stewart, Superintendent, United States Military Academy-Major Edward L. Kelly, Master of the Sword.

1936 – *Physical Training (Basic Field Manual-BFM–Volume 1, Chapter 4* - Army, published under the supervision of Major General William D. Connor, Superintendent, United States Military Academy.

1941 – *Physical Training (FM 21-20)*; prepared under the supervision of Robert L. Eichelberger, Superintendent, United States Military Academy (supersedes Vol. I, Ch. 4, BFM, March 26, 1936, and TR 115-5, Part II, 10 September, 1928).

1942 – *Physical Training (Training Circular- TC 87);* Washington: US Government Printing Office, 17 November 1942 (supplement to FM 21-20, 1941).

1942 – *Army Ground Forces Test* approved for all Soldiers-oriented toward physical combat skills.

1943 – *Physical Training–W.A.C. Field Manual (FM 35-20)*, 15 July, 1943.

1944 – *Physical Reconditioning (TM 8-292)*, War Department, December 1944–for the soldier who had been wounded or suffered from a prolonged illness.

1944 – *Physical Conditioning (Army Pamphlet–DA Pam 21-9);* US War Department, Washington: US Government Printing Office, May 1944; Physical Efficiency Test Battery first presented; PETB was oriented more towards combat readiness; designed by Bank/McCloy/Esslinger.

1946 – *Physical Training (FM 21-20);* US Government Printing Office: Washington, DC; revised the Physical Efficiency Test Battery: both outdoor and indoor tests specified; scoring standards changed; allowance made for age, 1 January 1946 (supersedes FM 21-20 (1941), TC 87 (1942), DA Pam 21-9 (1944).

1950 – *Physical Readiness Training (FM 21-20);* revised the Physical Fitness Test Battery; scoring standards changed. Physical Achievement Test added; designed to measure certain physical combat skills; both tests made mandatory for basic combat training, 30 November 1950 (supersedes FM 21-20, 1 January 1946).

1951 – *Change 1: Physical Readiness Training, FM 21-20,* 26 October 1951.

1954 – *Army Training Program–Male, (ATP 21-114)* - basic training program for personnel without prior service (revised in 1956, 1958, 1961, 1970).

1956 – *Physical Training - Women's Army Corps (FM 35-20)*, 25 January 1956 (supersedes FM 35-20, 15 July, 1943).

1957 – *Physical Training (FM 21-20)*; program/training materials were removed and published separately in TM 21-200; 8 October 1957 (supersedes FM 21-20, 30 November 1950, including C 1, 26 October 1951, and C 2, 15 September 1952; and Training Circular 21-3, 18 April 1957).

1957 – *Physical Conditioning (TM 21-200)*, Washington: US Government Publishing Office–extracted from FM 21-20, 30 November 1950, retained the Physical Achievement Test to measure combat-related physical fitness, 31 December 1957.

1958 – *Physical Fitness Seminar*, hosted by the United States Army Infantry School, Fort Benning, GA, 21-24 April, 1958.

1959 – *Change 1. TM 21-200–Physical Conditioning*, Washington: US Printing Office–established a 200-point minimum score for both 1957 tests.

1961 – *Change 2. TM 21-200–Physical Conditioning*–previewed the Physical Combat Proficiency Test (PCPT): entirely new test–40-yard low crawl, horizontal ladder, doge run and jump, grenade throw, and one-mile run; minimum score=300 pts; personnel over forty exempted; mandatory test for Army; first test to have total score=300 and component scores–had to pass all components.

1962 – *Physical Fitness Programs (DoD Directive 1308.1)*.

1963 – *Physical Fitness Program for Specialists and Staff Personnel (DA Pamphlet 21-1)*, Washington: US Government Printing Office–established an Army Minimum Physical Fitness Test–Male: mandatory for staff and specialist personnel under forty. PCPT made mandatory for medically fit personnel under forty years old.

1963 – *Physical Fitness Program for Women in the Army (DA Pamphlet 21-2)*, 7 January 1963; (supersedes).

1963 – *Army Physical Fitness Program (Technical Circular 21-1)*, Washington: US Government Publishing Office, 7 January 1963 including Change 3, 26 July 1963.

1963 – *Weight Control (AR 600-7)*, Washington: US Government Publishing Office (supersedes DA Circular 600-7, 10 September, 1962).

1965 – *Army Physical Fitness Program (AR 600-9)*, Washington: US Government Publishing Office, 5 January, 1965, (supersedes TC 21-1, 7 January 1963).

1965 – *Physical Fitness Program for Women in the Army (DA Pamphlet 21-2)*, 26 February 1965 (supersedes DA Pam 21-2, 7 January 1963; including Change 1, 26 July 1963).

1965 – *Physical Conditioning–Change 4 (TM 21-200)*, Washington: US Government Publishing Office–dodge run and jump standards were raised from 1-4 seconds; 26 May 1965.

1965 – *Physical Fitness Program for Specialists and Staff Personnel (Army Pamphlet 21-1)*, Washington: US Government Printing Office – 2nd revision, 25 February 1965 (supersedes DA Pam 21-1, 7 January 1963, including C2, 26 July 1963).

1965 – *Physical Training Women's Army Corps (FM 35-20)*; 2d revision, 2 September 1965 (supersedes FM 35-20, 25 January 1956).

1966 – *Continental Army Command Pamphlet 600-1*–Establishes the Inclement Weather Physical Fitness Test for basic, advanced, and combat supported trainees.

1969 - *Physical Readiness Training (FM 21-20)*. Physical fitness standards adjusted according to duty assignment; scoring standards modified. Minimum Fitness Test-Male: major revision of test events and scoring standards, 31 January 1969 (supersedes FM 21-20, 8 October 1957 and all changes; TM 21-200, 31 December 1957 and all changes).

1970 – *Physical Fitness Symposium*, hosted by the USAIS, Fort Benning, GA, 12-14 October 1970.

1973 – *Physical Readiness Training (FM 21-20)*, 30 March 1973 (supersedes FM 21-20, 31 January 1969).

1974 – *Army Physical Fitness Program (AR 600-9)*, 7 May 1974 (supersedes AR 600-9, 5 January 1965).

1975 – *Training: Army Training (AR 350-1)* Washington: US Government Publishing Office, 25 April 1975.

1975 – *Physical Training Women's Army Corps (FM 35-20)*, 17 February 1975 (supersedes FM 35-20, 2 September 1965, and DA Pam 21-2, 26 February 1965).

1975 – *Change 1. Physical Training Women's Army Corps (FM 35-20)*, 30 October 1975.

1976 – *The Army Physical Fitness and Weight Control Program (AR 600-9)*, 30 November 1976 (supersedes AR 600-9, 7 May 1974).

1980 – *The Revised Physical Training Program (APTP-1)*, US Army Infantry School, Fort Benning, GA–January, 1980–primary a primmer of MSE and CRE activities.

1980 – *Department of Defense Study of the Military Services Physical Fitness*; hosted by the Secretary of Defense, 17-19 June 1980; final report was published on 3 April 1983.

1980 – *Physical Readiness Training (FM 21-20)*, 31 October 1980 (supersedes FM 21-20, 30 March 1973, and FM 35-20, 17 February 1975).

1981 – *Training: Army Training (AR 350-1)*, 1 August 1981 (supersedes AR 350-1, 25 April 1975).

1981 – *Physical Fitness and Weight Control Programs (DoD Directive 1308.1)*, required all services to use body fat as the sole measure of obesity; obesity was defined as anything over 22%, 29 June 1981 (superseded DoD Directive 1308.1, 20 November 1962).

1982 – *US Army Soldier Physical Fitness Center* was formed at Fort Benjamin Harrison, IN.

1982 – *Committee on Military Nutrition Research* was formed by the US Army Assistant Surgeon General.

1982 – *The Army Physical Fitness Program (AR 350-15)*, 15 July 1982 (supersedes chapter 2 of AR 600-9, 30 November 1976).

1982 – *Commander's Handbook on Physical Fitness* (DA PAM 350-15), 15 October 1982.

1983 – *Department of Defense Committee on Physical Fitness Conference*, San Diego, CA, 24-25 February 1983.

1983 – *The Army Weight Control Program (AR 600-9)*, 1 February 1983 (supersedes AR 600-9, 30 November 1976).

1983 – *Training: Army Training (AR 350-1)*, 1 August 1983 (supersedes AR 350-1, 1 August 1981).

1983 – *US Military Fitness Planning Conference*, Carlisle Barracks, PA, 14 September, 1883.

1985 – *Physical Readiness Training (FM 21-20)*. 28 August 1985, (supersedes FM 21-20, 31 October 1980).

1985 – *The Army Physical Fitness Program (AR 350-15)*, 30 December 1985 (supersedes AR 350-15, 15 October 1982).

1986 – *The Army Weight Control Program (AR 600-9)*, 1 September 1986 (supersedes AR 600-9, 1 February 1983).

1986 – *Army Forces Training (AR 350-41)*, 26 September 1986; a new Army regulation; identifies training goals and philosophy, commander's responsibilities, and training requirements.

1987 – *The Army Weight Control Program (AR 600-9)*, 10 June 1987 (supersedes AR 600-9, 1 February 1983 and the original form published on 1 September 1986; includes Change 1, February, 1987 and Change 2, June, 1987.

1989 – *Army Physical Fitness Program (AR 350-15),* 3 November 1989 (supersedes AR 350-15, 30 December 1985).

1990 – *National Conference on Military Physical Fitness*, hosted by the President's Council on Physical Fitness and Sports, in cooperation with the National Defense University, 25-26 January 1990.

1992 – *Physical Readiness Training (FM 21-20),* 30 September 1992 (supersedes FM 21-20, 28 August 1985).

1993 – *Training in Units (AR 350-41),* consolidated several publications to provide a comprehensive policy for training in units, 19 March 1993, (supersedes AR 350-15, 3 November 1989, and AR 350-41, 26 September 1986).

1995 – *Physical Fitness and Body Fat Program (DoD Directive 1308.1)*; 20 July 1995 (supersedes 29 June 1981).

1995 – *Physical Fitness and Body Fat Program Procedures (DoD Directive 1308.3),* 30 August, 1995.

1998 – *Physical Readiness Training (FM 21-20).* 1 October 1998, (supersedes 30 September 1992).

1998 – *Training in Units (FORSCOM Regulation 350-1),* 15 October 1998.

2002 – *Training in Units (FORSCOM Regulation 350-1),* 25 October 2002 (supersedes FORSCOMR 350-1 1998).

2002 – *Physical Fitness and Body Fat Program Procedures (DoD Directive 1308.3)*, 5 November 2002 (supersedes 20 July 1995).

2003 – *Army Training and Education (AR 350-1),* established Army physical fitness policy; defined Army physical fitness test and height and weight standards as enrollment and graduation requirements for professional development schools; and provided guidance for physical fitness training in units, 9 April 2003 (supersedes AR 350-1, 1 August 1983, and AR 350-41, 19 March 1993).

2004 – *Physical Fitness and Body Fat Program (DoD Directive 1308.1),* 30 June 2004, (supersedes DoD Directive 1308.1, 20 July 1995).

2006 – *Ranger Warrior Athlete Physical Training (v.1.0)*, no date provided, established feasibility, acceptability, and suitability of the RAW program.

2006 – Army Weight Control Program (AR 600-9), 1 September 2006 (supersedes AR 600-9, 10 June 1987).

2006 – *Army Training and Leadership Development (AR 350-1)*, date (supersedes AR 350-1, 2003).

2007 – *Ranger Warrior Athlete Physical Training (v.2.0)*, no date provided (supersedes RAW v.1.0, no date provided).

2007 – *Army Training and Leader Development (AR 350-1)*, 3 August 2007 (supersedes AR 350-1, 2006); rapid action revision.

2008 – *Ranger Warrior Athlete Physical Training (v.3.0)*, 13 May 2008 (supersedes RAW v.2.0, no date provided).

2009 – *Eagle Tactical Athlete Program* Spring, 2009, developed by the University of Pittsburgh's Department of Sports Medicine and Nutrition; implemented with the 101st Airborne Corps, Fort Campbell, KY.

2009 – *Army Training and Leader Development (AR 350-1)* 18 December 2009 (supersedes AR 350-1, 2007).

2010 – *Army Physical Readiness Training (TC 3-22.20)*, (supersedes FM 21-20, 30 September 1992, and Change 1–FM 21-20, 1 October 1998).

2010 – *Ranger Warrior Athlete Physical Training (v.4.0)*, 13 April 2010 (supersedes RAW v.3.0, 13 May 2008).

Bibliography

Allen, Edward F. *Keeping Our Fighters Fit For War And After* (Written with the Cooperation of Raymond B. Fosdick). New York: The Century Co. 1918.

Armed Forces Health Surveillance Center. "Ambulatory Visits among Members of Active Components, US Armed Forces, 2008." *Medical Surveillance Monthly Report* 16:4 (April, 2009): 10.

"American Literary, Scientific, and Military Academy." *The American Journal of Education* 7:82 (1872): 857-864.

American Military History Volume I: The United States Army and the Forging of a Nation, 1775-1917. Edited by Richard W. Stewart. Washington, DC: Center for Military History, United States Army, 2005.

Anderson, William G. "The Early History of the American Association for HPER then Called the AAPE. *Journal of Health and Physical Education* 12(1) (1941): 3-4, 61-62.

"A New Commandant, F.A.S." *The Field Artillery Journal* 32:8 (August, 1942): 578.

Annual Reunion of the Association of Graduates, 1858.

Annual Reunion of the Association of Graduates, Necrology Report: John C. Kelton, No. 1519, Class of 1851, 1894, 9-18.

Annual Report of the President of Stanford University, 1943, 228–231.

Annual Report of the Board of Visitors to the United States Military Academy, Washington: US Government Printing Office, 1826.

Annual Report of the Board of Visitors to the United States Military Academy, Washington: US Government Printing Office, 1889.

Annual Report of the Superintendent of the United States Military Academy, Washington: US Government Printing Office, 1881.

Annual Report of the Superintendent of the United States Military Academy, Washington: US Government Printing Office, 1884.

Annual Report of the Superintendent of the United States Military Academy, Washington: US Government Printing Office, 1885.

Annual Reports of the War Department, Washington: US Government Printing Office; Vol. 1, Part 2 (1919): 1437-2012.

Appleman, Roy. *The US Army in the Korean War: South to the Naktong, North to the Yalu*, Washington, DC: Center for Military History, Department of the Army, 1992.

Ardmore Army Air Field (1942-1946):Chronological Reminders of the Past (November 27, 1943), www.oklahomahistory.net/airbase/1jogger.html (accessed 21 June 2011).

Ardmore Army Air Field (1942-1946): Chronological Reminders of the Past, Ardmore, OK. www.oklahomahistory.net/airbase/1jogger.html (accessed 10 September 2010).

"Army Heads Answer Militia Complaints." *New York Times*, 20 July, 1916.

"Army Physical Culture Institution May Have Far-Reaching Influence," *Miami News*, 5 October 1919.

"Army is Antiquated Declares General Bell," *New York Times*, December 25, 1908.

Astor, Gerald. *Battling Buzzards: The Odyssey of the 517th Parachute Regimental Combat Team*. New York: Dell Publishing, 1993.

Axtell, James. *The Making of Princeton University: from Woodrow Wilson to the Present*, Princeton, NJ: Princeton University Press, 2006.

Baker, Newton D. "Letter to President Woodrow Wilson v. Raymond Fosdick," in *The Papers of Woodrow Wilson*, Vol. 4, January 24-April 6, 1917, 505-506, edited by Arthur S. Link, Princeton: Princeton University Press, 1983.

Baker, Newton D. "Letter to President Woodrow Wilson–Mr. Fosdick and Army Recreation." in *The Papers of Woodrow Wilson*, Vol. 4, January 24-April 6, 1917, 527-528, edited by Arthur S. Link, Princeton: Princeton University Press, 1983.

Bank, Theodore. "The Army Physical Conditioning Program." *Journal of Health and Physical Education* 14:4 (1943): 195-197, 238, 240.

Bank, Theodore. "Trends Toward Separate Commission on Fitness." *Aim for Industrial Sports and Recreatio –A Sports World Digest (AIM)* 4:4 (1945): 22-23, 26.

"Bayonet Practice Again." *New York Times*, 25 June 1917.

Bean, William. B., Charles R. Park, David M. Bell, and Charles R. Henderson. *A Critique of Physical Fitness Tests,* Fort Knox, KY: Army Medical Research Lab, Report 56-1(07), 19 February 1947.

Beans, Harry C. "Sex Discrimination in the Military." *Military Law Review*–VOL. 67; Headquarters–Department of the Army, Pam 27-100-67 (Winter 1975): 19-83.

Beck, Belinda R. "Stress Fractures," *ACSM Current Comment*, American College of Sports Medicine, Indianapolis, IN, 2007 http://www.acsm.org (accessed 3 May 2011).

"Bell Beats Roosevelt," *New York Times*, February 5, 1908.

Bellafaire, Judith. *The Women's Army Corps: A Commemoration of World War II Service*; CHM Publication 72-15; www.history.army.mil; last updated 15 February 2005 (accessed 14 November 2011).

"Big Physical Training Play for the Army." *Pittsburgh Press*, October 5, 1919.

Blair, Clay. *The Forgotten War: America in Korea 1950-1953.* New York: Times Books, 1987.

Bovard, John., and Frederick Cozens. *Test and Measurements in Physical Education*. Philadelphia: W.B. Saunders Co., 1938.

Bowden, Sue, and Avner Offer. "Household Appliances and the Use of Time: The United States and Britain since the 1920s." *The Economic History Review* 47:4 (1994): 725-748.

Boykin, J.C. "Physical Training," in *Report of the Commissioner of Education for The Year 1891-1892*, 451-494. Washington: US Government Printing Office, 1894.

Boyle, R.H. "The Report that Shocked the President." *Sports Illustrated* (August 15, 1955): 30-33, 72-73.

Brame, Grace. *Receptive Prayer–A Christian Approach to Meditation*. St. Louis, Mo: CBP Press, 1985.

Brodie, Bernard, and Fawn Brodie. *From Cross Bow to H-bomb*; Bloomington: Indiana University Press, 1973.

Broekhoff, Jan. (1968) "Chivalric Education in the Middle Ages." *Quest* 11 (1968): 24-31.

Brosius, George. *Fifty Years Devoted to the Cause of Physical Culture, 1864-1914*. Milwaukee: Germania Publishing, 1914.

Brownell, C.L. "We Learned About Fitness from Them." *Journal of Health and Physical Education* 15:4 (April 1944): 182-184, 228.

Burrowes, Reynold A. *Revolution and Rescue in Grenada: an Account of the US Caribbean Invasion*. New York: Greenwood Press, 1988.

Butts, Edmund. *Manual of Physical Drill, United States Army*. New York: D. Appleton and Company, 1898.

Camp, Walter. "A Daily Dozen Set-up."*Outing* 73:2 (1918): 98,100.

Campbell, J.D. "Training for Sport Is Training for War: Sport and the Transformation of the British Army, 1860-1914.," *International Journal of the History of Sport*, 17: 4 (2000): 21-58.

Campbell, J.D. *The Army isn't all work": Physical Culture in the Evolution of the British Army, 1860-1920*; A Thesis Submitted in Partial Fulfillment of the Requirements for the Degree of Doctor of

Philosophy-Individualized in British History-The Graduate School, The University of Maine, December, 2003, 275.

Cannon, Michael W. "Task Force Smith: A Study in (Un)Preparedness and (Ir)Responsibility." *Military Review* 57 (February, 1988): 62-73.

"Capt. Sladen to Head West Point Cadets," *New York Times*, December 24, 1910.

Cardia, Emanuela. 2009. "Household Technology: Was It the Engine of Liberation?" University of Montreal. Unpublished manuscript. Current version April 2010, (http://www.cireq.umontreal.ca/personnel/ cardia_household_technology.pdf).

Cartledge, Paul. *Spartan Reflections*. Los Angeles: University of California Press, 2001.

Cazers, Gunars, and Glenn A. Miller. "The German Contribution to American Physical Education: A Historical Perspective." *The Journal of Physical Education, Recreation & Dance* 71:6 (2000): 344-348.

Chase, Constantine. *Physical Drill for Foot Troops*. 4th Artillery, US Army. Washington: US Government Printing Office, 1897.

Charlston, Jeffery A. "Disorganized and Quasi-Official but Eventually Successful: Sport in the US Military, 1814-1914." *International Journal of the History of Sport* 19:4 (2002): 70-88.

Clias, Phokion H. Captain. *An Elementary Course of Gymnastic Exercises*. 4th ed. London: Sherwood, Gilbert, And Piper, 1825.

Clute, Penelope D. "The Plattsburg Idea." *New Your Archives* 5:2 (Fall 2005): 10-15.

Coffman, Edward. *The Old Army: A Portrait of the American Army in Peacetime, 1784-1898*. New York: Oxford University Press, 1986.

Cole, James, and Oliver Schoomaker. *Military Instructors Manual (special emphasis on Chapter 3: Physical Training)*. New York: Edwin N. Appleton, 1917.

Combat Fitness Handbook. Australian Army, Land Warfare Procedures–General–LWP-G 7-7-4, Commonwealth of Australia (Australian Army), 2009.

Cook, Paul J. *How Did a Lack 0f Strategic and Operational Vision Impair the Army's Ability to Conduct Tactical Operations in Korea in the Summer Of 1950?* Master's thesis, US Army Command and General Staff College; Fort Leavenworth, KS, 2002.

Cooper, Ken *Aerobics*. New York: M. Evans (distributed in association with Lippincott, Philadelphia, 1968.

Cooper, Pamela. *The American Marathon*. Syracuse, New York: Syracuse University Press, 1999.

Crampton, C. Ward. *Fighting Fitness: A Preliminary Training Guide*. New York: McGraw-Hill Book Co, 1944.

Crosby, Alfred. *Epidemic and Peace, 1918*. Westport, CT: Greenwood Press, 1976.

Cypher, Dorothea. "Urgent Fury: The US Army in Grenada." In *American Intervention in Grenada: The Implications of Operation "Urgent Fury"*. edited by Peter M. Dunn and Bruce W. Watson, 99-108. Boulder, CO: Westview Press, 1985.

Davies, William J. *Task Force Smith–A Leadership Failure?* Study Project, Carlisle Barracks, PA: US Army War College, 1992.

Degen, Robert. *The Evolution of Physical Education at the United States Military Academy*, Master thesis, University of Wisconsin, Madison, 1967.

Delafield, Richard. *Report on the Art of War in Europe in 1854, 1855, 1856*. Washington: George W. Bowman, Printer, 1860.

D'Eliscu, Francois. *How to Prepare for Military Fitness*. New York: W. W. Norton & Company, 1943.

Department of Defense. *Conduct of the Persian Gulf War: Appendix R-Role of Women in the Theater of Operations*. Washington, DC (April, 1992): 647-649.

Department of Defense. *Directive on Physical Fitness and Weight Control Programs* (Directive No. 1308.1), Washington DC, 1981.

Department of Defense. *Study of the Military Services Physical Fitness*. Washington DC, 3 April 1981.

Department of the Army. *Army Forces Training (FM 350-41)*. Washington, DC: US Government Printing Office, 1986.

Department of the Army. *Army Physical Readiness Training–TC 3-22.20*. Washington: US Government Printing Office, March 2010.

Department of the Army. *Army Training and Education (AR 350-1)*. Washington: US Government Printing Office, 9 April 2003.

Department of the Army. *Army Training and Leader Development – Army Regulation 350-1*. Washington: US Government Printing Office, 13 January 2006.

Department of the Army. *Army Training and Leader Development – Army Regulation 350-1*. Washington: US Government Printing Office, 18 December 2009.

Department of the Army. *Army Physical Fitness Program (AR 600-9)*. Washington, DC: US Government Printing Office, 1965.

Department of the Army. *Army Physical Fitness Program (AR 600-9)*. Washington, DC: US Government Printing Office, 1971.

Department of the Army. *Army Physical Fitness and Weight Control Program (AR 600-9)*. Washington, DC: US Government Printing Office, 1976.

Department of the Army. *Army Physical Fitness Program (AR 600-9)*. Washington, DC: US Government Printing Office, 1974.

Department of the Army. *Army Physical Fitness Program (FM 350-15)*. Washington, DC: US Government Printing Office, 1982.

Department of the Army. *Army Physical Fitness Program (FM 350-15)*. Washington, DC: US Government Printing Office, 1985.

Department of the Army. *Army Physical Fitness Program (FM 350-15)*. Washington, DC: US Government Printing Office, 1989.

Department of the Army. *Army Physical Fitness and Weight Control Program (AR 600-9)*. Washington, DC: US Government Printing Office, 1976.

Department of the Army. *Army Weight Control Program (AR 600-9)*. Washington, DC: US Government Printing Office, 1983.

Department of the Army. *Army Weight Control Program (AR 600-9)*. Washington, DC: US Government Printing Office, 1987.

Department of the Army. *Army Weight Control Program (AR 600-9)*. Washington, DC: US Government Printing Office, 2006.

Department of the Army. "Basic Field Manual, Vol. I, Chapter 4." *Physical Readiness Training (FM 21-20)*. Washington, DC: US Government Printing Office, 1936.

Department of the Army Historical Summary–Fiscal Year 1977. Edited by Karl E. Cocker. Washington, DC: Center of Military History, 1979.

Department of the Army Historical Summary–Fiscal Year 1979. Edited by Edith M. Boldan, Washington, DC: Center of Military History, 1982.

Department of the Army Historical Summary–Fiscal Year 1980. Edited by Lenwood Y. Brown. Washington, DC: Center of Military History, 1983.

Department of the Army Historical Summary: Fiscal Year 1981. Edited by Christine O. Hardyman. History, Washington, DC: Center of Military Department of the Army, 1988.

Department of the Army Historical Summary–Fiscal Year 1988. Edited by Cherly Morai-Young. Washington: Center of Military History, United States Army, 1993.

Department of the Army Historical Summary–Fiscal Year 1989. Edited by Vincent H. Demma. Washington: Center of Military History, United States Army, 1998.

Department of the Army Historical Summary, Fiscal Years 1990 and 1991. Edited by Scott W. Janes. Washington: United States Army, Center for Military History, 1997.

Department of the Army. *Medical Services Standards of Medical Fitness (AR 40-501, C35)*. Washington, DC: US Government Printing Office; 1987 (first published in December, 1960).

Department of the Army. M*emorandum of Understanding between the US Army Soldier Support Center and the US Army Infantry Center*, Subject: Army Physical Fitness System, signed 8 April 1982, Lieutenant General Julius Becton, Deputy Commander for Training.

Department of the Army. *Physical Conditioning (TM 21-200)*. Washington: US Government Printing Office; extracted from FM 21-20, 1957.

Department of the Army. *Physical Fitness Program for Women in the Army (DA Pamphlet 21-2).Washington: US Government Printing Office,* 7 January 1963.

Department of the Army. *Physical Fitness Program for Women in the Army (DA Pamphlet 21-2)*. Washington: US Government Printing Office, 26 February 1965.

Department of the Army. *Physical Fitness Training Program for Specialist and Staff Personnel (DA PAM 21-1),* Washington: US Government Printing Office, 7 January 1963 including Change 3, 26 July 1963.

Department of the Army. *Physical Readiness Training (FM 21-20)*. Washington, DC: US Government Printing Office, 1941.

Department of the Army. *Physical Readiness Training (FM 21-20)*. Washington, DC: US Government Printing Office, 1946.

Department of the Army. *Physical Readiness Training (FM 21-20)*. Washington, DC: US Government Printing Office, 1950.

Department of the Army. *Physical Readiness Training (FM 21-20)*. Washington, DC: US Government Printing Office, 1957.

Department of the Army. *Physical Readiness Training (FM 21-20)*. Washington, DC: US Government Printing Office, 1969.

Department of the Army. *Physical Readiness Training (FM 21-20)*. Washington, DC: US Government Printing Office, 1973.

Department of the Army. *Physical Readiness Training (FM 21-20)*. Washington, DC: US Government Printing Office, 1980.

Department of the Army. *Physical Readiness Training (FM 21-20)*. Washington, DC: US Government Printing Office, 1985.

Department of the Army. *Physical Fitness Training (FM 21-20)*. Washington, DC: US Government Printing Office. 1992.

Department of the Army. *Physical Fitness Training (FM 21-20)*. Washington, DC: US Government Printing Office, 1998.

Department of the Army. *Physical Training-Women's Army Corps (FM 35-20)*. Washington, DC: US Government Printing Office, 1956.

Department of the Army. *Physical Training-Women's Army Corps (FM 35-20)*. Washington, DC: US Government Printing Office, 1965.

Department of the Army. *Physical Training-Women's Army Corps (FM 35-20)*. Washington, DC: US Government Printing Office, 1975.

Department of the Army. *Standards of Medical Fitness (AR 40-501)*. Washington: US Government Printing Office 1960 (Changes to AR 40-501 occur almost annually up to 1987 (Change 35); after 1987 AR 40-501 was revised in 1998, 2008, 2010, 2011); the most current revision was published on 4 August 2011).

Department of the Army. *The Army Physical Fitness Program (AR 350-15)*. Washington: US Government Printing Office, 1982.

Department of the Army. *The Commander's Handbook on Physical Fitness (Pamphlet 350-15)*. Washington, DC: US Government Printing Office, 1982.

Department of the Army. "The Inclement Weather Physical Fitness Test." *Continental Army Command Pamphlet 600-1*. Fort Monroe: US Continental Army Command, 1966.

Department of the Army. *The Individual's Handbook on Physical Fitness (Pamphlet 350-18)*. Washington, DC: US Government Printing Office, 1983.

Department of the Army. *Training: Active Duty Training for FORSCOM Units-FORSCOM Regulation 350-1*. Fort McPherson, Georgia: United States Army Forces Command, 25 October 2002.

Department of the Army. *Training in Units (FM 350-41)*. Washington, DC: US Government Printing Office, 1993.

Department of the Army. *Training: Training in USAREUR–USAREUR Regulation 350-1*. Heidelberg, Germany: United States Army Europe Command, 22 July 2002.

Department of the Army. *Weight Control (AR 600-7)*. Washington: US Government Printing Office 1963.

Department of the Army. *Weight Control (AR 600-7)*. Washington: US Government Printing Office 1965.

Department of the Army. *Your Individual Physical Fitness*. Fort Benning, GA: US Army Infantry School, no date.

Gustave Dore, trans. *The Works of Rabelais (with notes and illustrations)–Book 1: Gargantua and His Son Pantagruel*. Derby: The Moray Press, 1894; later translated into English by Sir Thomas Urquhart of Cromarty and Peter A. Motteux.

Draper, George. (1918) Memorandum for the Chief of Staff, July 26, 1918, file # 7541-117; 296/165, NA; as reported in Jennifer D. Keene, *Doughboys, The Great War and the Remaking of America*, 26. Baltimore: Johns Hopkins University Press, 2003.

Drew, George. (1945) "A Historical Study of the Concern of the Federal Government for The Physical Fitness of Non-Age Youth with Reference to the Schools, 1790-1941." *Research Quarterly* October (1945): 202.

Dubik James. M., and T.D. Fullerton. "Soldier Overloading in Grenada." *Military Review* 66 (January, 1987): 38-47.

Easter, William. *Marine Corps PFT: Not Equal, Not Fair*. paper completed for the Expeditionary Warfare School, US Marine Corps, Command and Staff College, Marine Corps University, 2076 South Street, Marine Corps Combat Development Command, Quantico, VA, 22134-5068, 2009.

Eichna, Ludwig, William Bean, and William Ashe. *Comparison of Tests of Physical Fitness*. Fort Knox: Army Ground Forces Medical Research Laboratory, Project No. 5-5-29, File: 749.2-12, 1944.

Eisenberg, Christina. (1996) "Charismatic Nationalist Leader: Turnvater Jahn." *International Journal of the History of Sport* 13:1 (March 1996): 14–27.

Ellis, O.O., and E.B. Garey. *The Plattsburg Manual–A Handbook for Military Training*. New York: The Century Co., 1917.

Emerson, D.A., and Joy Hills. *The Victory Corps Program: A Wartime Program for High Schools*. Issued by Rex Putnam, Superintendent of Public Instruction, Salem, OR, January 1943.

Eckerle, Greg "Veteran Warren Evans Shares His War Stories." Evansville Currier & Press, 14 April 2008; http://www.courierpress.com/news/2008/apr/14/stranger-than-fiction (accessed 29 February 2012).

Farrow, Edward. *A Military System of Gymnastic Exercises and a System of Swimming* (prepared under the instructions of the Superintendent, for the use of the cadets of the United States Military Academy and military colleges). New York: Metropolitan Publishing Company, 1881.

Farrow, Edward. *Farrow's Manual of Military Training*. New York: Scientific American Publishing Co., 1920.

Fehrenbach, Theodore. *This Kind of War: A Study in Unpreparedness*. New York: The MacMillan Company, 1963.

Finlayson, Kenneth. *An Uncertain Trumpet: The Evolution of US Army Infantry Doctrine, 1919-1941*. Westport, CT: Greenwood Press, 2001.

"First Women Take Off." *Army Times*, May 17, 1993.

Flavius, Josephus. *The War of the Jews*. 78 AD; available at: http://www.sacred-texts.com/jud/ josephus/index.htm (accessed 11 April 2012).

Flint, Roy K. "Task Force Smith and the 24th Division: Delay and Withdrawal, 5-19 July 1950." In *America's First Battles 1776-1965*, edited by Charles E. Heller and William A. Stoff, 266-299. Lawrence, KS: University Press of Kansas, 1986.

Forbes, Clarence. *Greek Physical Education*. New York: The Century Company, 1929.

Ford, Edward. (1954) "The "de Arte de Gymnastica" of Mercuriale, *Australian Journal of Physiotherapy* 1:1 (October 1954): 30-32.

Forman, Sidney. *West Point: A History of the United States Military Academy*. New York: Columbia University Press, 1951.

"Former Michigan Quarterback Considered for Texas Coach: Has Colorful, Fighting Career," *San Antonio Express*, 10 January 1934.

Fosdick, Raymond B., and Edward F. Allen. "Athletics for the Army" *The Century Magazine* 96:3 (July 1918): 367-374.

Fosdick, Raymond B. *Chronicle of a Generation: An Autobiography* (specifically Chapter 8: Training Camps in World War I). New York: Harper, (1958): 142-186.

Fosdick, Raymond B. "Fit to Fighting–And After." *Scribner's Magazine* 63:4 (April 1918): 415-423

Fosdick, Raymond B. "The Commission on Training Camp Activities." *Proceedings of the Academy of Political Science in the City of New York* 7:4 (February, 1918): 163-170.

Fosdick, Raymond B. "The War and Navy Departments Commission on Training Camp Activities." *Annals of the American Society of Political and Social Science* 79 (September 1918): 130-142.

Fox, Don. *Patton's Vanguard: The Unites States Army Fourth Armored Division*. Jefferson, NC: McFarland & Company, Inc., Publishers; 2003.

Foxley, Barbara, trans. *Emile (On Education) by Rousseau, Jean-Jacques.* The Project Gutenberg EBook Series, 18 July 2002.

France, Robert. *Introduction to Physical Education and Sports Science*. Clifton Park, New York: Delmar, Cengage Learning, 2009.

Franklin, Benjamin. *Proposals Relating to the Education of Youth in Pensilvania*. National Humanities Center Resource Toolbox, Becoming American: The British Atlantic Colonies, 1690-1763, 1774.

Friedl, Karl, James A. Vogel, Matthew W. Bovee, and Bruce H. Jones. *Assessment of Body Weight Standards in Male and Female Army Recruits*, Natick, MA: US Army Research Institute of Environmental Medicine Technical Report No. T15-90, 1989.

Friedl, Karl. "Body Composition and Military Performance: Origins of the Army Standards." In *Body Composition and Physical Performance–Applications for the Military Services*; edited by Bernadette M. Marriott and Judith Grumstrup-Scott, 31-55. Washington: DC-National Academy Press, 1992.

"General Order, No. 53." *The American Annual Cyclopedia and Register of Important Events of the Year 1862, Volume II* (by order of Major General Jackson on 28 May, 1862), New York: D. Appleton & Company, 1863.

"General Bell's Career." *New York* Times, 26 March, 1917.

Gerber, Ellen. *Innovators and Institutions in Physical Education*. Philadelphia: Lea & Febiger, 1971.

Goldman, Nancy. "The Changing Role of Women in the Armed Forces." *American Journal of Sociology* 78(4) (1973): 892-911.

Goldstein, Marcus. "Physical status of men examined through selective service in World War II." *Public Health Reports* 66:19 (11 May, 1951): 587-609.

Graham, Stanley. *Life of the Enlisted Soldier on the Western Frontier: 1815-1845*. Masters Thesis, North Texas State University, Denton, TX, 1972.

Grant, Michael. *A Short History of Classical Civilization*. London: Weidenfeld & Nicolson, 1991.

Green, Peter. *Classical bearings: Interpreting ancient history and culture*. London: Thames & Hudson, 1989.

Greene, Francis. *Physical Fitness and Physical Training in Korea – Survey of USMA gradates*; unpublished; 22 October 1951.

Hagen, Monys. "Sport, Domestic Strength, and National Security." In *Work, Recreation, and Culture*, edited by Martin H. Blatt and Martha K. Norkunas, 73-99. New York: Garland Publishing Inc., 1996.

Hartwell, Edward. "Physical Training in American Colleges and Universities." *Report to the Commission of the US Stated Bureau of Education, No. 5-1885*. Washington: US Government Printing Office–including a report titled "Physical Training in Germany" (Appendix), 1886.

Hastings, Max. *The Korean War*. New York: Simon and Schuster, 1987.

Hawkins, John. *A Manual of Physical Exercises*. Indianapolis: s.n., 1909.

Hearings on H.R. 1975-First Deficiency Appropriations Bill for 1943. Subcommittee of the Committee on Appropriations, United States Senate, 78th Congress, Washington, DC: US Government Printing Office, 1943.

Hearings on H.R. 1975-First Deficiency Appropriations Bill for 1943. Subcommittee of the Committee on Appropriations, United States House of Representatives, 78th Congress, Washington, DC: US Government Printing Office, 1943.

Hearing on S.875-A Bill to Provide for the Preparation of High School Students for Wartime Service. Subcommittee of the Committee on Appropriations, Hearings 41-42; US Senate, 78th Congress, 1st Session, Committee on Education and Labor, Washington, DC: US Government Printing Office, 1943.

Heinrichs, Allison M. "University of Pittsburgh Strengthens Army Training." *Tribune-Review*, 23 August, 2009. (assessed at: http://www.pittsburghlive.com/x/pittsburghtrib/news/pittsburgh/s_639635.html)

Hesse-Lichtenberger, Ulrich. *Tor! The Story of German Football*, London: WSC Books Ltd, 2003.

Hertling, Mark. *Physical Training and the Modern Battlefield: Are We Tough Enough?* Fort Leavenworth, KS: School of Advanced Military Studies Monograph, US Army Command and General Staff College, 1987.

Higgs, Robert, and Michael Braswell. *An Unholy Alliance: The Sacred and Modern Sports*. Macon, GA: Mercer University Press, 2004.

High School Victory Corps. Hearings before the Committee on Education and Labor; United States Senate on S.875–Bill to provide for the preparation of high-school students for wartime service. Washington: US Government Printing Office, 14 April, 1943.

Hodgdon, James. "Body Composition in the Military Services: Standards and Methods." In *Body Composition and Physical Performance–Applications for the Military Services*, edited by Bernadette M. Marriott and Judith Grumstrup-Scott, 50-70. Washington, DC: National Academy Press, 1992.

Hodgdon, James. *A History of the US Navy Physical Readiness Program from 1976 to 1999.* Arlington, VA: Office of Naval Research, 18 August, 1999.

Holm, Jeanne. *Women in the Military: An Unfinished Revolution.* Navato, CA: Presidio Press, 1982 (revised in 1992).

Hooker, J.T. *The Ancient Spartans*. London: J.M. Dent, 1980.

Hooker, Richard. "Presidential Decision Making and Use of Force: Case Study Grenada." *Parameters* Summer (1991): 61-72).

House, Jonathan. "Review of 'After the Trenches: The Transformation of US Army Doctrine, 1918-1939', by W. 0. Odom." *Journal of Military History* 63:4 (1999): 1000-1001.

House, Jonathan. *Toward Combined Arms Warfare: A Survey of 20th-Century Tactics, Doctrine, and Organization*. Research Survey No. 2, Combat Studies Institute, Fort Leavenworth, KS: US Army Command and General Staff College, 1984.

Idone, Frank. *US Army Exercises: Rearranged for General Use*, New York: Richard K. Fox, 1904.

"Induction Statistics." www.sss.gov/induct.htm (accessed 24 Sept 2010).

"J. Franklin Bell, Army Unfit, Says General Bell," *New York Times*, May 24 1908.

Jahn, Friedrick and Ernst Eiselen. *Die Deutsche Turnkunst.* Berlin: Preis and Thaler, 1816.

Jones Lieutenant General, Anthony R. *AR 15-6 Investigation of the Abu Ghraib Prison and 205th Military Intelligence Brigade*, Department of the Army, 23 August 2004.

Karpovich, Peter, and R. A. Weiss. "Physical Fitness of Men Entering the Army Air Forces." *Research Quarterly* 17:3 (1946): 184-192.

Karpovich, Peter. "Exercise." *Annual Review of Physiology* 9:1 (1947): 149-162.

Keene, Jennifer. *Doughboys, The Great War and The Remaking of America*. Baltimore: Johns Hopkins University Press, 2003.

Keene Jennifer. *World War I*. Westport, CT: Greenwood Press, 2006.

Keene Jennifer. *The United States and the First World War*; New York: Longman Press; 2000.

Kelly, Jack. "Training to prevent injuries gains strength at an Army base." *Pittsburgh Post-Gazette*, 02 September 2009. (accessed at: http://old.post-gazette.com/pg/09245/994728-114.stm#ixzz1rfPzqmJC)

Kennedy, John F. *Remarks by Senator John F. Kennedy on Defense Department Appropriations Bill to the Senate on June 17, 1954*. JFK Presidential Library and Museum, 1954.

Kennedy, John F. "The Soft American." *Sports Illustrated* 12:26 (December 26, 1960): 14-17.

Knapik, Joseph J., Jeffery Staab, Michael Bahrke, Katy Reynolds, James Vogel, and John O'Connor. *Soldier Performance and Mood States Following a Strenuous Road March*. Natick, MA: US Army Research Institute of Environmental Medicine, 1990.

Knapik, Joseph J., Louis Banderet, Michael Bahrke, John O'Connor, Bruce Jones, and James Vogel. *Army Physical Fitness Test (APFT): Normative Data on 6022 Soldiers* (Technical Report No. T94-7). Natick, MA: US Army Research Institute of Environmental Medicine, 1994.

Knapik, Joseph J., Phillip Ange, Katy Reynolds, and Bruce Jones. "Physical Fitness, Age, and Injury Incidence in Infantry Soldiers." *Journal of Occupational* Medicine 35:6 (June 1993): 598-603.

Knapik, Joseph J., Michelle Canham-Chervak, Keith Hauret, Mary Jo Laurin, Edward Hoedebecke, Stephen Craig, and Scott J. Montain. "Seasonal Variations in Injury Rates during US Army Basic Combat Training." Annals of Occupational Hygiene 46:1 (2002): 15-32.

Knapik, Joseph J, Michelle Canham-Chervak, Edward Hoedebecke, William C. Hewitson, Keith Hauret, Christy Held, and Marilyn A. Sharp. "The Fitness Training Unit in US Army Basic Combat Training: Physical Fitness, Training Outcomes, and Injuries." *Military Medicine* 166:4 (2001) 356-361.

Koehler, Herman J. *Manual of Callisthenic Exercises*. Washington, DC: US Government Printing Office, War Department, 1892.

Koehler, Herman J. (1904) "The Physical Training of Cadets." In *The Centennial of the United States Military Academy at West Point, New York–1802-1902*, Washington: Government Printing House; Volume I (1904): 893-908.

Koehler, Herman J. *Manual of Gymnastic Exercises: Prepared for Use in Service Gymnasiums*. Washington DC: US Government Printing Office, War Department, 1904.

Koehler, Herman J. *Manual for Physical Training for use in the United States Army*. New York: Military Publishing Company, War Department, 1914.

Koehler, Herman J. *Extracts From the Manual for Physical Training for Use in the United States Army*. Washington, DC: US Government Printing Office, War Department, 1918.

Koehler, Herman J. *Koehler's West Point Manual of Disciplinary Training*. New York: E. P. Dutton & Company, 1919.

Kraus, Hans, and Bonnie Prudden. "Muscular Fitness and Health." *Journal of the American Association for Health, Physical Education, Recreation* 24:10 (December, 1953): 17-19.

Kraus, Hans. and Ruth P. Hirshland. "Minimum Muscular Fitness Tests in School Children." *Research Quarterly*, 25 (1954): 177-178.

Krause, Michael D. "History of US Army Soldier Physical Fitness." In *National Conference on Military Physical Fitness-Proceedings Report*, edited by Lois A. Hale, 20-23. Washington, DC: National Defense University, (1990).

LaGrange, Fernand. *Physiology of Bodily Exercise*. New York: D. Appleton and Co. 1890.

Lacy, F. E. Colonel. War Department: Memorandum for the Chief of Staff–Subject: Physical and Bayonet Training." In "News and Notes." *American Physical Education Review* 24:7:152 (October 1919): 418-420.

Ladd, John P. *US Army Physical Fitness Testing: Past, Present and Future*, Student paper written for the Communicative Arts Program, March, 1971.

Lang, Will. "Lucian Truscott." *Life Magazine* (2 October 1944): 96-108.

Larkin, Christopher. P. "Combat Fitness a Concept Vital to National Security." Paper-Master of Science Degree, Department of Defense: Joint Forces Staff College, 18 June 2010.

Laurens, John. *The Army Correspondence of Colonel John Laurens in the Years 1777-8,* New York: Bradford Club, 1867.

LeBoeuf, Maureen K., and Whitfield B. East. "Case No. 2: Physical Readiness and Assessment." In *The Future of the Army Profession*; edited by Lloyd J. Matthews, 469-487, Boston: McGraw Hill Primis Custom Publishing, 2006.

Leland, Anne, and Mari-Jana Oboroceanu. "American War and Military Operations Casualties: Lists and Statistics." *Congressional Research Service*, 7-5700, RL32492, 26 February 2010.

Leonard, Fred E. "The Beginning of Modern Physical Training in Europe." *American Physical Education Review* 9:2 (1904): 89-110.

Leonard, Fred. E. "Per Heinrich Ling, and His Successors at the Stockholm School of Gymnastics." *American Physical Education Review* 9:4 (1904) 226-244.

Leonard, Fred E. "The Transition from Medieval to Modern Times-Chapters in the History of Physical Training." *American Physical Education Review* 10:3 (1905): 189-202.

Leonard, Fred E. *Pioneers of Modern Physical Training*, New York: Association Press, 1915.

Leonard, Fred E. *History of Physical Education*; Philadelphia: Lea & Febiger, 1923.

Leonard, Fred E., and George B. Affleck. *A Guide to the History of Physical Education*; Philadelphia: Lea & Fibiger, 1947.

Link, Arthur S. *Woodrow Wilson and the Progressive Era, 1910-1917*. New York: Harper and Row, 1954.

Little, L. L. "There is No Limit to Human Endurance." *Outing* November (1918): 113-117.

Locke, John. *Some Thoughts Concerning Education*. London: Printed for A. and J. Churchill, 1693

Lovett, Charles C. *Olympic Marathon: A Centennial History of the Games' Most Storied Race*. Westport, Conn: Praeger, 1997.

Lowman, C. Thomas. "Does Current Army Physical Training Doctrine Adequately Prepare Soldiers For War?." MA thesis, Fort Leavenworth, KS: Command and General Staff College, 2010.

MacArthur, Douglas. *Reminiscences*. New York, NY: McGraw Hill Book Company, 1964.

MacLaren, Archibald. *A Military System of Gymnastic Exercises, and a System Of Fencing, for the Use of Instructors*. London: Her Majesty's Stationary Office, 1868.

MacLaren, Archibald. *A System of Physical Education–Theoretical and Practical*. Oxford: Clarendon Press Series, 1869.

Magee, James C. "Relationship of the Health of Civilians to the Efficiency of the Army." *American Journal of Public Health* 30 (November 1940): 1283-1290.

"Manual of Military Gymnastics." *Army and Navy Journal* III:24:128 (1866): 376-377.

Marshall, S.L.A. "First Wave at Omaha Beach." *The Atlantic* (November, 1960); http://www.theatlantic.com/magazine/archive/1960/11/first-wave-at-omaha-beach/3365/ (accessed 2 March 2012).

Marshall, S.L.A. *The Soldier's Load and the Mobility of a Nation*. Quantico: The Marine Corps Association, 1980.

Mason, Samuel. W. *Manual of Gymnastic Exercises for Schools and Families*, 4th Ed. Boston: Crosby and Nichols, 1863.

Matthews, David O. "A Historical Study of the Aims, Contents, and Methods of Swedish, Danish, and German Gymnastics." *Proceedings National College Physical Education Association for Men*. 72nd Conference, (January, 1969): 145.

McClary, William J. *Captain Alden Partridge, Superintendent of West Point during Its Formative Years-The Truth about the Man behind the Myth*. Paper completed for LD 720–American Military History, United States Military Academy, 2001.

McClellan, George B. *The Seat of War in Europe* (Report to the Secretary of War), Washington: A.O.P Nicholson, Printer, 1857.

McCloy, Charles H. *Tests and Measurements in Health and Physical Education*. New York: F.S. Crofts & Co., 1939.

McElroy, Mary. "A Sociohistorical Analysis Of US Youth Physical Activity And Sedentary Behaviors." In *Physical Activity and Sedentary Behavior–Challenges and Solutions*, edited by Alan L. Smith and Stuart J.H. Biddle, 59-78, Champaign, IL: Human Kinetics Inc., 2008.

McGugan, Stephen. *The Cadet Physical Fitness Test: Overachieving Or Overdemanding?*, Paper completed for LD720, American Military History, West Point, NY, 1997.

McMillian, Danny "Ranger Athlete Warrior Program: A Systemic Approach to Conditioning." *Infantry* 96:3 (May-June 2007): 5-8.

McNeese, Tim. *The Battle of the Bulge*, Philadelphia: Chelsea House Publishers, 2004.

"Medal of Honor for Colonel Bell," *New York Times*, 29 November 1899.

Merkel, Udo. "Politics of Physical Culture and German Nationalism: Turnen versus English Sports and French Olympians: 1871-1914." *German Politics & Society* 21:2 (Summer 2003) 69-96.

Mercurialis, Hieronymus. *De Arte De Gymnastica Libri Sex; Venetiss: APVD Ivntas*, 1601.

Miller, Nathan. *Theodore Roosevelt: A Life*. New York: Quill–William Morrow, 1992.

"Millions Taught to Box in Army," *New York Times*, May 11, 1919.

Mitchell, Brian P. *Weak Link: The Feminization of the American Military*. Washington: Regnery Gateway, 1989.

Mitchell, Brian P. *Women in the Military: Flirting With Disaster*. Washington, DC: Regnery Publishing, Inc., 1998.

Moore, Stephen, and James Carter. *The Strongest Economy in a Generation–If You're a Government Worker*. 15 November 1996, on http://www.cato.org/pub_display.php?pub_id=6254 (accessed March 15, 2011).

Montaigne, Michel De. *The Education of Children* (1580). Translated by L. E. Rector. New York: D. Appleton and Company, 1899.

Morden, Bettie. J. *The Women's Army Corps, 1945-1978*. Washington: Center of Military History, Unites States Army, 2000 (especially Chapter XIII–Women in the Army: 367-398).

"Move to Close Army School Scored." *The Times-News* (Hendersonville, NC), October 5, 1953.

"Muldoon Curing General Bell," *New York Times*, October 14, 1907.

Mustion, Richard. P. "Sustaining Our Army Then and Now." In *Professional Bulletin of the United States Army Sustainment* PB700-09-06 41:6 (November-December 2009): 25-29.

Muukkonen, Martti. "Orandum Est Ut Sit Mens Sana In Corpore Sano–Formation of the Triangle Principle of the YMCA." Paper presentation to the TUHTI Seminar of the Finnish Youth Research Society. Helsinki, 20 September 2001.

Nash, Willard Lee. *A Study of the stated aims and purposes of the Departments of Military Science and Tactics and Physical Education in the land-grant colleges of the United States*, Doctoral Dissertation, Teachers College, Columbia University, NY, 1934.

National Conference on Military Physical Fitness–Proceedings Report. Edited by Lois Hale. Washington, DC: National Defense University, US Department of Health and Human Services, 1990.

"Neuromuscular Research Laboratory Newsletter," Department of Sports Medicine and Nutrition, University of Pittsburgh, 1:2 (2009): 4.

Nye, David E. *Electrifying America: Social Meanings of a New Technology, 1880-1940*. Cambridge, Mass: MIT Press, 1990.

O'Connor, John S., Michael S. Bahrke, and Robert G. Tetu. "1988 Active Army Physical Fitness Survey." *Military Medicine* 155:12 (1990): 579-585.

Odom, William O. *After The Trenches: The Transformation of US Army Doctrine, 1918-1939*. College Station: Texas A&M Press, 1999.

"Official Army Register for 1907," 59th Congress, 2nd Session, December 3, 1906; Washington: US Government Printing Office, House Document, Volume 100, 4 March 1907.

"Official Register of the Officers and Cadets of the United States Military Academy,"
West Point, NY: USMA Press and Bindery, June, 1905.

"Official Register of the Officers and Cadets of the United States Military Academy,"
West Point, NY: USMA Press and Bindery, June, 1906.

Oldfield, E.A.L. *History of the Army Physical Training Corps*. Aldershot: Gale & Polden LTD, 1955.

Ogorkiewicz, Richard. M. *Armor: A History of Mechanized Forces*. New York: Frederick A. Praeger, Publisher, 1960.

Orvis, Bruce R., Laurie L. McDonald, Michael G. Mattock, M. Rebecca Kilburn, and Michael G. Shanley. *Ensuring Personnel Readiness in the Army Reserve Components*, Santa Monica, CA: The Rand Corporation, 1996.

Paine, Jeffery, James Uptgraft, and Ryan Wylie. *CrossFit Study*, Fort Leavenworth, KS: Command and General Staff College, May, 2010.

Paine, Ralph D. "The Gospel of the Turn Verein." *Outing* 46:2 (May, 1905): 174-182.

Park, Roberta. J. "Research Note: Edward M. Hartwell and Physical Training at the Johns Hopkins University, 1879-1890." *Journal of Sport History* 14:1 (1987): 108-119.

Park, Roberta. J. "Physiologists, Physicians And Physical Educators: Nineteenth Century Biology and Exercise." *Journal of Sport History* 14 (1987): 29-60.

Parkes, E. A. *On Personal Care of Health*, London: Society for Promoting Christian Knowledge, 1886.

Partridge, Alden. "Individual and Corporate Institutions for Military Instruction." *The American Journal of Education* 7:82 (1872): 834-848.

Partridge, Alden. "Lecture on Education." In *The Art of Epistolary Composition and Discourse on Education*, edited by Francois Peyre-Ferry's, 263-280, Middletown, Conn.: E & H. Clark, 1826.

Partridge, Alden. *A Journal of an Excursion Made by the Corps of Cadets of the American Literary, Scientific and Military Academy.* Concord: Hill and Moore, June, 1822

Pemrick, Michael D. *Physical Fitness and the Seventy-Fifth Ranger Regiment: The Components of Physical Fitness and the Ranger Mission.* Master of Military Art and Science Thesis, US Army Command and General Staff College, Fort Leavenworth, KS, 1999.

Pfister, Gertrud. "The Role of German *Turners* in American Physical Education." *International Journal of the History of Sport* 26:13 (2009): 1893–1925.

Pfister, Gertrud. "Cultural Confrontations: German Turnen, Swedish Gymnastics and English Sport–European Diversity in Physical Activity from a Historical Perspective." *Culture, Sport, Society* 6:1 (2003): 61-91

Physical Activity and Health: A Report of the Surgeon General (1999). US Department of Health and Human Services; Superintendent of Documents, PO Box 371954, Pittsburgh, PA 15250–7954, S/N 017–023–00196–5; http://www.cdc.gov/nccdphp/sgr/index.htm (accessed 15 July 2011).

"Physical and Employment Standards." Australian Defense Force: Point of Contact–Major Ryan Holmes, March 2011.

"Physical Fitness and Musculoskeletal Injury." In *Assessing Fitness for Military Enlistment: Physical, Medical, and Mental Health Standards*, edited by Paul R. Sackett and Anne S. Mavor, 66-108, Washington, DC: The National Academies Press, 2006.

"Physical Fitness Policies and Programs." In *Assessing Readiness in Military Women: The Relationship of Body Composition, Nutrition, and* Health. published by the Committee on Body Composition, Nutrition, and Health of Military Women; Committee on Military Nutrition Research; Food and Nutrition Board, 61-85; Washington, DC: National Academic Press; 1998.

"Physical Fitness Program – Editorial." *The Journal of the American Medical Association*, 125:12 (22 July 1944): 850 (unsigned, however often attributed by several to Colonel Leonard Rowntree).

Physical Fitness Seminar Report. Fort Benning: United States Army Infantry School (Osgard, J.L., Secretary), 21-24 April, 1958.

Physical Fitness Symposium Report. Fort Benning: United States Infantry School (Frandsen, H. F., Secretary), 12-14 October, 1970.

"Physical Training for Army Officers and Men," *New York Evening Post*, October 6, 1919.

Pilcher, James. E. "The Building of the Soldier." *The United Service* 7:4 (April, 1892): 321-337.

Pollock, Michael L., Glenn A. Gaesser, Janus D. Butcher, Jean-Pierre Després, Rod K. Dishman, Barry A. Franklin, and Carol Ewing Garber. "Position Stand: The Recommended Quantity and Quality of Exercise for Developing and Maintaining Cardiorespiratory and Muscular Fitness, and Flexibility in Healthy Adults," *Medicine & Science in Sports and Exercise* 30:6 (June 1998): 500-511.

Preventing Injuries in the US Military: The Process, Priorities, and Epidemiologic Evidence. Injury Prevention Report No. 12-HF-04MT-08, Aberdeen Proving Ground, MD: Army Center for Health Promotion and Preventive Medicine, December 2008.

Proceedings of the Annual Meeting of the American Association of Physical Education. New York: Adelphi University, 1885.

Rabelais, François. *Gargantua and His Son Pantagruel.* Book 1, Chapter 1.23,1535.

Ranger Athlete Warrior (RAW) Manuals/Materials:

RAWPT, v.2.0. Fort Benning, GA: 75th Ranger Regiment, 2006.

RAW PT, v.3.0. Fort Benning, GA: 75th Ranger Regiment, 2008.

RAW PT, v.4.0. Fort Benning, GA: 75th Ranger Regiment, 2010.

Further, Faster, Harder (RAW Historical Briefing Slides). Fort Benning, GA: 75th Ranger Regiment, 1 September 2011.

Raycroft, Joseph. *Mass Physical Training for use in the Army and Reserve Officer Training Corps.* Washington: US Infantry Association, 1920.

Reagor, Michael J. "Herman J. Koehler: The Father of West Point Physical Education, 1985–1923." *Assembly*, 51:3 (Jan 1993): 16-19.

Reiser, Stanley J. "The Emergence of the Concept of Screening for Disease." *The Milbank Memorial Fund Quarterly, Health and Society* 56:4. (1978): 403-425.

Report of the Commission. Appointed under the eighth section of the act of Congress of June 21, 1860, to Examine into the Organization, System of Discipline, and Course of Instruction, West Point: United States Military Academy, 13 December 1860.

Reports Of A Curriculum Study–To Recommend Changes in the USMA Curriculum: 1857-1859. USMA Archives, 1859.

Rice, Emmett A. *A Brief History of Physical Education.* New York: A. S. Barnes and Company, 1936.

Rice, Emmett A., John L. Hutchinson, and Mabel E. Lee. *A Brief History of Physical Education*. New York: The Ronald Press Co, 1958.

"Roosevelt Led 60 on A Bully Tramp," *New York Times*, November 8, 1908.

Roosevelt, Theodore. *America and the First World War*. New York: Charles Scribner's Sons, 1915.

Rowntree, Leonard G. "National Program for Physical Fitness." *The Journal of the American Medical Association* 125:12 (22 July 1944): 821-827.

Ruscio, Bruce, Jack Smith, Paul Amoroso, Jerry Aslinger, Steve Bullock, Bruce Burnham, et al. *DOD Military Injury Prevention Priorities Working Group: Leading Injuries, Causes and Mitigation Recommendations*. Washington, DC: Office of the Assistant Secretary of Defense for Health Affairs, Clinical and Program Policy, February 2006.

Ryan, Allan J. "A Medical History of Gymnastics." *Journal of the American Medical Association* 162:12 (1956): 1112-1115.

Saunders, Mark. "1982 US Army Year of Physical Fitness". *Soldier Support Journal* 147 (May/June, 1982): 4-7.

Schaible, Charles Henry. *An Essay on the Systematic Training of the Body*. London: Trubner and Co., Ludgate Hill, 1878.

Schoy, Michael. *General Gerhard Von Scharnhorst: Mentor of Clausewitz and Father of the Prussian-German General Staff*. unpublished, March, 1809.

Schwarzkopf, H. Norman. *It Doesn't Take a Hero*. New York: Bantam Books, 1992.

Scott, Hugh. "Comments on Compulsory Military Service," War Department Annual Reports, 1916. Washington, DC: US Government Printing Office, 1917), Volume I, 155-162 (Reprint in *The Military Draft: Selected Readings on Conscription*, edited by Martin Anderson, 515-25, Stanford: Hoover Institution Press, 1982).

Selective-Service Act: Hearings before the Committee on Military Affairs, House of Representative, Sixty-fifth Congress, The Bill Authorizing the President to Increase Termorarly the Military Establishment of the United States (April 7, 14, and 17, 1917), Washington: US Government Printing Office, 1918.

Spencer, Lyle M., and Robert K. Burns. *Youth Goes to War*, Chicago: Science Research Associates, 1943.

Stansbury, Edgar B. "The Physical Fitness Program of the Army Air Forces." *The Journal of Health and Physical Education* 14:9 (1943): 463-504.

Stelpfug, Peggy A., and Richard Hyatt. "Home of the Infantry: The history of Fort Benning." In *Historical Chattahoochee Commission: National Infantry Association*, 396:400, Macon, GA: Mercer University Press, 2009.

Stewart, M.B. *The Physical Development of the Infantry Soldier*. Menasha, WI: George Banta Press, 1913.

Stille, Charles J. "The Life and Services Of Joel R. Poinsett, The Confidential Agent In South Carolina Of President Jackson During The Nullification Troubles Of 1832." Reprinted from *The Pennsylvania Magazine of History and Biography* (1888).

Studies in Citizenship for the Recruit, US Army Training Manual No. 1, Washington, DC: US Government Printing Office, 1922.

Studies in Citizenship for the Recruit–Military Training Camps US Army Training Manual No. 2, Washington, DC: US Government Printing Office, 1922.

Sturgeon, Julie, and Janice Meer. *The First 50 Years 1956-2006 – The President's Council on Physical Fitness and Sports Revisits Its Roots and Charts Its Future*, (no date): 40-53, http://www.fitness.gov/ about/history_narrative/index.html (accessed 15 September 2011)

Sullivan, Gordon R. "A Trained and Ready Army: The Way Ahead." *Military Review* 71:11 (November, 1991): 2-9.

The Plattsburger. New York: Wynkoop, Hallenbeck, Crawford Co., 1917.

"The Retirement of Colonel Herman Koehler." *The Pointer* 1 (22 October 1923): 4.

"The US Army in Vietnam." In *American Military History*, edited by Vincent H. Demma, 619-693. Washington, DC: Center of Military History, United States Army, 1898.

Thomas, David E. "Selection of the Parachutist." *Military Surgeon Magazine* 91 (1942): 81-83 and *Military Review* 86 (1942): 64.

Tomasi, Louis F., P. Rey Regualos, Gene Fober, and Matthew Christenson. *Age and Gender Performance on the US Army Physical Fitness Test*. Fort Benning, GA: Army Physical Fitness School, 1995.

Townsend, Stephen J. "The Factors of Soldier's Load." Master's thesis, Command and General Staff College, Fort Leavenworth, KA, 1994.

TRADOC Information Pamphlet: An Imminent and Menacing Threat to National Security. Fort Monroe, VA: TRADOC Public Affairs Office, 2008."

"Transition, Change, And The Road To War, 1902–1917," In *American Military History Volume I: The United States Army and the Forging of a Nation, 1775-1917*, edited by Richard W. Stewart, 365-386. Washington, DC: Center for Military History, United States Army, 2005.

Truscott, Lucian. *Command Missions, A Personal Story*. New York: Dutton, 1954.

Turnbull, George. *Observations upon Liberal Education, In All Its Branches*. London: Printed for A Milar (1742), edited with introduction by Terrance O. Moore, Indianapolis: Liberty Fund, 2003.

Tuttle, Jr., William. "Part Two: The American Family on the Home Front." In *World War II and the American Home Front*, prepared by Marilyn M. Harper, Project Manager & Historian, 51- 79. Washington, DC: The National Historic Landmarks Program, Cultural Resources, National Park Service, US Department of the Interior, October 2007.

Ugland, Richard M. "Education for Victory: The High School Victory Corps and Curricular Adaptation during World War II." *History of Education Quarterly* 19:4, (1979): 435-451.

United States Army Physical Fitness School Archived Historical Documents (unpublished):

"History of the Present APFT," (no date, unsigned), 1-12.

"World War II," (1987, unsigned), 33-41.

"Soldier Physical Fitness Center: An Historical Review," (no date, unsigned), 42-52.

"Physical Fitness and the Modern Army: 1980 Onward," (no date, unsigned), 53-69.

"Why Physical Fitness is Important to the Modern Army," (1987, unsigned), 70.

USAF Aerobics Physical Fitness Program–Pamphlet 50-56. Washington, DC: US Government Printing, 1966.

Urwin, Gregory J.W. *United States Infantry: An Illustrated History 1775-1918*, New York: Sterling Publishing Company, 1988.

Victory Corps Series. Published by the Officer of Education and the Federal Security Agency, Washington: US Government Printing Office.

Pamphlet 1 – "High School Victory Corps," (1942).

Pamphlet 2 – "Physical Fitness through Physical Education," (1942).

Pamphlet 3 – "Physical Fitness through Health Education," (1943).

Pamphlet 4 – "Guidance Manual," (1943).

Pamphlet 5 – "Community War Services," (1943).

Pamphlet 6 – "Service in the Armed Forces," (1944).

"Victory through Fitness"–National War Fitness Conference." *Journal of Health and Physical Education* 14:4, (1942): 131.

Von Hassell, Agostino, and Ed Breslin. *Patton: The Pursuit of Destiny*. Nashville: Nelson, 2010.

Vogel, James A., James E. Wright, John F. Patton III, Dan S. Sharp, James Dawson, and Mary Pat Eschenback. *A System for Establishing Occupationally-Related Gender-Free Physical Fitness Standards (Report No. T 5/80)*. Natick, MA: US Army Research Institute of Environmental Medicine, April 1980.

Vorschriften uber das Turnen der Infanterie. Gr. 8v0. Berlin: Mittler u. Sohn,1876.

Waldron, William H. *Army Physical Training*, New York: Henry Holt and Co, 1919.

"Wants Mexico Cleaned Up–Senator Falls Fears Conflict with European Army There." *New York Times*, 22 March 1916.

War Department Annual Report (1840): 32.

War Department Annual Report (1847): 81-82.

War Department Annual Report (1849): 186.

War Department Annual Report (1858): 14, 762, 788.

War Department. *Basic Field Manual: Volume I (Field Service Pocketbook–Chapter 4–Physical Training)*. Washington, DC: US Government Printing Office, 1936.

War Department. *Commission on Training Camp Activities*. Washington: US Government Printing Office. 1917.

War Department. *Field Physical Training of the Soldier: Special Regulations No. 23*. Washington, DC: US Government Printing Office, 1917

War Department. *Physical Conditioning–Pamphlet 21-9*. Washington: US Government Printing Office, 1944.

War Department. *Physical Training: Part I and Part II: Training Regulations No. 115-5*. Washington, DC: US Government Printing Office, 1928.

War Department. *General Orders and Circulars-1906*, Washington: US Government Printing Office, 1-3 (1907): 251.

War Department. *W.A.C. Field Manual Physical Training-FM 35-20*. Washington: US Government Printing Office, 1943.

Warfighter Support: Observations on DOD's Ground Combat Uniforms. US Government Accounting Office Report: GAO-10-669R Warfighter Support, May 28, 2010.

Watson, J. Madison. *Manual of Calisthenics: A Systematic Drill Book*. New York: E. Steiger & Co, 1882.

Webb, Lester A. *Captain Alden Partridge and the United States Military Academy, 1806-1833*. Northport, Ala: American Southern, 1965.

Whitfield, Richard W. *History of the US Army Artillery and Missile School*–Volume 3: 1945-1957. Fort Sill, OK: US Army Field Artillery School, 1957.

Whitlock, Joseph E. *How To Make Army Force Generation Work for the Army's Reserve Components*; Paper prepared for the Army War College Fellowship at the Institute for Advanced Technology at The University of Texas at Austin, August, 2006.

Wiley, Bell I., and William P. Govan. *History of the Second Army (Study No. 16)*. Washington: Historical Section, Army Ground Forces, 1946.

Winjum, Arte R.T. *Manual of Physical Exercises: A Health Hand-book*. Battle Creek, MI, by the author, 1909.

Wood, William. *Manual of Physical Exercises*, New York: Harper & Brothers, 1867.

Woodhull, Alfred A. *Notes on Military Hygiene for Officers of the Line*. New York: John Wiley & Sons, 1898.

Women Content in Units Force Development Test (MAXWAC Test). Alexandria, VA: US Army Research Institute for the Behavioral Sciences, 3 October 1977.

Worden, William L. *General Dean's Story as Told by William F. Dean*; New York: The Viking Press, 1954.

Wright, Robert K. *The Continental Army*, Washington, DC: Center for Military History, US Army, 1983.

Yebra, David J. *Colonel Herman J. Koehler: The Father of Physical Education at West Point*; paper written for LD 720: American Military History, United States Military Academy, 1998.

Figures Bibliography

Figure 1. Jahn's Turnplatz 8
 This drawing shows one of the earliest Turnplatz in Germany (1811); public domain, per Mr. Ed Thomas; www.ihpra.org.

Figure 2. MacLaren's 12 Apostles–Gymnasium, Oxford (April, 1861) 12
 Photo was taken in 1861–later published in Oldfield, E.A.L, History of the Army Physical Training Corps (Aldershot: Gale & Polden LTD, 1955), 2; in 1971 The Aldershot News (owned G/P) was acquired by the Surrey Advertiser Group, which later became part of the Guardian Group of newspapers. Robert Maxwell gained control of BPC and Gale & Polden with it in 1981, and named his new Company Maxwell Communications. In November 1981 Gale & Polden finally closed. Robert Maxwell died in 1991 and in 1992 Maxwell Communications collapsed, abandoning © privileges.

Figure 3. US Turnvereine Team–Frankfort 1880. 35
 Published in 1880–public domain.

Figure 4. USMA Physical Education under Herman Koehler 39
 Property of United States Military Academy, NY; public domain.

Figure 5. US Army's First PRT Manual–Herman Koehler 40
 Public Domain–Government Publication.

Figure 6. Milwaukee Bundesturnfest–1893 ....…... 41
 George Brosius, Fifty Years Devoted to the Cause of Physical Culture, 1864-1914 (Milwaukee: Germania Publishing, 1914), p. 39, photo published prior to 1923–public domain.

Figure 7. Roosevelt and Wood at the Plattsburg Training Camp (1916) 50
 Please find attached the CCHA agreement granting permission for use of the image you requested which includes President Theodore Roosevelt and General Leonard Wood. The CCHA board was happy to approve of the use, with no fee. Tricia Davies, Director/Curator, Clinton County Historical Association, 98 Ohio Avenue, Plattsburgh, NY 12903, director@clintoncountyhistorical.org www.clintoncountyhistorical.org.

 This photo is available in the Library of Congress' Digital Library with no known restrictions. See information: title: Honorable Theodore Roosevelt and General Wood, date created/published: c1920 January 15, medium: 1 photographic print, reproduction number: LC-USZ62-28470 (black

&white film copy negative), LC-USZC4-11865 (color film copy transparency), rights advisory: no known restrictions on publication, call number: PRES FILE-Roosevelt, Theodore—As Ex-President [item] [P&P], repository: Library of Congress Prints and Photographs Division, Washington, DC, 20540, http://hdl.loc.gov/loc.pnp/pp.print.

Figure 8. WWI Recruiting Posters for Plattsburg and the Army (1917) 53
Available through NARA/LOC–published prior to 1923–public domain.

Photo #1: Title: Are you trained to do your share? Plattsburg, date created/published: [1917], rights advisory: no known restrictions on reproduction, repository: Library of Congress Prints and Photographs Division, Washington, DC, 20540.

Photo #2: Paus, Herbert Andrew, artist. "The United States Army builds men. Apply nearest recruiting office," c1919. From Library of Congress Prints and Photographs Division, Washington, DC, http://www.loc.gov/pictures/item/94514699/.

Figure 9. Secretary of War Newton Baker drawing the First Draft Number (1917) 55
Drawing The First Number: after he had been blindfolded, Mr. Baker, Secretary of War, plunged his hand into the large glass jar containing the 10,500 numbers enclosed in capsules. He drew one forth and passed it to a clerk who opened it and announced the number "258." Thus the drawing began. The date was 20 July 1917. Photograph Copyright 1917 by Committee on Public Information (now in public domain). http://www.gjenvick.com/Military/WorldWarOne/TheDraft/SelectiveServiceSystem/1917-07-20-Draft- DrawingTheFirstNumber.html.

Figure 10. WWI Army Physical Training Formation 56
Raycroft, Joseph. Mass Physical Training for use in the Army and Reserve Officer Training Corps. Washington: US Infantry Association, 1920.

Figure 11. Boxing Instruction and Contests–WWI Training Camps................. 58
Photo #1 Title: Boxing Instruction During Basic Training. Photo is from Raycroft (1920, 85)–US Government Publication.

Photo #2 Title: Boxing Barracks, 311th Supply Trains, Camp Grant (1918). Photo is from the New York Public Library (pre 1923). Image Title: Boxing in barracks, 311th Supply Trains, Camp Grant, depicted date: [1918?], digital ID: 117132, record ID: 136623, digital item published: 2-3-2004; updated 3-25-2011; public domain.

Photos #3 Title: Boxing at Camp Greene, Charlotte, NC (1918). Photo is from: Charlotte Mecklenburg Library; approved by phone Jane Johnson, Librarian 15 March 2012. Source: Robinson-Spangler Carolina Room, Public Library of Charlotte and Mecklenburg County, 310 North Tryon Street, Charlotte, NC 28202, #704.416.0150. Accreditation: "Courtesy of the Robins-Spangler Carolina Room–Charlotte Mecklenburg Library."

Photo 4 Title: World's Largest Boxing Class, 337th Infantry Brigade, 27 June 1918. Photo is from the Library of Congress; Title: World's largest boxing class, 1st, 2nd and 3rd Bat's. [sic] of 337th Infantry Brigade conducted by Billy Armstrong, 27 June 1918. Related names: Mock, T. F., copyright claimant, date created/published: 27 June 1918, medium: 1 photographic print : gelatin silver ; 7.5 x 47.5 in., reproduction number: —, rights advisory: no known restrictions on publication. No renewal found in Copyright Office. Call Number: PAN US Military-Army no. 205 (E size) [P&P], repository: Library of Congress Prints and Photographs Division Washington, DC 20540.

Figure12. WWI Combat Readiness Training 59

All 5 photos are from the digital collection at the New York Public Library–open source, public domain.

Photo #1 Title: Wire Entanglement Negotiation Drills. Image title: Scene at student officers training camp at Fort Sheridan, IL; showing attack wave jumping barbed wire entanglements; depicted date: 1917, digital ID 117158, record ID: 136737.

Photo #2 Title: Trench Negotiation Drills. Image title: Trenches at student officers training camp, Fort Sheridan. Start of infantry attack; depicted date: [1917-1918] digital ID: 117192, record ID: 136788.

Photo #3 Title: Bayonet Charge from Trench. Image title: Bayonet charge out of a trench; depicted date: [1917-1918], digital ID: 117194, record ID: 136790.

Photo #4 Title: Casualty Evacuation Drills. Image title: Rescue from "no man's" land. Scene at student officers training camp, Fort Sheridan, IL; depicted date: 1917, Digital ID: 117161, record ID: 136740.

Photo #5 Title: Rush Drills with Rifle. Photo #5 image title: Soldiers running in a field; depicted date: 1917-1918, digital ID: 117188, record ID: 136784.

Figure 13. Post WWI PRT Manuals (Raycroft and Koehler) 61

Figure 14. Obstacle Course Run–Post WWI 65

Raycroft, Joseph. Mass Physical Training for use in the Army and Reserve Officer Training Corps. Washington: US Infantry Association, 1920.

Figure 15. Studies in Citizenship for Recruits 67

Figure 16. Renault Light Tank (1917) 69

Photo # 3: American troops going into the Forest of Argonne, France. Author: unknown or not provided, record creator: Department of Defense, Department of the Army, Office of the Signal Officer (18 September 1947- 28 February 1964, date: 26 September 1918, permission: this image is the work of a US Army Soldier or employee, taken or made during the course of the person's official duties. As a work of the US federal government, the image is in the public domain.

Figure 17. John B. Kelly, Chair–National Physical Fitness Council 81

Photo #2: is from the University of Pennsylvania Archives–open source: http://imagesvr.library.upenn.edu/cgi/i/image/imageidx?type=detail&cc=p ennarchive&entryid=X20050915004&viewid=1&sstrt=&hits=&q1=&cat 1=&thsz=&txsz=&slsz=1&med=&quality=thumbnail&ts=&c=pe nnarchive.

Figure 18. Physical Efficiency Matrix 84

Department of the Army. Physical Readiness Training (FM 21-20). Washington, DC: US Government Printing Office, 1941.

Figure 19. WWII Physical Readiness Training 85

Photo 1: Air Service Command PT Formation (1943). Photo is from FM 21-20 (1941); Department of the Army. Physical Readiness Training (FM 21-20). Washington, DC: US Government Printing Office, 1941.

Photo 2: Darby's Rangers Training (1942). A personal photo from the collection of Mr. Warren Evans; permission by phone on 19 March 2012, from Mr. Warren Evans and confirmed with his daughter "Connie" same date. Mr. Warren's son provided an updated permission for the publication.

Photo 3: Obstacle Course Training, Fort Jackson, SC (1943). A NARA photo: figure 126, obstacle course at Fort Jackson, SC, 28 April 1943 (NARA College Park, RG 111-SC WWII, Box 155, Photo SC173955), http://www.denix.osd.mil/cr/upload/05-265_Miscellaneous_Training_ Sites.pdf.

Photo 4: Commando Training, Camp Carson, CO (1943). A NARA photo: Commando training at Camp Carson, Colorado: 24 April 1943, ARC Identifier 197168, Franklin D. Roosevelt Library, Hyde Park, NY.

Figure 20. Obstacle Course Test (1941) 86
   Department of the Army. Physical Readiness Training (FM 21-20). Washington, DC: US Government Printing Office, 1941.

Figure 21. Rescuing Soldiers during Normandy Invasion (1944) 87
   Photo is part of the Army Signal Corps Collection posted by US National Archives (NARA).

Figues 22. Colonel Theodore Paul "Ted" Bank 88
   A "crop" from the 1920 University of Michigan football team photo; permission from: karen jania, sent: Thursday, 23 February 2012 10:11 AM, to: East, Whitfield, subject: Re: Fwd: Copyright question:

   Thank you for contacting the Bentley Historical Library for permission to use the image of Ted Bank, as the image is located within our holdings. The Bentley Historical Library is pleased to give you permission to use the requested image from the records of the University of Michigan Athletic Department in your monograph on the History of Army Physical Readiness Training. Please be aware that any further use of this material, whether in print or digital form (including use on a website) constitutes another use and that permission should be requested from us again, listing this new project. Please use the name of the collection, as well as Bentley Historical Library, University of Michigan, in your citation. If it is at all possible, we would be very interested in obtaining a copy of your monograph. Source: Karen L. Jania, Reference Archivist. "1920 Michigan Football Portrait" is cleared for use, Karen Jania provided an updated permission for the publication.

Figure 23. Victory Through Fitness–The Victory Corps 93
   Photo is the cover of a US Government publication.

Figure 24. Women's Army Corps Fitness (1943) 94
   Photo was taken from: War Department, W.A.C. Field Manual Physical Training-FM 35-20, Washington: US Government Printing Office, 1943.

Figure 25. Women's Army Corp (WAC) Physical Training 95
   Photo #1 Title: WASP Pilot Physical Training (1942). Physical Education training classes of WASPS at Avenger Field, Sweetwater, TX, 17 August 1944-NARA.

   Photo #2 Title: WACs Physical Training in Barracks. Time/Life – for personal, non commercial use; http://images.google.com/hosted/life/58c044a93a2b942a.html, WACs doing daily calisthenics exercises.

Location: Fort Des Moines, IA, date: 1942, photographer: Maria Hansen, Size: 1259 x 1280 pixels.

Photo #3 Title: WACs Performing Calisthenics (1942). Searching–ed Thomas (www.ihpra.org).

Photo #4 Title: Obstacle Course Training to Increase Agility. http://www.history.army.mil/books/wwii/Wac/ch09.htm, PHYSICAL TRAINING at an Army Air Forces Training Command base in 1943, "WACS Physical Training in Barracks." This photo is deemed Public Domain.

Figure 26. WAC Combat Readiness Training …….............................. 96

All four photos were taken from the Army Training Film (TF 35 3838), produced in 1967; http://www.youtube.com/watch?v=cUJyG7J8-44.

Figure 27. Army Air Corps Physical Training, Miami Beach (c. 1943) 100

Title: Soldiers performing training exercises on the beach during WWII- Miami Beach, Florida; image number RC04847, year: between 1939 and 1945, courtesy of: State Archives of Florida , source: approved by Mr. Adam Watson.

Figure 28. WWII Combat Readiness Training ………................................ 105

All four photos are from the Library of Congress:

Photo #1: Title: Camp Edwards, Massachusetts. In perfect steeplechase form, these soldiers of the anti-aircraft training center fling themselves over the five-foot rail fence. Par for the course is three and a half minutes; created/published: 1942(?), reproduction number: LC-USW33-000255-ZC (black &white film negative), rights advisory: no known restrictions on images made by the US government; images copied from other sources may be restricted.

Photo #2: Title: Camp Edwards, Massachusetts. Swinging across fifteen feet of horizontal ladders are soldiers of the anti-aircraft training center. This is the next-to-the-last obstacle on the course and comes at a time when a man's wind is coming hard and his arms are feeling fatigue. A fall here means a wetting to the unlucky soldier; created/published: 1942, reproduction number: LC-USW33-000256-ZC (black & white film negative), rights advisory: no known restrictions on images made by the US government; images copied from other sources may be restricted.

Photo #3: Title: Camp Edwards, Massachusetts. A hard-running leap takes these artillerymen over one of the obstacles on the obstacle course at the anti-aircraft training center. Here we see the different phases of the jump; one man has just landed on the sandbags; two are in the air; and another man is gathering himself for the spring across; Created/Published: 1942(?), reproduction number: LC-USW33-000257-ZC (black & white film negative), rights advisory: no known restrictions on images made by the US government; images copied from other sources may be restricted.

Photo #4: Title: Camp Edwards, Massachusetts. Up and over an eight-foot wall go seven soldiers of the anti-aircraft training center. The ropes are used only by the shorter warriors who cannot otherwise reach the top. Note the full equipment on each soldier; created/published: 1942(?), reproduction number: LC-USW33-000254-ZC (black & white film negative), rights advisory: no known restrictions on images made by the US government; images copied from other sources may be restricted.

Figures 29. Bayonet and Unarmed Combat Instruction 106

Photo is the property of USMC: Corporal Alvin "Tony" Ghazlo, the senior bayonet and unarmed combat instructor at Montford Point, demonstrates a disarming technique on his assistant, Private Ernest "Judo" Jones. Between 1942 and 1947, approximately 20,000 black recruits received training at Montford Point Camp; http://www.marinecorpstimes.com/news/2011/09/marine-montford-marines-added-to-crucible-091011. Source: the photo is public domain and you're welcome to use it. Please credit to Marine Corps. V/r; source: Captain Gregory A. Wolf, USMC Media Officer, Division of Public Affairs, Pentagon, Washington DC.

Figure 30. Exercises from the Kraus-Weber Test 121

Mr. Ed Thomas (www.ihpra.org/chapter_3.htm) has confirmed that this .jpeg is in the public domain and has given permission to use.

Figure 31. US Physical Fitness Program manual (1963) 128

Figure 32. Army Special Forces Rappel training (1963) 131

Photo is from NARA: Figure 157. Special Forces rappelling training tower at Fort Bragg, NC, 18 September 1963 (NARA College Park, RG 111-SC post-1955, Box 385, Photo SC609492).

Figure 33. Physical Fitness Readiness Training.. 132

All four photos were taken from a You Tube copy of a 1967 US Army training film (TF7–3856); http://www.youtube.com/watch?v=OXZ6dTo2Ksk.

Photo #1 Title: Bend and Twist.

Photo #2 Title: Knee Bender.

Photo #3 Title: Push-up.

Photo #4 Title: Formation Run.

Figure 34. Strength and Circuit in Basic Combat Training 134
    All four photos were taken from a You Tube copy of a 1967
    US Army training film (TF7–3856); http://www.youtube.com/
    watch?v=OXZ6dTo2Ksk.

Figure 35. Combat Readiness Physical Training (1967) 135
    All four photos were taken from a You Tube copy of a 1967
    US Army training film (TF7–3856); http://www.youtube.com/
    watch?v=OXZ6dTo2Ksk.

    Photo #1 Title: Rifle Drills, photo #2 Title: Log Drills, photo #3 Title: Guerilla/Grass Drills, photo #4 Title: Double-time Formation Runs.

Figure 36. Combat Obstacle Course Training (1967) 136
    All four photos were taken from a You Tube copy of a 1967
    US Army training film (TF7–3856); http://www.youtube.com
    watch?v=OXZ6dTo2Ksk.

Figure 37. Physical Combat Proficiency Test (1969) 138
    All four photos are still photos taken from a 1967 US Army Training file; Photos 1-3 were provided by Andy Erickson from www.CriticalPast.com. Photo 4: was taken from a You Tube copy of a 1967 US Army training film (TF7–3856); http://www.youtube.com/watch?v=OXZ6dTo2Ksk.

    Photo #1 Title: Horizontal Ladder Test, photo #2 Title: Run, Dodge, Jump Test, photo #3 Title: 150-yard Man Carry, photo #4 Title: 40-yard Low Crawl.

Figure 38. Combatives Training during Basic Training (Fort Knox, 1967) 139
    These four photos are all from Marshall Gagne's private collection–email permission; "Master Barror sent this email to me but the pictures wouldn't go. Feel free to use any picture you want and I appreciate that you will mention me." Marshall Gagne. Marshall Gagne has approved the use of all 4 photos for the publication.

Figure 39. Kenneth Cooper and Arthur Jones (c. 1975) 140
    Photo #1 Title: Kenneth H. Cooper, MD, MPH, Founder and Chairman of Cooper Aerobics at Cooper Clinic (c. 1970). Ken Cooper photo (email): Attached please find two photos you may use for your monograph. These photos were taken of Kenneth H. Cooper, MD, MPH, Founder and Chairman of Cooper Aerobics at Cooper Clinic in Dallas in the 1970s. Please let me know if you need anything else. Source: Christine (Buzzetta) Witzsche, Communications Manager, Cooper Aerobics, Health and Wellness, cooperaerobics.com.

Photo 1 of "Kenneth Cooper." Permission has been received and they would like the photo description to read: "Kenneth H. Cooper, MD, MPH, Founder and Chairman of Cooper Aerobics." Credit line should read: Photo courtesy of Cooper Aerobics.

Photo #2 Title: Arthur Jones, Founder of Nautilus, Inc taken during the Colorado Experiment, Fort Collins (1973). Arthur Jones photo (email):

From: John Turner , To: theflyingwej, Sent: Thu, Mar 15, 2012 6:38 pm, Subject: Photo permission.

Good evening William. I spoke with Mr. East and informed him the photo in question was taken at Fort Collins, Colorado in 1973. He advised me that he has a publishing deadline and there is no profit motive attached to the periodical. Do you have any objection to the Army's request? John Turner, www.arthurjonesexercise.com <http://www.arthurjonesexercise.com/>.

----- Forwarded Message -----

From: theflyingwej, To: mr.nautilus, Sent: Thursday, March 15, 2012 6:50 PM, Subject: Re: Photo permission, I hereby grant permission for him to use the photo. Permission based upon shot having been taken by Inge, Arthur having inherited from her, and I having inherited from Arthur. WEJ (William E. Jones–Arthur Jones' son–"owner" of photo.")

Photo 2 of Arthur Jones has been approved. Credit Line should read: Photo courtesy of www.arthurjonesexercise.com.

Figure 40. Women's Army Corp PRT (FM 35-20, 1975) 142
All four photos were taken from a You Tube copy of a 1963 US Army training film (TF35–3400): http://www.youtube.com/watch?v=bZTuLO-RkRE.

Figure 41. WAC Combat Readiness Training (FM 35-20, 1975) 144
All Photos are from: Department of the Army. Physical Training-Women's Army Corps (FM 35-20), Washington, DC: US Government Printing Office, 1975.

Figure 42. Message from President Ronald Reagan-PAM 350-18 (1983) 150
Photo from government publication (1983).

Figure 43. Introduction to DPAM 350-18 (1983) 157
Photo from government publication (1983).

Figure 44. Ranger-Athlete-Warrior-Task-Matrix ..…..................................... 187

"Slide" was originally published in a .PPT slide packet produced by the 75th Ranger Regiment entitled "RAW Introduction–Further, Faster, Harder"; also may be found in another format in: McMillian, Danny. "RANGER ATHLETE WARRIOR: A Systematic Approach to Conditioning;" Infantry (May/Jun 2007; 96, 3), 5.

Figure 45. OER/OIF Physical Readiness Training 190

Photos 2 & 3 are from DIVIDS Media services (governmental agency)–no permissions required: RE DVIDS Media, request-accessing.

Photo #1: is from an article in http://www.army.mil/article/44021/flight-school-leaders-incorporate-crossfit-to- diversify-pt/.

Photo #2: Soldiers stationed at the National Training Center lift perform the Step Up exercise during a Physical Readiness Training familiarization course at Fort Irwin, Calif., March 2010. The exercise is part of the Army's new PRT program which is designed to improve trunk strength, stability, and movement in the battlefield; date taken: 10 March 2011, photo ID:376594 , VIRIN: 110310-O-#####-862, location : Fort Irwin, CA.

Photo #3: Company commanders with 1st Brigade Combat Team, 4th Infantry Division, lift weights during the weight lifting portion of the 'Raider Six' physical training with Colonel Jeffrey Martindale, commander of 1BCT, 4th Infantry Division, 24 December, in the Kandahar province; date taken: 24 December 2010, photo ID:353379, location: Kandahar, AFB.

Photo #4 is from the photo files, Department of Physical Education, United States Military Academy, West Point, New York.

Figure 46. OER/OIF Combat Readiness Training 192

Photo #1 and 5 came from Fort Jackson, Basic Combat Training website (training photos): http://www.jackson.army.mil/sites/bct/.

Photos 2,3,4,6 all came from DIVIDS Media services (governmental agency)–no permissions required: RE DVIDS Media, request-accessing.

Photo #2: 1-73 Cavalry's "Stress Shoot" competition at Fort Bragg, NC, July 15; date taken: 07.15.2009, photo ID:188099, VIRIN:090715-A-#####-002, location: Fort Bragg, NC.

Photo #3: the obstacle course at Camp Rilea during the 1st Squadron, 82 Cavalry Regiment, Spur Ride contest; date taken:19 March 2011, photo ID: 442847, VIRIN: 110319-A-#####-095, location: Salem, OR.

Photo #4: US Army Soldiers conduct simulated medical training during the Cultural Support Assessment; date taken: 12 May 2011, photo ID:4248, location: Camp Mackall, in Hofman NC.

Photo #6: Army Soldiers conduct a ruck march during the Cultural Support Assessment and Selection program; date taken: 8 May 2011, photo ID:424890, location: Fayetteville, NC.

Figure 47. Physical Work Capacity Continuum 210
Author made.

Figure 48. Unit Formation Run 213
Photo was obtained from DIVIDS Media–government agency, no permission required. Soldiers with the 525th Military Police Battalion participate in a formation run at Joint Task Force Guantanamo, 7 July 2010 ; photo ID:297440, VIRIN:100707-F-#####-060, location: Guantanamo Bay, Cuba.

www.ingramcontent.com/pod-product-compliance
Lightning Source LLC
Chambersburg PA
CBHW082112230426
43671CB00015B/2673